Spinal Cord Medicine: Evidence-Based Diagnosis and Treatment of Spinal Cord Injuries

Spinal Cord Medicine: Evidence-Based Diagnosis and Treatment of Spinal Cord Injuries

Editor: Carson Diaz

AMERICAN
MEDICAL PUBLISHERS
www.americanmedicalpublishers.com

AMERICAN
MEDICAL PUBLISHERS
www.americanmedicalpublishers.com

Cataloging-in-Publication Data

Spinal cord medicine : evidence-based diagnosis and treatment of spinal cord injuries / edited by Carson Diaz.
p. cm.
Includes bibliographical references and index.
ISBN 978-1-63927-810-7
1. Spinal cord--Diseases. 2. Spinal cord--Wounds and injuries. 3. Spinal cord--Wounds and injuries--Diagnosis.
4. Spinal cord--Wounds and injuries--Treatment. 5. Spinal cord--Diseases--Diagnosis. 6. Spinal cord--Diseases--Treatment.
7. Evidence-based medi I. Diaz, Carson.
RD594.3 .S65 2023
616.83--dc23

American Medical Publishers,
41 Flatbush Avenue,
1st Floor, New York,
NY 11217, USA

ISBN 978-1-63927-810-7 (Hardback)

Contents

Preface

Every book is initially just a concept; it takes months of research and hard work to give it the final shape in which the readers receive it. In its early stages, this book also went through rigorous reviewing. The notable contributions made by experts from across the globe were first molded into patterned chapters and then arranged in a sensibly sequential manner to bring out the best results.

The spinal cord is a thin, long and tubular structure made up of nervous tissue. It extends from the medulla oblongata in the brainstem to the lumbar region of the vertebral column. Impairment to the spinal cord results in temporary or permanent changes in its functioning. There are several symptoms of spinal cord injury (SCI), such as loss of muscle function, loss of sensation and difficulty in breathing. An X-ray, MRI or CT scan might be utilized to evaluate whether or not there is damage in the spinal column and the place wherever it is situated. The treatment of SCI concentrates on the prevention of additional injury and helping persons suffering from SCI to lead an active and productive lifestyle. Some conditions of SCI can be managed with medications, to relieve muscle stiffness and pain in addition to medications for improving sexual functioning, bladder control and bowel control. This book is meant for students who are looking for an elaborate reference text on the diagnosis and treatment of spinal cord injuries. It will prove to be immensely beneficial to students and researchers in this field.

It has been my immense pleasure to be a part of this project and to contribute my years of learning in such a meaningful form. I would like to take this opportunity to thank all the people who have been associated with the completion of this book at any step.

Editor

1

The Effect of Functional Electrical Stimulation and Therapeutic Exercises on Trunk Muscle Tone and Dynamic Sitting Balance in Persons with Chronic Spinal Cord Injury

Margot Bergmann [1,*], Anna Zahharova [1], Märt Reinvee [2], Toomas Asser [3], Helena Gapeyeva [1] and Doris Vahtrik [1]

1 Institute of Sport Sciences and Physiotherapy, University of Tartu, 51008 Tartu, Estonia; anna_zahharova@mail.ru (A.Z.); helena.gapeyeva@ut.ee (H.G.); doris.vahtrik@ut.ee (D.V.)
2 Institute of Technology, Estonian University of Life Sciences, 51006 Tartu, Estonia; mart.reinvee@emu.ee
3 Institute of Clinical Medicine, University of Tartu, 50406 Tartu, Estonia; toomas.asser@ut.ee
* Correspondence: margot.bergmann@ut.ee

Abstract: *Background and objectives:* Functional electrical stimulation (FES) has shown good results in improving static and dynamic sitting balance in persons with spinal cord injuries. There is limited information about how regular surface FES combined with therapeutic exercise (TE) affect dynamic sitting balance and muscle tone. The objective of this study was to evaluate the effectiveness of a six-week physical therapy program consisting of FES and TE on muscle tone and sitting balance in persons with spinal cord injury (SCI). It was also important to explore the relationship between muscle tone and dynamic sitting balance. The third objective was to assess the change of characteristics over a six month period, when no intervention was carried out. *Material and methods:* Five men with SCI were alternately allocated to two study groups: SCI_FES+TE and SCI_TE. Eight healthy control group participants were recruited to collect reference data. SCI participants' intervention lasted for six weeks in their homes. SCI_FES+TE conducted exercises with FES applied on erector spinae (ES) and rectus abdominis (RA) muscles. SCI_TE conducted exercises only. Muscle oscillation frequency (MOF; characterizing muscle tone) and limits of stability (LOS; characterizing sitting balance) were measured. A crossover study design was used. The time between the initial intervention and the crossover was seven months (ClinicalTrials registration ID NCT03517787). *Results:* MOF in SCI_FES+TE increased by 6.0% for ES and 6.1% for RA muscles. LOS of flexion increased 30.1% in SCI_FES+TE. Increase in lateral directions was similar for both study groups. Moderate to high negative correlation was found between MOF and LOS. After seven months, MOF of ES decreased 0.8%, MOF or RA decreased 1.4%, LOS of flexion decreased 31.9%, and LOS of lateral flexion to the left decreased 46.4%. *Conclusions:* The six-week therapy program combining FES and TE increased trunk muscle tone and dynamic sitting balance in flexion more than TE alone. Higher antagonist muscle tone negatively affects dynamic sitting balance and center of pressure (COP) trajectory distance in various directions. After seven months, a slight decline in trunk muscles tone values and an extensive decrease in sitting balance values were noticed.

Keywords: spinal cord injury; functional electrical stimulation; therapeutic exercise; muscle tone; dynamic sitting balance

1. Introduction

Traumatic spinal cord injury (SCI) may lead to long-term disability, which can have an impact on a person's psychological, social, and physical well-being, and therefore, also on quality of life [1,2]. Among other factors, an SCI sufferer's quality of life depends on the person's dynamic sitting balance and the ability to sit unsupported [3,4], together with upper extremity function [5]. Due to the changes in sensation, muscle paralysis, and presence of spasticity, persons with SCI can have severely impaired postural control and balance [6,7]. As tonic activation of trunk muscles is required to maintain an upright sitting position and phasic activation is required to maintain the position while resisting balance disturbances [8], paralysis of trunk muscles is one of the most important factors affecting sitting balance [4]. Trunk, hip, and lower extremity muscle synergies are responsible for postural stability, thus, the paralysis of these muscles causes impairment of sitting balance [9]. Stretch reflexes, intermuscular reflexes, and intrinsic muscle properties are also responsible for trunk stability [10].

A muscle's structure is composed of connective tissue and muscle fibers—both affect muscle tone [11]. The tone itself results from neural and non-neural (intrinsic) aspects [12]. Muscle oscillation frequency (MOF; Hz) describes the intrinsic tension of the muscle in the resting or passive state. Muscle tone reflects the possibility to restore the muscle's physiological properties between contractions, and is measured without any voluntary contraction [11,13]. Muscle tone is altered in neurological conditions [12], including persons with SCI. It is difficult to assess muscle tone in clinical settings, as different scales (e.g., Modified Ashworth scale and Tardieu scale) are subjective and laboratory techniques (e.g., ultrasound imaging and magnetic resonance elastography) are not clinically feasible [12,13]. Muscle tone can be assessed using myotonometry [11–13]. The MyotonPRO device has shown good reliability in assessing person with SCI, therefore, it can be used to measure muscle properties over time [13].

Physical therapy programs for persons with SCI typically incorporate therapeutic exercises (TE), along with practicing functional activities in a seated position. Therapy follows the principles of motor re-learning [6,14]. Strength training is commonly used to improve muscle activation, but in the case of SCI, functional electrical stimulation (FES) can also be applied to improve muscle recruitment [15]. FES is used to elicit muscle contractions in upper motor neuron lesions, and thus, provide increases in trunk stability [3,15].

Despite the importance of persons with SCI having seated postural stability, only a few biomechanical studies have analyzed quantitative data [9]. Force plates are mainly used to register the center of pressure (COP) displacement [16], however, force-sensing surfaces underneath the left and right buttock have also been used [9]. There is limited information examining links between intrinsic muscle tension and sitting balance, and on whether a physical therapy program of concurrent FES and TE influences both characteristics. The objective of the study was to evaluate the effectiveness of a six-week physical therapy program consisting of FES and TE on muscle tone and sitting balance in persons with SCI. It was also important to explore the relationship between muscle tone and dynamic sitting balance. The third objective was to assess the changing of characteristics over a seven-month period, when no intervention was carried out.

2. Materials and Methods

This crossover trial was conducted at the University of Tartu between March 2017 and October 2018. The study protocol is registered in the United States National Library of Medicine (ClinicalTrials.gov), ID NCT03517787, protocol ID Spinaal. All applicable institutional and governmental regulations concerning the ethical use of human volunteers were followed during this research. The current study was approved by Research Ethics Committee of the University of Tartu (permit number: 263/T-4, 17.10.2016). All patients signed a written informed consent for participation in the study.

2.1. Participants

Data from 18 participants were transmitted from the university hospital to the main author of the study. The suitability for the study was initially specified with a telephone interview, followed by consultation with a neurosurgeon who confirmed that the participant can be included in the study. Inclusion criteria for the study participants were: (1) age 18–55 years; (2) chronic SCI (≥12 months' post injury) [17]; (3) traumatic origin of the injury located in the cervical region, resulting in tetraplegia; (4) scoring of B or C by American Spinal Injury Association Impairment Scale (AIS); (5) able to sit unsupported on a custom-made chair. Participants were excluded from the study if they had cardiopulmonary insufficiency, cardiac pacemaker, oncological disease, epilepsy, open wounds, or metal implants in the area where FES was planned to be performed. Eleven participants were excluded from the study due to inadequacy of inclusion criteria. Seven were alternately allocated to SCI_FES+TE and SCI_TE study groups, but due to health complications during the first six-week intervention, two more participants had to be excluded from the study. A total of five SCI participants completed the study. Participants were alternately assigned to two groups: group 1 performed simultaneous TE and FES on erector spinae (ES) and rectus abdominis (RA) muscles, while group 2 performed only TE. As the crossover study design was used, randomization was used for only the first intervention. After seven months, participants enrolled in the opposite intervention group, ensuring that both groups had equal sample sizes. In the current study, the groups were marked accordingly: SCI_FES+TE, SCI_TE, and control group (CG). Due to the small sample size and crossover study design, participants were the same in both SCI study groups. Participants who were initially assigned to FES+TE group were assigned seven months later to TE group, and vice versa. Anthropometric data was measured only once as a baseline, and the same data were used seven months later.

Eight control group (CG) participants were recruited from the employees of the University of Tartu, whose gender and age were matched with SCI participants' respective characteristics. Inclusion criteria for CG participants were a sedentary lifestyle and that they were not supposed to be physically active during leisure time. Exclusion criteria were the same for CG as they were for the SCI participants. Participants' demographic data, duration, and classification of SCI are presented in Table 1.

Table 1. Participants' anthropometric data, duration, and classification of spinal cord injury.

Variable	SCI	CG
Participants (*n*)	5	8
	Age (years)	
Mean ± SD 95% CI	39.2 ± 7.1 30.4, 48.0	30.3 ± 7.9 17.7, 42.8
	Weight (kg)	
Mean ± SD 95% CI	76.9 ± 26.6 46.3, 107.4	90.5 ± 14.4 67.6, 113.4
	Height (cm)	
Mean ± SD 95% CI	183.0 ± 8.8 172.1, 193.9	184.9 ± 5.3 180.5, 189.4
	BMI (kg·m^{-2})	
Mean ± SD 95% CI	23.0 ± 7.7 13.4, 32.7	24.3 ± 4.1 20.8, 27.7
	Time Post Injury (years)	
Mean ± SD 95% CI	10.8 ± 6.0 3.4, 18.2	N/A
Level of the injury	C5–C6	N/A
AIS—B/C (*n*)	4/1	N/A

Abbreviation: SCI—spinal cord injury; CG—control group; AIS—American Spinal Injury Association Impairment Scale; BMI—body mass index; CI—confidence intervals; N/A—not applicable. Data include mean and standard deviation (SD).

2.2. *Intervention*

The therapy program consisted of eight different exercises aimed at improving sitting balance and upper body posture. The program lasted for 6 weeks and therapy was carried out twice a week. Twelve repetitions were performed for each exercise, with 3 sets performed for the first 3 weeks and 4 sets for the last three. SCI participants' training and data collection were conducted in their homes. Exercises were conducted in their own wheelchair with the guidance of a physical therapist. CG carried out only one round of therapy to collect reference data. Training and data collection for CG took place on the university premises. SCI_TE performed exercises only, while SCI_FES+TE performed the same exercises, but additionally FES was delivered.

FES was used to induce muscle contraction in ES and RA. A preset program from a T-One Rehab (I-Tech Medical Division, Martellago, Italy) four-channel FES device was selected to deliver transcutaneous electrical stimulation using 5 × 5 cm self-adhesive gel electrodes (I-Tech Medical Division, Martellago, Italy). The preset program was chosen because the overall aim was that participants could continue the training using the same parameters. The program was selected mainly according to the frequency parameters. Lower frequency parameters postpone fatigue and discomfort [18], and they are also in compliance with previous studies [19]. Electrodes were placed on the thoraco-lumbar area of the ES and RA muscles bilaterally. ES and RA muscles were chosen for stimulation as these muscles have been shown to contribute significantly to trunk stability [20]. The FES program consisted of three phases: warm-up, work phase, and recovery. Characteristics of the program were obtained from the user manual [21]. The pulse frequency was set to 3 Hz for warm-up and recovery phases. Both warm-up and recovery lasted for 5 min throughout the six-week program. During the work phase, the frequency alternated according to the following scheme: one cycle includes pulses of 8 Hz for 18 secs, then pulses of 2 Hz for 2 secs, and finally pulses of 18 Hz for 10 secs, with a pulse duration of 275 μs. The work phase lasted for 30 min for the first three weeks and for 40 min for the last three weeks. The intensity of the current was individually increased to the level at which strong visible muscle contraction was obtained, but with no unpleasant sensation reported by the participants. Muscles were activated simultaneously to generate co-activation, and therefore, to stiffen the trunk. To maintain correct alignment of the upper body during stimulation, the intensity of the current for one muscle was bilaterally equal.

2.3. *Outcome Measures*

2.3.1. Muscle Tone

The natural oscillation frequencies (MOF) for ES and RA muscles were measured in a sitting position on a custom-made adjustable chair, so that the participant had 90° of flexion in hip, knee, and ankle joints. Participants were asked to sit in a relaxed position, so that the measurements were taken with the muscles in a relaxed state. Measurement was carried out using a MyotonPro device (Myoton AS, Tallinn, Estonia) (Figure 1). Measurement points were marked on skin using a permanent marker by an experienced physical therapist, according to the MyotonPro user manual [22]. Measurement points of muscle belly for ES were marked at the L2 vertebrae level and for RA 2 cm bilaterally below the umbilicus. Measurements were performed prior to the first and last therapy session. Pre-pressure of 0.18 N was applied to a muscle, followed by a short duration (15 ms) mechanical impulse with a quick release of 0.40 N. The mechanical force applied to a muscle was 0.58 N (pre-load + impulse), hence, the minimal force did not cause residual mechanical deformation nor neurological reaction [22]. Each parameter was measured five times and the mean value was calculated and accepted for statistical analysis. If the coefficient of variation was more than 4%, the measurement was repeated.

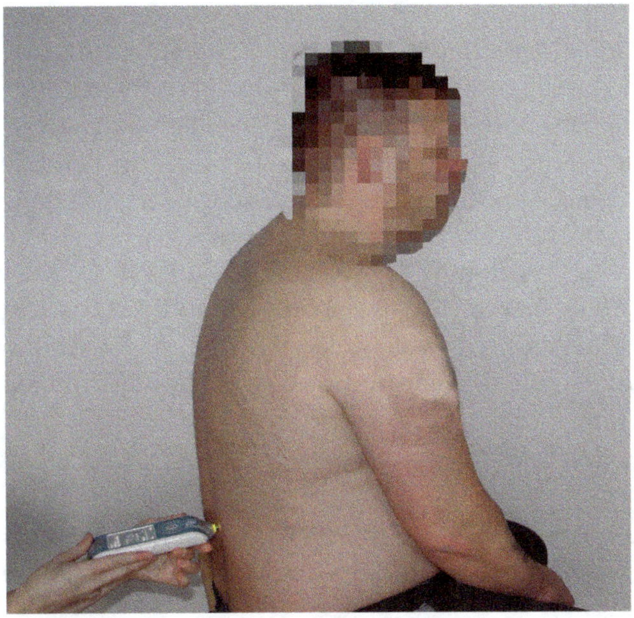

Figure 1. Measurement of erector spinae muscle oscillation frequency at L2 disc level using a MyotonPRO device.

2.3.2. Dynamic Sitting Balance

Limits of stability (LOS; cm) were used to assess participants' dynamic sitting balance. LOS can be defined as the maximum distance that a participant is able to move their COP in various directions while remaining stable and without changing the configuration of the base of support (BOS) [23]. Multidirectional LOS has been used to describe dynamic sitting balance in individuals with SCI [24].

Sitting balance parameters were measured with a CONFORMat sensor model 5530 (Tekscan, Inc., South Boston, USA) body pressure measurement system. The system was calibrated according to the manufacturer's guideline prior to the testing, and then mounted on an adjustable chair. The chair height was individually adjusted considering the height of the participant. After sitting on the chair, the participants were instructed to keep their sitting area in contact with the chair and then to consecutively tilt their torso forward as far as possible in flexion, and then to the right (R) and left (L) in lateral flexion. Each motion cycle in the three directions was separated with a three second stabilization break. Three attempts were performed in each direction and mean data were accepted for statistical analysis. During the motions, the COP coordinates were acquired using the CONFORMat Research 7.20 software (Tekscan, Inc., South Boston, MA, USA) with a sample rate of 100 Hz. The COP data was then processed with Matlab (MathWorks, Inc., Natick, MA, USA) script to register the range of COP anterior–posterior and medio–lateral displacement in centimeters. In the current study, all analyzed dynamic sitting balance measures (cm) were normalized to participants' body height (cm), and measured supine from cranium to calcaneus (LOS/body height).

MOF and LOS data from the last therapy session of the first intervention period were compared with the data obtained during the first therapy session of the second intervention period after a seven month break to see whether there had been a decline in the values.

2.4. Statistical Analysis

Data analysis was performed using IBM SPSS software (version 20, IBM Corporation, New York, NY, USA). Descriptive statistics were used to explain the demographics and SCI characteristics. As the sample size was very small, nonparametric tests were used for analyses. The Kruskal–Wallis H test was used to compare data between groups. Dunn´s post-hoc tests with Bonferroni correction were carried out for pairwise correction after a significant Kruskal–Wallis H test. As data from control group were collected for reference values, the baseline measures were also used for comparison of data with the SCI groups after the intervention. The Wilcoxon sign rank test was used for pre- and post-intervention comparison within one study group. The Wilcoxon test was also used to compare the outcome measures after the seven month break period. For the comparison after the seven month break period, all SCI participants formed one group ($n = 5$). Spearman's rank correlation coefficient was calculated to assess the relationship between muscle tone and sitting balance. The relationship was calculated only at baseline. Data from the SCI participants' ($n = 5$) first appointment were used for the analyses. The following correlation coefficient ranges were considered: 0.0–0.3 was considered negligible, 0.3–0.5 low; 0.5–0.7 moderate; 0.7–0.9 high; and 0.9–1.0 very high correlation [25]. A probability value (p-value) less than 0.05 was considered to be statistically significant. Hedges's g value with 95% confidence intervals (CI) was calculated to describe the effect size of the intervention. A value of 0.2 was considered small, 0.5 medium, and over 0.8 was considered a large and substantial difference [26].

3. Results

As crossover study design was used, where data from 5 SCI participants were included for analysis for both intervention groups. The representation of the study design is presented in Figure 2.

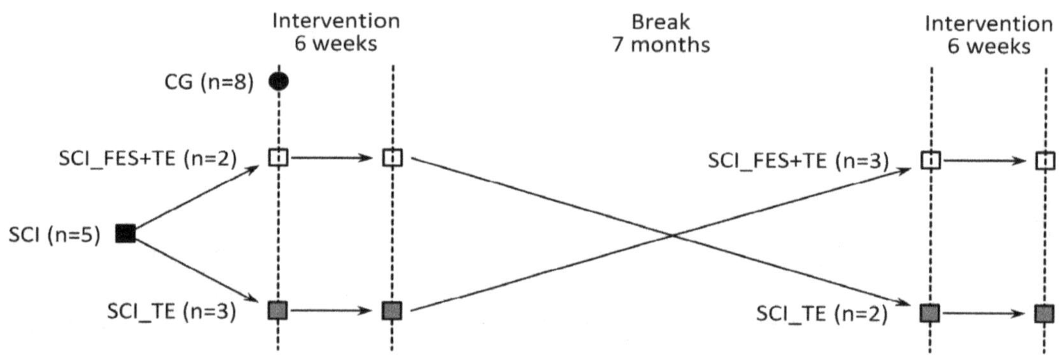

Figure 2. Schematic representation of crossover study design.

3.1. Muscle Tone

Results for muscle tone are presented in Table 2. Mean values for left and right body side were calculated and used for analysis.

After six weeks of intervention, MOF of ES increased 6.0% in SCI_FES+TE ($p = 0.138$), but decreased by 1.1% in SCI_TE ($p = 0.500$). Effect size values show that the therapy had a substantial effect on the SCI_FES+TE group. There was no significant difference of ES muscle tone between the three groups pre- ($p = 0.989$) and post-intervention ($p = 0.553$).

After six weeks of intervention, MOF of RA increased 6.1% in SCI_FES+TE group ($p = 0.225$) and 2.7% in SCI_TE group ($p = 0.345$). The therapy had a small effect on RA muscle tone in the SCI_FES+TE group. There was no significant difference of RA muscle tone between the three groups pre- ($p = 0.542$) and post-intervention ($p = 0.329$).

Within group comparison revealed that prior to the intervention, the MOF of ES was significantly higher than the MOF of RA in each of the three groups (SCI_FES+TE and SCI_TE $p = 0.043$; CG $p = 0.018$). After the intervention, a significant difference remained between MOF of ES and RA (SCI_FES+TE and SCI_TE $p = 0.043$; CG $p = 0.018$).

After the seven month break period, the MOF of ES decreased by 0.8% ($p = 0.686$, g = 0.16, 95% CI −1.08, 1.4). MOF or RA decreased by 1.4% ($p = 1.000$, g = 0.08, 95% CI −1.16, 1.32) in SCI participants.

Table 2. Mean (SD) pre- and post-intervention results for muscle tone (muscle oscillation frequency) and dynamic sitting balance (normalized limits of stability) with effect size (95% confidence interval) data.

	SCI_FES+TE (n = 5)			SCI_TE (n = 5)			CG (n = 8)
	Pre-Intervention	**Post-Intervention**	**Effect Size**	**Pre-Intervention**	**Post-Intervention**	**Effect Size**	**Reference Value**
Muscle Oscillation Frequency (Hz)							
ES	17.10 (1.05)	18.13 (1.07)	−0.88, (−2.18, 0.42)	17.56 (0.97)	17.36 (1.06)	0.18, (−1.06. 1.4)	16.99 (3.36)
RA	12.14 (1.37)	12.88 (2.04)	−0.38, (−1.64, 0.87)	12.34 (1.44)	12.88 (2.04)	−0.17, (−1.41, 1.0)	11.44 (1.66)
Limits of Stability (cm, Normalized to Body Height)							
Flexion	0.018 (0.016)	0.023 (0.023)	−0.23, (−1.47, 1.02)	0.022 (0.016)	0.020 (0.013)	0.12, (−1.12, 1.36)	0.049 (0.010)
Lateral flexion R	0.022 (0.015)	0.023 (0.017)	−0.06, (−1.3, 1.18)	0.021 (0.013)	0.021 (0.012)	−0.00, (−1.24, 1.24)	0.039 (0.008)
Lateral flexion L	0.018 (0.014)	0.022 (0.016)	−0.24, (−1.48, 1.00)	0.020 (0.010)	0.025 (0.011)	−0.43, (−1.68, 0.82)	0.038 (0.007)

Abbreviations: SCI—spinal cord injury; CG—control group; FES—functional electrical stimulation; TE—therapeutic exercise; ES—m erector spinae; RA—rectus abdominis; R—right; L—left.

3.2. *Dynamic Sitting Balance*

Results for dynamic sitting balance are presented in Table 2.

After six weeks of intervention, LOS of flexion increased 31.3% in SCI_FES+TE ($p = 0.465$), but decreased by 12.1% in SCI_TE ($p = 0.345$). Pre-intervention LOS of flexion was significantly lower for SCI_FES+TE ($p = 0.022$) as compared to CG. There was no statistical difference between SCI_TE and CG values pre-intervention ($p = 0.056$). Post-intervention LOS of flexion was not statistically different between SCI_FES+TE and CG ($p = 0.059$), but values for SCI_TE were significantly lower ($p = 0.049$) as compared to CG.

After six weeks of intervention, LOS of lateral flexion R increased 5.0% in SCI_FES+TE ($p = 0.686$) and 2.7% in SCI_TE ($p = 0.465$). Pre-intervention LOS of lateral flexion R was significantly lower ($p = 0.049$) for SCI_FES+TE as compared to CG. There was no statistically significant difference between the three study groups post-intervention ($p = 0.054$).

After six weeks of intervention, LOS of lateral flexion L increased 20.1% in SCI_FES+TE ($p = 0.686$) and 21.3% in SCI_TE ($p = 0.500$). Therapy had a small effect on both study groups. Prior to intervention, LOS of lateral flexion L was significantly lower for SCI_FES+TE ($p = 0.042$) and SCI_TE ($p = 0.020$) as compared to CG. After the intervention, no significant differences appeared between groups ($p = 0.116$).

After the seven month break period, LOS of flexion decreased by 31.9% ($p = 0.138$, $g = 0.34$, 95% CI -0.9, 1.59), LOS of lateral flexion R decreased by 27.3% ($p = 0.225$, $g = 0.4$, 95% CI −0.86, 1.65), and LOS of lateral flexion L decreased by 46.4% ($p = 0.043$, $g = 0.99$, 95% CI −0.33, 2.30).

3.3. *Relationship between Muscle Tone and Dynamic Sitting Balance*

A high negative correlation was found between MOF of ES and LOS of lateral flexion L. A moderate negative correlation was found between MOF of ES and LOS of flexion together with lateral flexion to R, and also between MOF of RA and LOS of flexion and lateral flexion R in SCI group ($p > 0.05$). Other analyzed correlation coefficients showed negligible to low correlation between muscle tone and dynamic sitting balance. Correlation values are presented in Table 3.

Table 3. Spearman's rank correlation coefficient for muscle tone and dynamic sitting balance. SCI participants' pre-intervention data were used in correlation analysis.

	Muscle Oscillation Frequency	
Limits of Stability	**ES**	**RA**
	SCI Group	
Flexion	−0.600	−0.500
Lateral flexion R	−0.600	−0.500
Lateral flexion L	−0.700	−0.300
	CG group	
Flexion	−0.252	0.120
Lateral flexion R	−0.071	0.286
Lateral flexion L	−0.333	−0.190

Abbreviation: SCI—spinal cord injury; CG—control group; ES—erector spinae; RA—rectus abdominis; R—right; L—left.

4. Discussion

Important findings of the study were as follows: combined therapy of FES and TE had a greater effect on increasing SCI participants' muscle tone and improving their dynamic sitting balance than TE only; higher antagonist muscle tone had a negative impact on COP displacement characterizing dynamic sitting balance; after the seven month non-therapy period, trunk muscle tone and sitting balance characteristics decreased.

Spasticity is defined as "a motor disorder characterized by a velocity-dependent increase in tonic stretch reflexes (muscle tone) with exaggerated tendon jerks" [27]. Trunk muscle tone has to be high enough to resist gravity, but should be low enough to allow movement [28]. In the case of SCI, spasticity could also affect truncal muscles, causing abnormal posture [29]. In the current study, comparison between SCI participants and CG trunk muscle tone in a resting position showed that SCI participants' MOF of ES and RA muscles was only slightly higher than in controls. There may have been more differences in tone characteristics if the measurements had been made during trunk muscles contractions, as the spasticity is velocity dependent, meaning the increase in muscle tone could only occur during movements.

One of the rehabilitation goals for SCI patients is to decrease spasticity, but it should be done within a limit, whereby the positive effect of spasticity still occurs [29]. Otherwise, it could be more difficult for SCI participants to sit unsupported and to perform daily activities. FES is usually used to decrease spastic muscle tone in spinal cord lesions [30], but the current study showed that resting tone does not differ between groups. A decrease in muscle tone was noted only in ES in the SCI_TE group, but the muscle tone characteristics were not significantly different between groups. It has been found that decrease in muscle tone while using FES occurs only when the muscle tone is initially high enough [31]. As the muscle tone was already low for the subjects, no further decrease was obtained. In the current study, increase in muscle tone was greater when FES was used. Although the increase was not statistically significant, the effect size values showed that the therapy had a substantial effect on ES muscle tone in the SCI_FES+TE group. This phenomenon may have occurred because therapeutic exercise and FES can also increase muscle tone. Similar results have also been obtained in previous research [32]. In a previous study, SCI participants' thigh muscles were stimulated and the results showed an increase in resting muscle tone; therefore, the results are consistent with the current study. The increase in muscle tone has to be monitored during therapy, as the results of current study revealed that higher muscle tone has a negative impact on dynamic sitting balance. Therefore, if antagonist muscle tone is too high, the COP distance is reduced. Muscle tone has to be kept in an optimal state, whereby it does not interfere with movement but still helps to maintain posture against gravity.

Tonic and phasic muscle activity is needed for postural control, but as SCI participants' muscles are partially or completely de-innervated [4] and the sensory information transmitted to the brain is decreased [33], their sitting balance is also decreased. Using FES in combination with TE showed better results in improving LOS of flexion. Changes were not significantly different, and although the percentage change (31.29%) was quite extensive, the effect size values revealed that the therapy had a small effect on LOS of flexion. Initially, there was a statistically significant difference between SCI_FES+TE and CG, but the increase in LOS of flexion was so extensive that the significant difference disappeared. LOS of R and L lateral flexion increased similarly in the two study groups. Although there was a slight increase in both study groups, effect size values demonstrated that there was almost no effect of the therapy on either group. However, the increase in SCI_FES+TE was still enough that the significant difference between SCI and CG groups disappeared. The reason why the results were not significantly better for the lateral flexion while using FES could be that FES stiffens the body, but during the exercises participants were supposed to move their trunk in different directions. In some cases, participants stated that stimulation was an interference and that it turned on at the wrong time; the participant wanted to move, but stimulation was keeping their trunk in place. Therefore, using stimulation that is not synchronized with exercises could be more beneficial for improving static sitting balance. The small increase in LOS of lateral flexion was probably because only ES and RA were stimulated. Activation of the quadratus lumborum muscle with stimulation has previously showed good results in mediolateral stability and side leaning positions [15]. Flexion and lateral flexion were used because most everyday activities are conducted in these directions. As participants were supported from behind while sitting in a wheelchair, the LOS of extension was not measured.

After the seven month break period, MOF of ES and RA decreased slightly, but the decrease in LOS characteristics in flexion and lateral flexion directions was extensive. However, a significant decrease was only noted in LOS of lateral flexion. The reason why MOF characteristics changed by only slightly over time could be that muscle tone is controlled by neural factors to a large extent [11,12]. Therefore, in the case of a central nervous system lesion, it is difficult to alter muscle tone over a long period of time with only exercises. Regular therapy could have an effect on muscle tone via intrinsic factors that the tone also depends on [11,12], but only during the time that therapy is conducted; the results do not increase over time. Participants' dynamic sitting balance can be improved with training. Even if the participant has a severe lesion, other muscles can compensate for the movement, and to some extent, participants' functional abilities can be improved. Therefore, the training had a bigger effect on LOS in different directions. However, during the seven month break period, when participants did not use FES or conduct exercises and did not use these maximum LOS values during their everyday activities, the results decreased. This shows that in order to keep the results, or even improve them, SCI participants need to exercise regularly, as the decrease in functional abilities is extensive over time.

Correlation analyses showed that in the SCI group, there was a low to moderate negative relationship between LOS directions and muscle tone. This finding indicates that the higher the muscle tone is, the smaller the LOS values are. This provides information for physical therapists, showing that while improving participants' dynamic sitting balance, attention has to be paid to antagonist muscle tone.

The main limitation of the current study was the small sample size. Due to strict demands on participants and the limited region of the study, it was difficult to include enough participants. As the participants were very heterogeneous and the sample size was small, more research needs to be conducted to generalize the results.

5. Conclusions

A six week therapy program including combined FES and TE increases trunk muscle tone and dynamic sitting balance in flexion more than TE alone. Higher antagonist muscle tone negatively affects dynamic sitting balance and COP trajectory distance in various directions. After a seven month break period, a slight decline in trunk muscles tone values and extensive decrease in sitting balance values was noticed.

Author Contributions: Conceptualization, M.B. and D.V.; methodology, M.B., D.V., H.G., and M.R.; formal analysis, M.B. and M.R.; investigation, M.B., A.Z., and T.A.; resources, D.V., H.G., M.R., and T.A.; data curation, M.B. and M.R.; writing—original draft preparation, M.B.; writing—review and editing, A.Z., M.R., H.G., T.A., and D.V.; supervision, D.V.

Acknowledgments: The authors gratefully acknowledge Aleko Peipsi and Myoton AS for providing us with the MyotonPRO device used for experiments. The authors also acknowledge all of the study participants who agreed to take part in the research.

References

1. Sabre, L.; Pedai, G.; Rekand, T.; Asser, T.; Linnamägi, U.; Kõrv, J. High Incidence of traumatic spinal cord injury in Estonia. *Spinal Cord* **2012**, *50*, 755–759. [CrossRef] [PubMed]
2. Singh, A.; Tetreault, L.; Kalsi-Ryan, S.; Nouri, A.; Fehlings, M.G. Global prevalence and incidence of traumatic spinal cord injury. *Clin. Epidemiol.* **2014**, *6*, 309–331. [PubMed]
3. Kukke, S.N.; Triolo, R.J. The effects of trunk stimulation on bimanual seated workspace. *IEEE Trans. Neural Syst. Rehabil. Eng.* **2004**, *12*, 177–185. [CrossRef] [PubMed]
4. Milosevic, M.; Masani, K.; Kuipers, M.J.; Rahouni, H.; Verrier, M.C.; McConville, K.M.; Popovic, M.R. Trunk control impairment is responsible for postural instability during quiet sitting in individuals with cervical spinal cord injury. *Clin. Biomech.* **2015**, *30*, 507–512. [CrossRef] [PubMed]
5. Anderson, K.D. Targeting recovery: Priorities of the spinal cord-injured population. *J. Neurotrauma* **2004**, *21*, 1371–1383. [CrossRef] [PubMed]
6. Abou, L.; de Freitas, G.R.; Palandi, J.; Ilha, J. Clinical Instruments for Measuring Unsupported Sitting Balance in Subjects with Spinal Cord Injury: A Systematic Review. *Top. Spinal Cord Inj. Rehabil.* **2018**, *24*, 177–193. [CrossRef] [PubMed]

7. Tse, C.M.; Chisholm, A.E.; Lam, T.; Eng, J.J.; SCIRE Research Team. A systematic review of the effectiveness of task-specific rehabilitation interventions for improving independent sitting and standing function in spinal cord injury. *J. Spinal Cord Med.* **2018**, *41*, 254–266. [CrossRef]
8. Masani, K.; Sin, V.W.; Vette, A.H.; Thrasher, T.A.; Kawashima, N.; Morris, A.; Preuss, R.; Popovic, M.R. Postural reactions of trunk muscles to multi-directional perturbations in sitting. *Clin. Biomech.* **2009**, *24*, 176–182. [CrossRef]
9. Gauthier, C.; Gagnon, D.; Grangeon, M.; Jacquemin, G.; Nadeau, S.; Masani, K.; Popovic, M.R. Comparison of multidirectional seated postural stability between individuals with spinal cord injury and able-bodied individuals. *J. Rehabil. Med.* **2013**, *45*, 47–54. [CrossRef]
10. Feldman, A.G. The relationship between postural and movement stability. *Adv. Exp. Med. Biol.* **2016**, *957*, 105–120.
11. Rusu, L.; Cosma, G.; Calina, M.L.; Dragomir, M.M.; Marin, M. Evaluation of two muscle training programs by assessment of the muscle tone. *Sci. Sports* **2015**, *30*, e65–e72. [CrossRef]
12. Agyapong-Badu, S.; Warner, M.; Samuel, D.; Stokes, M. Measurement of ageing effects on muscle tone and mechanical properties of rectus femoris and biceps brachii in healthy males and females using a novel hand-held myometric device. *Arch. Gerontol. Geriatr.* **2016**, *62*, 59–67. [CrossRef] [PubMed]
13. Ko, C.Y.; Choi, H.J.; Ryu, J.; Kim, G. Between-day reliability of MyotonPRO device for the non-invasive measurement of muscle material properties in the lower extremities of patients with a chronic spinal cord injury. *J. Biomech.* **2018**, *17*, 60–65. [CrossRef] [PubMed]
14. Boswell-Ruys, C.L.; Harvey, L.A.; Barker, J.J.; Ben, M.; Middleton, J.W.; Lord, S.R. Training unsupported sitting in people with chronic spinal cord injuries: A randomized controlled trial. *Spinal Cord* **2010**, *48*, 138–143. [CrossRef] [PubMed]
15. Ho, C.H.; Triolo, R.J.; Elias, A.L.; Kilgore, K.L.; DiMarco, A.F.; Bogie, K.; Vette, A.H.; Audu, M.L.; Kobetic, R.; Chang, S.R.; et al. Functional electrical stimulation and spinal cord injury. *Phys. Med. Rehabil. Clin. N. Am.* **2014**, *25*, 631–654. [CrossRef] [PubMed]
16. Rath, M.; Vette, A.H.; Ramasubramaniam, S.; Li, K.; Burdick, J.; Edgerton, V.R.; Gerasimenko, Y.P.; Savenko, D.G. Trunk Stability Enabled by Noninvasive Spinal Electrical Stimulation after Spinal Cord Injury. *J. Neurotrauma* **2018**, *35*, 2540–2553. [CrossRef] [PubMed]
17. Gao, K.L.; Chan, K.M.; Purves, S.; Tsang, W.W.N. Reliability of dynamic sitting balance tests and their correlations with functional mobility for wheelchair users with chronic spinal cord injury. *J. Orthop. Transl.* **2014**, *3*, 44–49. [CrossRef]
18. Doucet, B.M.; Lam, A.; Griffin, L. Neuromuscular electrical stimulation for skeletal muscle function. *Yale J. Biol. Med.* **2012**, *85*, 201–215.
19. Ibitoye, M.O.; Hamzaid, N.A.; Hasnan, N.; Abdul Wahab, A.K.; Davis, G.M. Strategies for rapid muscle fatigue reduction during FES exercise in individuals with spinal cord injury: A systematic review. *PLoS ONE* **2016**, *11*, e0149024. [CrossRef]
20. Milosevic, M.; McConville, V.; Seidic, E.; Masani, K.; Kvan, M.J.; Popovic, M.R. Visualization of trunk muscle synergies during sitting perturbations using self-organizing maps (SOM). *IEEE Trans. Biomed. Eng.* **2012**, *59*, 2516–2523. [CrossRef]
21. I-Tech Medical Division. *Electrotherapy Model T-One Rehab*; MNPG236 Rev.0 of 21/06/16; User manual; I-Tech Medical Division: Martellago, Italy, 2016.
22. Myoton AS. *MyotonPRO Digital Palpation*; User manual; Myoton AS: Tallinn, Estonia, 2016.
23. Lemay, J.F.; Gagnon, D.H.; Nadeau, S.; Grangeon, M.; Gauthier, C.; Duclos, C. Center-of-pressure total trajectory length is a complementary measure to maximum excursion to better differentiate multidirectional standing limits of stability between individuals with incomplete spinal cord injury and able-bodied individuals. *J. Neuroeng. Rehabil.* **2014**, *11*, 8. [CrossRef] [PubMed]
24. Gauthier, C.; Gagnon, D.; Jacquemin, G.; Duclos, C.; Masani, K.; Popovic, M.R. Which trunk inclination directions best predict multidirectional-seated limits of stability among individuals with spinal cord injury? *J. Spinal Cord Med.* **2012**, *35*, 343–350. [CrossRef] [PubMed]
25. Mukaka, M.M. Statistics Corner: A guide to appropriate use of Correlation coefficient in medical research. *Malawi Med. J.* **2012**, *24*, 69–71. [PubMed]

26. McGough, J.J.; Faraone, S.V. Estimating the size of treatment effects: Moving beyond P values. *Psychiatry* **2009**, *6*, 21–29. [PubMed]
27. Lance, J.W. The control of muscle tone, reflexes, and movement: Robert Wartenbeg Lecture. *Neurology* **1980**, *30*, 1303–1313. [CrossRef] [PubMed]
28. Bobath, B. *Adult Hemiplegia Evaluation and Treatment*, 3rd ed.; Butterworth-Heinemann: Oxford, UK, 1990.
29. Naro, A.; Leo, A.; Russo, M.; Casella, C.; Buda, A.; Crespantini, A.; Porcari, B.; Carioti, L.; Billeri, L.; Bramanti, A.; et al. Breakthroughs in the spasticity management: Are non-pharmacological treatments the future? *J. Clin. Neurosci.* **2017**, *39*, 16–27. [CrossRef] [PubMed]
30. Krause, P.; Szecsi, J.; Straube, A. Changes in spastic muscle tone increase in patients with spinal cord injury using functional electrical stimulation and passive leg movements. *Clin. Rehabil.* **2008**, *22*, 627–634. [CrossRef]
31. Lo, H.C.; Tsau, K.H.; Su, F.C.; Chang, G.L.; Yeh, C.Y. Effects of a functional electrical stimulation-assisted leg-cycling wheelchair on reducing spasticity of patients after stroke. *J. Rehabil. Med.* **2009**, *41*, 242–246. [CrossRef]
32. Douglas, A.J.; Walsh, E.G.; Wright, G.W. The effects of neuromuscular stimulation on muscle tone at the knee in paraplegia. *Exp. Physiol.* **1991**, *76*, 357–367. [CrossRef]
33. Shin, S.; Sosnoff, J.J. Spinal Cord Injury and Seated Postural Control: A Test of the Rambling and Trembling Hypothesis. *Mot. Control* **2017**, *21*, 443–456. [CrossRef]

2

Filling the Gap: Neural Stem Cells as a Promising Therapy for Spinal Cord Injury

Inês M. Pereira [1,2], Ana Marote [1,2], António J. Salgado [1,2] and Nuno A. Silva [1,2,*]

1 Life and Health Sciences Research Institute (ICVS), School of Medicine, University of Minho, Campus de Gualtar, 4710-057 Braga, Portugal; inesmiguelmarquespereira@gmail.com (I.M.P.); anammarote@gmail.com (A.M.); asalgado@med.uminho.pt (A.J.S.)

2 ICVS/3B's—PT Government Associate Laboratory, Braga/Guimarães, Portugal

* Correspondence: nunosilva@med.uminho.pt

Abstract: Spinal cord injury (SCI) can lead to severe motor, sensory and social impairments having a huge impact on patients' lives. The complex and time-dependent SCI pathophysiology has been hampering the development of novel and effective therapies. Current treatment options include surgical interventions, to stabilize and decompress the spinal cord, and rehabilitative care, without providing a cure for these patients. Novel therapies have been developed targeting different stages during trauma. Among them, cell-based therapies hold great potential for tissue regeneration after injury. Neural stem cells (NSCs), which are multipotent cells with inherent differentiation capabilities committed to the neuronal lineage, are especially relevant to promote and reestablish the damaged neuronal spinal tracts. Several studies demonstrate the regenerative effects of NSCs in SCI after transplantation by providing neurotrophic support and restoring synaptic connectivity. Therefore, human clinical trials have already been launched to assess safety in SCI patients. Here, we review NSC-based experimental studies in a SCI context and how are they currently being translated into human clinical trials.

Keywords: spinal cord injury; cell-based therapies; induced pluripotent stem cells; neural stem cells; clinical trials

---

1. An Overview on Spinal Cord Injury

Spinal cord injury (SCI) is one of the most disabling and devastating neurological injuries. It is recognized as a global health issue priority due to its impact on patient quality of life, complexity, and expensive medical care (Global Burden of Disease Study 2016 [1]). In 2016, the number of new SCI cases was 0.93 million (0.78–1.16 million) with a prevalence of 27.04 million (24.98–30.15 million) cases. Although the global incidence is similar between genders, men have higher incidence when compared with women at ages 20–40 years. Moreover, as the global population tends to grow and the health care systems to improve, it is expected an increase in the absolute number of people living with SCI [1]. Upon trauma, SCI patients can be stratified according to the spinal cord level affected, from higher cervical lesions that lead to partial or full tetraplegia (paralysis of the four limbs) to lower lesions that lead to paraplegia (paralysis of the lower limbs) [2]. Moreover, SCI etiologies can be subdivided into non-traumatic and traumatic injury. Non-traumatic SCI occurs when an acute or chronic disease (such as tumor, infection, or degenerative disc disease) causes the primary injury in the spinal cord, while traumatic SCI results from an external physical impact sufficient to damage the spinal cord (for instance, originated by a car crash, falls, violence or sports-related accident). Curiously, it was estimated that falls are the main cause, accounting for more than 50% of the total incidence [1].

1.1. From Acute to Chronic Phase

SCI can be described as a two-phase process: an initial acute phase divided in the "primary injury" and the "secondary injury"; and the chronic phase [3,4]. The "primary injury" depicts the time when the spinal cord is actually lesioned. Regarding the secondary events, it can occur over the time course of minutes to weeks, relying on a complex biological cascade of events that may aggravate the neurological outcomes. Finally, the onset of the chronic phase can occur days to months after the primary injury and continues throughout the patient's life. Figure 1 represents the typical biological events of each phase.

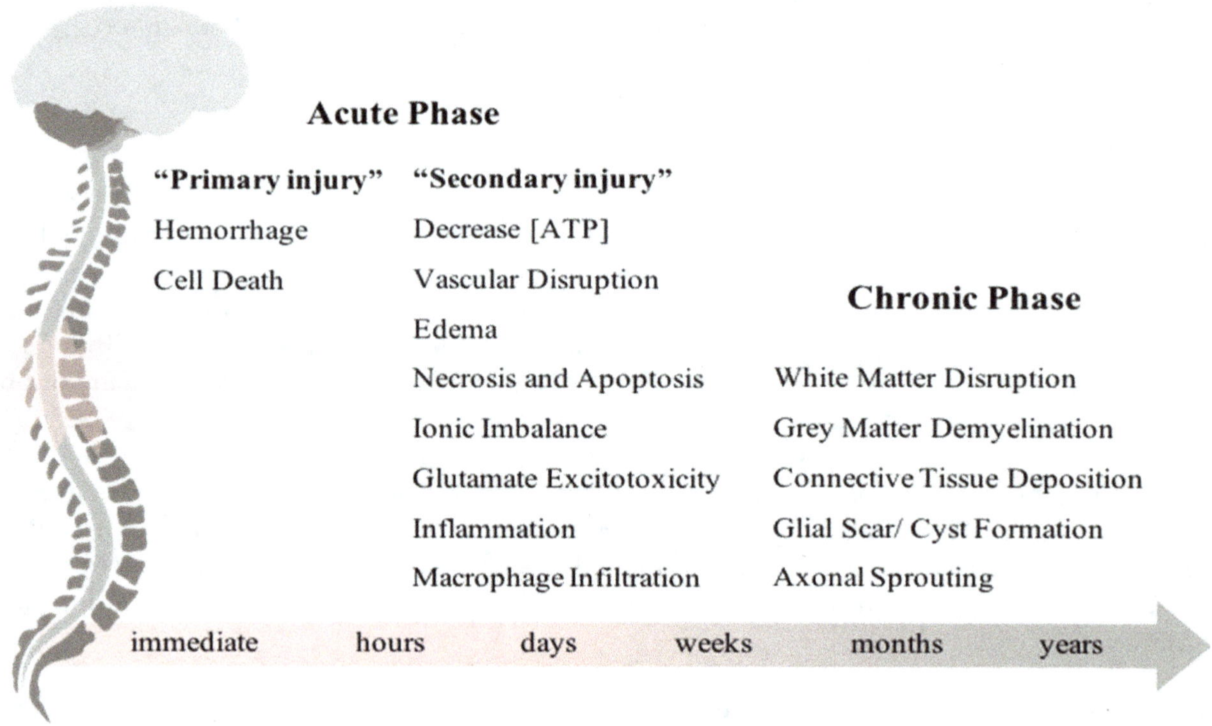

Figure 1. Underlying biological events during acute and chronic phases after spinal cord injury. The primary insult to the spinal cord immediately leads to a cascade of events that comprises the "secondary injury". Weeks to months after the acute phase, the chronic phase is established and it may last throughout the patient's life.

The pathophysiology behind each phase has been extensively studied allowing us a better understanding of the biochemical and cellular events that occur after injury. The initial impact leads to immediate hemorrhage and cell death. Then, the "secondary injury" takes place, which was first suggested by Dr. Allen, in Philadelphia (1911). In his work, Dr. Allen reported improvements in the motor function of lesioned dogs after successfully removing the inflammatory fluid [5]. Thenceforth, extensive work has been developed to dissect the potential events that could be exacerbating the lesion severity during the acute phase [6]. These include vascular disruption, ischemia, edema [7–9], cell death (necrosis and apoptosis) [10], excitotoxicity, ionic imbalance [11,12], and a dysfunctional inflammatory response [13–15].

During the chronic phase there is dissolution of the grey matter, white matter demyelination, deposition of connective tissue, and the formation of the glial scar. In addition to all these physiological complications, many SCI patients also experience the development of pain syndromes [11] and mood disorders, like depression [16,17]. The glial scar is driven by reactive gliosis of astrocytes, microglia/macrophages, pericytes, and extracellular matrix molecules, acting as a physical barrier that limits axonal growth [18–21]. Myelin-associated proteins and proteoglycans are among the most inhibitory molecules in the central nervous system (CNS). Nogo-A, myelin-associated glycoprotein

(MAG), and the chondroitin sulphate proteoglycans (CSPGs) have been the most studied ones [22–24]. Interestingly, several authors have already demonstrated that blocking such inhibitors in a SCI animal model leads to axonal regeneration and functional recovery [25–27].

Despite the inhibitory environment, after the injury, the spinal cord and the brain tend to reorganize and establish new circuits in a process called neuronal plasticity. Hollis and coworkers (2016) demonstrated that after a C5 dorsal column lesion in rats the motor cortex was able to remap when continuous training was performed. Moreover, when observing SCI patients, significant alterations in the brain reorganization were shown. In comparison with the control group, SCI patients showed a reduction in the sensorimotor cortex patterning activation under functional magnetic resonance imaging (fMRI) [28]. When looking to the spinal cord itself, several studies suggest that physical activity is one of the most critical influencers in neuronal plasticity. Regarding human studies, physical therapy is currently applied to incomplete SCI patients with positive results in patients' recovery.

Overall, SCI is a multi-dynamic process with no effective treatment mainly due to the failure of the CNS to successfully regenerate the damaged neuronal circuits. Therefore, researchers have been exploring novel therapies that can be translated into clinical meaningful recovery.

1.2. Clinical Management After SCI

Despite the major efforts currently made to develop new therapies for SCI, there is still no effective treatment. Numerous studies have reported some positive results in preclinical SCI models, however, translation to patients is still questionable and controversial. Typically, after trauma, the patient is completely immobilized and is constantly monitored to prevent possible complications, such as respiratory dysfunctions, cardiovascular aberrations, and hypoxia [29]. After stabilization, clinicians surgically decompress the spinal cord and control the lesion site [30].

The anti-inflammatory methylprednisolone sodium succinate (MPSS) was the first-line drug treatment for SCI patients [31]. Now spanning 50 years, a cordial discussion remains open regarding MPSS administration, safety, dosage, and time-administration [32,33]. Although neuroprotective effects were observed in preclinical studies as well as neurological improvements after its administration, the heightened risks of infection and death are a real concern for patients under MPSS treatment. In fact, the most recent guidelines from the Congress of Neurological Surgeons/American Association of Neurological Surgeons discouraged the administration of MPSS in acute SCI. Therefore, MPSS is not a viable long-term therapeutic choice, highlighting the need to develop new treatments targeting specific events that occur during the acute and/ or the chronic phase.

1.3. Novel Treatments for SCI

Pharmacologically, new neuroprotective alternatives have been targeting secondary events such as inflammation and excitotoxicity. Among them, minocycline and riluzole are two examples that are already under clinical trials. Minocycline, a semisynthetic tetracycline antibiotic, is classified as a neuroprotective agent by improving the exacerbated inflammatory microenvironment observed during secondary SCI [34]. After positive motor outcomes observed during phase I/II clinical trial, the pharmacological administration of minocycline was further encouraged to be tested in a phase III clinical trial (Minocycline in Acute Spinal Cord Injury (MASC)—NCT01828203) [35]. Riluzole, a benzothiazole anticonvulsant, showed to be able to block the abnormal glutamatergic transmission in neuronal synapses [36]. Preclinical studies strongly pointed out for a beneficial effect in neurological tissue preservation and motor recovery [37,38]. Consequently, and after the positive effects reported during the phase I/IIa clinical trial, riluzole is now involved in an international phase II/III multi-center clinical trial (Riluzole in Acute Spinal Cord Injury Study (RISCIS)—NCT01597518) [39,40].

Fibroblast growth factor-2 (FGF-2; or basic fibroblast growth factor) has been implied in different biological processes, such as limb and nervous system development, wound healing, and tumor growth, due to its function in cell proliferation and survival [41]. Regarding SCI, different reports have evidenced a role for FGF-2 in spinal cord neural stem and progenitor cells proliferation, angiogenesis, and glial cavitation reduction. While some SCI animal models shown hind limb improvements after intrathecal injection of FGF-2, other studies do not report any functional recovery benefits after treatment. Still, a human clinical trial is now being conducted to assess safety and efficacy of a specific biodegradable device with heparin-activated FGF1 in traumatic SCI patients (NCT02490501). The aim of the study is to develop a regenerative treatment option by taking advantage of the crucial role of FGF1 in neuroprotection and axon regeneration of the CNS [41,42].

Cytokines also exhibit interesting characteristics that can promote morphological and functional recovery of the spinal cord after trauma. The most widely studied cytokine for SCI treatment is the Glycoprotein Granulocyte Colony-Stimulating Factor (G-CSF), known to reduce inflammatory cytokine expression and to promote survival of ischemic cells [43]. Moreover, in a nonrandomized phase I/IIa clinical trial the administration of G-CSF demonstrated to be safe, leading to some improvements in the American Spinal Cord Injury Association (ASIA) scale [44,45]. Another promising cytokine for SCI treatment is interleukin-4 (IL-4). This cytokine is able to activate macrophages to a phenotype associated with repair [46]. Preclinical studies have demonstrated neuroprotection and motor recovery after the administration of IL-4 [47,48].

Besides these molecular approaches, stem cell-based therapies have shown great potential over the past decades, based on the rationale that transplanted cells can differentiate and substitute the lost tissue. Moreover, stem cell-based treatments can also modify the microenvironment and regenerate the damaged circuits. However, there are also some challenges inherent to cell transplantation, including: the choice of the cellular source, the establishment of differentiation protocols, and the monitoring of cell grafts survival and integration.

Regarding stem cell transplantation, encouraging results have already been reported for spinal cord repair, being particularly relevant for neuronal and glial replacement, remyelination, connectivity restoration, stimulation of precursor cells, as a bridge of cysts/cavities, and for improving the expression of beneficial neurotrophins/cytokines. A wide plethora of different cell-types has already been tested and transplanted into the injured spinal cord, both in animals and humans, including Schwann cells [49], olfactory ensheathing glia [50], skin-derived precursors [51], mesenchymal stem cells (MSCs) [52], oligodendrocyte progenitor cells (OPCs) [53], and neural stem/progenitor cells (NS/PCs) [54]. Although all cell-types have intrinsic advantages but also limitations, the focus of the present review is directed for NSC-based therapies.

2. Stem Cells in SCI: Past, Present, and Future

2.1. From the Embryo to A Structured Spinal Cord

The human embryonic development of the nervous system is a complex and highly tuned-process. During the embryonic period, the primary three germ layers (ectoderm, mesoderm, and endoderm) are established as the basis of the various systems and organs of the body through numerous mitotic divisions. As illustrated in Figure 2, from a solid mass of totipotent cells—morula—the embryo develops into the blastocyst. The blastocyst is a pluripotent structure that consists of a cellular outer layer of trophoblasts and an inner Embryonic Stem Cell (ESC) population, the inner cell mass (ICM) [55]. From the ICM cells adjacent to the cavity, a new layer of flat cells is formed, the hypoblast, while the rest of them remain relatively undifferentiated and are termed as epiblast. Subsequently, the blastocyst becomes attached to the endometrium of the uterus, and epiblast cells migrate ventrally along the median plane to form the primitive streak. Embryonic cells begin to differentiate, replacing the hypoblast by the endoderm whereas the remaining part of the epiblast arises to the ectoderm [56]. This process is termed as gastrulation where the monolayered blastula forms a bilayer gastrula with the well-defined primary layers. It is from the ectoderm the notochordal process began, that which will ultimately will arise into the nervous system [57,58].

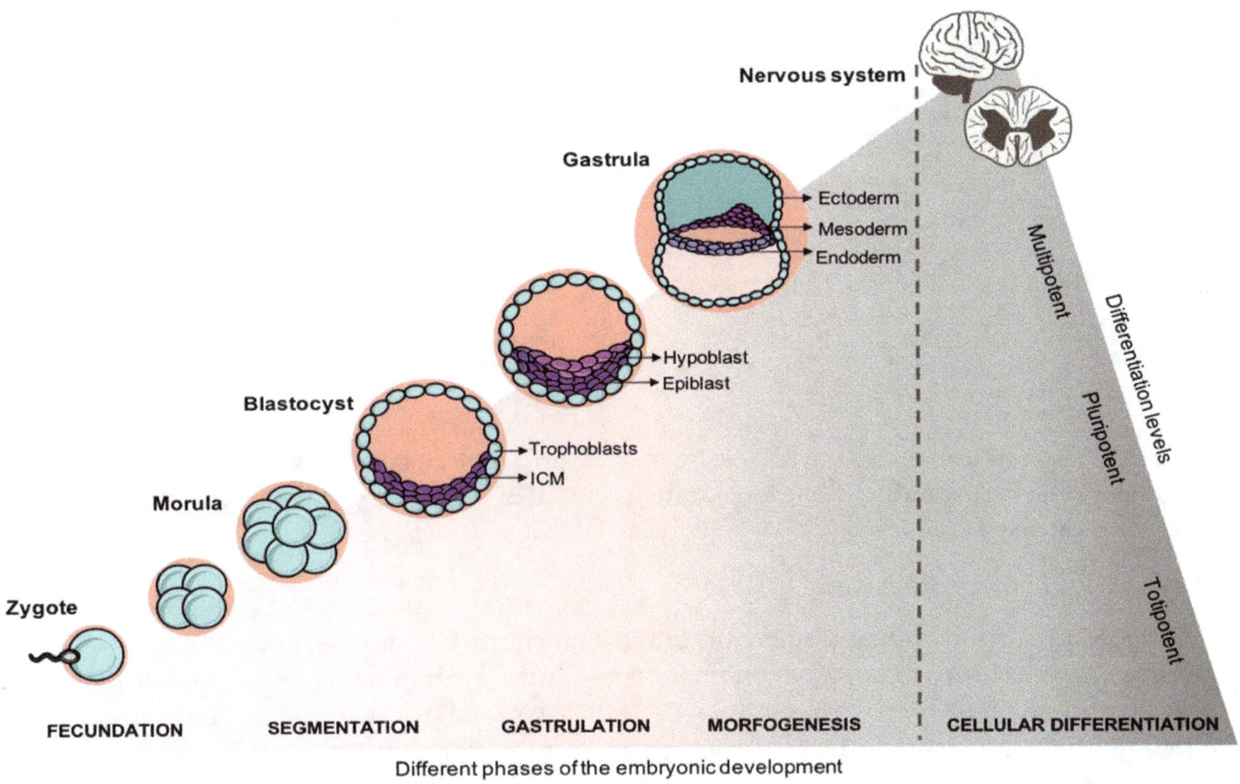

Figure 2. Embryonic development and cellular differentiation. After fecundation, the entire embryogenesis is spatially and temporally coordinated dynamically shifting the gene expression, cell growth, and cellular differentiation.

At approximately the 23rd day of development, the neural plate is already observed in the embryo initiating the neurulation process. As the neural plate begins to roll-up, it develops into the neural tube and consequently to the neural crest [58]. During this period, ESC-derived epiblast-like cells are redefined as neuromesodermal progenitors (NMPs) and are the cellular source for spinal cord development [59,60]. Timed and spatial expression pattern of *TBX6* and *SOX2* genes in NMPs drive cells into their mesoderm or neural fate [61]. Further, other specific patterning genes regulate the neural subtype fate of neural stem cells (NSCs) along the rostral-caudal and dorsoventral axis, in a concentration-dependent manner. While retinoic acid (RA) is highly involved in the activation of rostral homeobox (*HOX*) genes (*HOX1-5* paralog) responsible for a more broad brainstem-to-rostral cervical spinal cord identity, the balance between WNT and FGF signals induces a more caudal neuroaxis spinal HOX gene expression (*HOX6-9* paralog), specifically for a cervical and thoracic spinal cord identity [62–64]. Once the neurulation process is concluded, cells begin to differentiate into mature neurons, being the motor neurons the first ones to develop. Architectonic organization of the spinal cord becomes more and more complex and neurons, non-neurons, and fibers become myelinated for the development of the major tracts of the spinal cord. Fully maturated, the spinal cord is composed by the white matter (mostly myelinated axons) surrounding the gray matter (mostly interneurons, cell bodies, and glial cells). In the white matter the axons are organized in fiber tracts that run longitudinally through the spinal cord, ascending tracts transmit information from the periphery to the CNS and the descending tracts relay information from the brain to the rest of the body.

2.2. Historical Perspective of Cell-Based Research

Over the past decades, we have been witnessing to unprecedented and groundbreaking progress in cell-based research (Figure 3). The potential of such tools has been capturing the attention of the scientific community, clinicians, as well as the general public. The idea of innovative cell-based therapies to treat a wide spectrum of human diseases and traumas has been inspiring researchers.

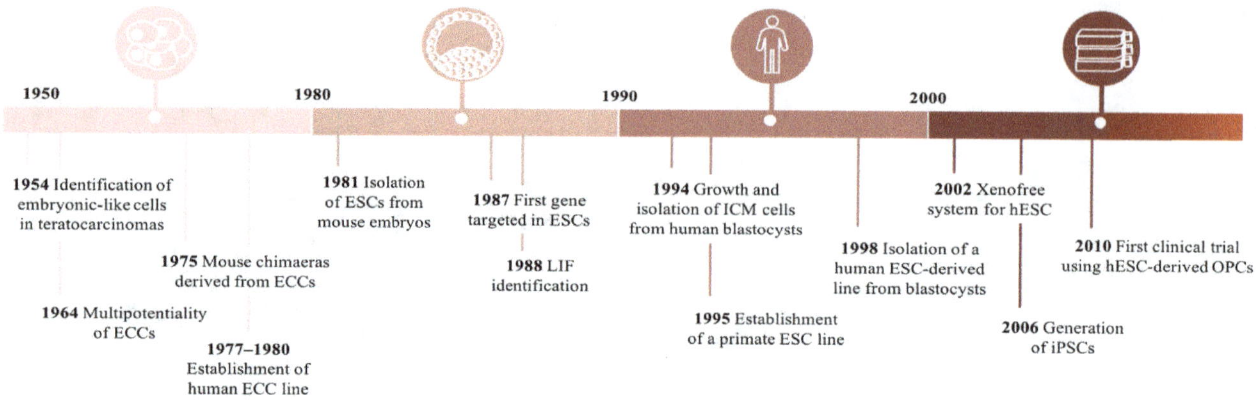

Figure 3. Timeline of embryonic stem cell (ESC)-based research. ICM: inner cell mass; OPC: oligodendrocyte progenitor cells; iPSCs: induced pluripotent stem cells; hESCs: human embryonic stem cells; ECCs: embryonal carcinoma cells.

2.2.1. Finding Embryonic Stem Cells

Cell-based research turning point begun in the 20th-century when Stevens and Little (1954) were deciphering the complexity of teratocarcinomas. These tumors contained a relatively undifferentiated cell-type known as "Embryonal Carcinoma Cells" (ECCs), long suspected as the stem cell of the tumor [65]. In the following decade, an emerging interest regarding ECCs was notorious, culminating in some important findings, namely: (1) a single tumor-derived cell is able to differentiate into all the heterogeneous cell types that are typically found in a teratocarcinoma [66]; (2) ECCs can be continuously expanded in vitro when co-cultured with inactivated mouse embryonic fibroblasts (MEFs); (3) after blastocyst ECC injection a chimeric mouse can be generated [67,68]; and (4) differentiation into any embryonic germ layer [69,70].

The ECCs therapeutic potential was compromised due to their tumorigenic potential and aneuploidy karyotype. In an attempt to overcome this drawback, in 1981 two independent laboratories reported the isolation and establishment of ESCs from early mouse embryos [71,72]. By resorting to pre-implanted blastocysts, Evans, Kaufman, and Martin surgically removed the ICM, a sharp source of pluripotent cells, and culture it on fresh feeder layers under conditioned medium. As a result, they obtained a normal diploid ESC line that could differentiate into all mature cell-types from the three germ layers in vitro, and in vivo [71,72]. In 1984, Andrews et al. and Thompson et al. resorted to Tera-2, the oldest extant cell line established from a human teratocarcinoma, to isolate and derive genetically identical clone cells. They observed that clones were highly adapted to culture overgrowth and could maintain their differentiation potential. Moreover, under retinoic acid exposure, clones were capable of differentiating into neuron-like cells and other somatic cell-types [71–73]. As the knowledge regarding pluripotency mechanisms improved, the derivation and differentiation protocols began to be more refined. For instance, Matsui et al. (1992) enhanced the long-term culture of ESCs by adding bFGF to the culture medium [74].

Considering the advances in animal derived-ESCs, the isolation and culture of human pluripotent cells became an exciting challenge at the time. In 1993, Bongso et al. described for the first time the development and maintenance of ICM cultures and the following isolation of ES-like cells from its center. Cells maintained a normal karyotype and stemness-like morphology, however, a limited number of clusters differentiated into fibroblasts [75]. In 1998, two groundbreaking works were reported the establishment of embryonic germ cell (EGC) and ESC lines isolation from a human source [76,77]. Shamblott et al. reported the isolation of PGCs from gonadal ridges and mesenteries at 5–9 weeks post-fertilization, which after a period of 7–21 culture days were positive for alkaline phosphatase activity and also for a commonly panel of immunological markers (SSEA-1, SSEA-3, SSEA-4, TRA-1–60, and TRA-1–81) used to characterize ESCs and EGCs [76]. Later, Thomson and his co-workers announced the derivation and establishment of ESCs in non-human primates. After several passages, the cells retained a normal karyotype, high levels of telomerase activity and typical pluripotency markers expression [77]. To obtain ESCs, researches were using blastocyst which is an embryonic structure that derives after fecundation which implies the use of human embryos. As expected, this idea started to provoke some discussion in the media due to the ethical and religious concerns involved. Despite the controversy, in the following years, different groups developed several ESC lines improving in vitro culture approaches and differentiation protocols. Traditionally, MEF feeders were used to support ESCs growth, however, the relevance of ESCs for a therapeutic approach motivate the reassessment of these support systems, considering the high risk of pathogens cross-transference from the animal feeder cells. A novel xeno-free system was suggested by Richards et al., (2002) with all animal-based products discarded, empowering the potential application of ESCs into the clinic [78].

Therefore, the first clinical trial using human ESC-derived OPCs was approved in 2010 (NCT01217008) [79,80]. The cells were transplanted into patients with spinal cord injury (SCI) and no major complications were reported regarding toxicity, allodynia, or tumor formation [81]. A phase I/IIa dose-escalation study was then initiated in 2014 (NCT02302157), and considering the updates from the responsible biotech company, OPCs were successfully engrafted into the spinal cord of patients. Moreover, some motor improvements were observed, but the official data for the entire study is expected to be published in the first quarter of 2019.

In conclusion, some convergent points stood out and common ESCs characteristics were established among the scientific community: (1) source of pluripotent cell population; (2) maintenance of a stable and diploid karyotype; (3) indefinite propagation in a primary embryonic state; (4) differentiation into any mature cell-type of the three embryonic germ layers; and (5) expression of specific nuclear and cytoplasmic markers of pluripotency [82]. All these characteristics put ESCs forward as good candidates for a wide range of applications, including as a platform for organogenesis studies through the generation of complex tissues such as, the patterned neural tube [83], cerebral organoids [84], and a mature spinal cord [85].

2.2.2. Searching for Pluripotency in Adult Tissues

Despite the excitement created around the ESCs therapeutic potential some issues were hampering their translation to the clinics, mainly, ethical concerns, tumorigenic potential, and impossibility for autologous transplantation. Adult stem cells, such as mesenchymal stem cells, were a viable alternative, however, their differentiation potential is limited. Thus, further efforts were pursued to find a source of pluripotent stem cells (PSCs).

Unexpectedly, in 1962 Gurdon et al. reported the full development of a complete *Xenopus organism* by transferring the nucleus from a somatic cell to an enucleated egg [86]. Although in a very primitive way, Gurdon et al. explored for the first time the concept of reprogramming somatic cells into pluripotent cells. These developments paved the fundamentals of somatic cell nuclear transfer (SCNT) technique which allows the production of genetically suitable cells and tissues. Particularly, it was through SCNT that the famous "Dolly the sheep" was produced, a live offspring capable to mature into adulthood [87]. Despite the notable progress in SCNT research, human experiments were still intolerable due to the ethical concerns [88].

Therefore, additional methodologies were explored to generate PSCs such as: parthenogenesis [89], cell fusion [90], direct somatic cell reprogramming [91], and testis-derivation [92], (see the Muller and Lengerke (2009) review [93]). Among all, when pros and cons are balanced direct somatic cell reprogramming shows to be the most promising technique opening up unprecedented opportunities for regenerative medicine. The groundbreaking report was originally published by Takahashi and Yamanaka in 2006 where they remarkably demonstrated the generation of induced PSCs (iPSCs) from mouse skin fibroblasts. After a full genomic screening, Takahashi and Yamanaka filtered 4 out of 24 genes as pivotal transcriptional factors for the induction and maintenance of iPSCs in an ES-like state: Oct3/4, Sox2, c-Myc, and Klf4 (Figure 4). As a proof of concept, the particular features of ESCs were also present in iPSCs, namely: (1) resembling morphology and growth properties; (2) expression of specific gene markers; (3) tumor formation after transplantation in nude mice; (4) tissue differentiation from all the primary germ layers in the tumor; and (5) complete embryonic development after mouse blastocysts injection [91]. Overall, Takahashi, and Yamanaka created important foundations in regenerative medicine by producing autologous cells and thus, avoiding the need for immunosuppressive agents after transplantation. This pioneering work was the base for the recognition in 2012 with the Nobel Prize in Physiology or Medicine award for Shinya Yamanaka.

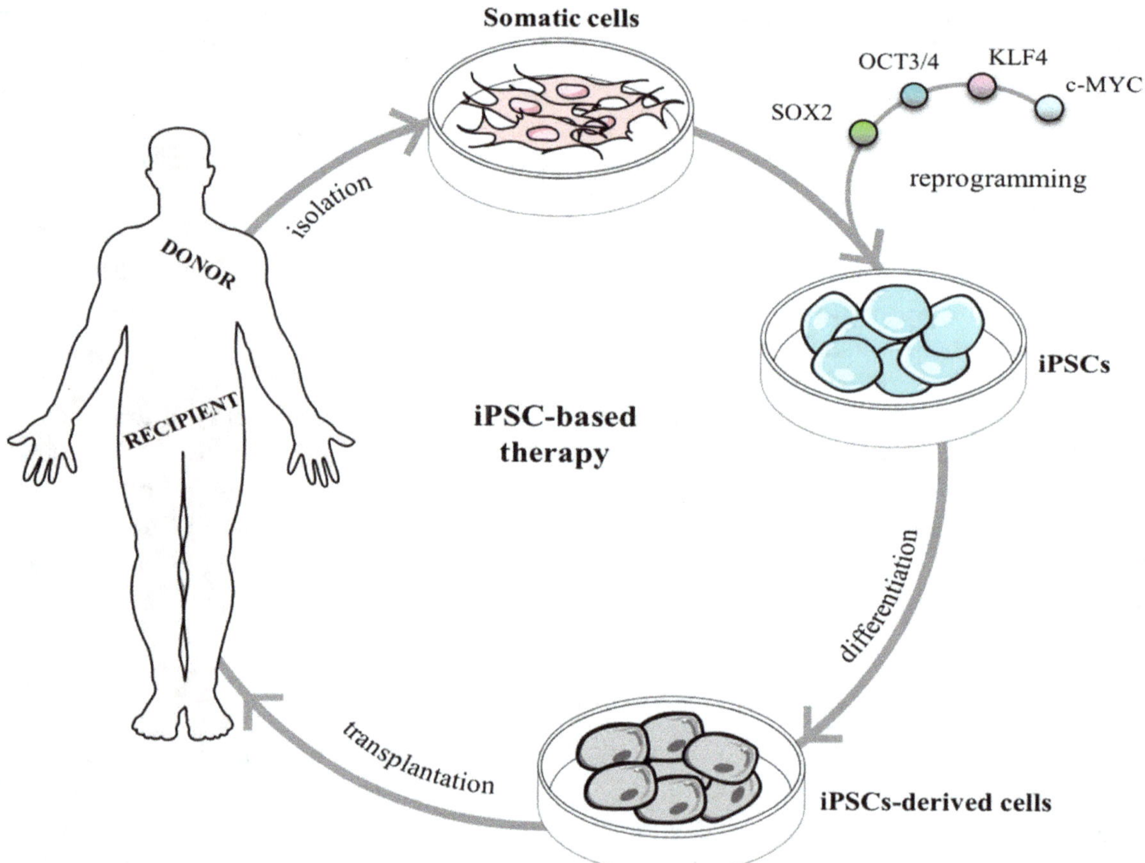

Figure 4. Somatic cells reprogramming using Takahashi and Yamanaka's factors (SOX2, OCT3/4, KLF4, c-MYC) to induced pluripotent stem cells (iPSCs). Induced PSCs can further be used as a novel therapeutic strategy for cell transplantation.

Despite all the benefits, there are some inherent limitations of iPSCs that must be kept in mind to ensure safety (Table 1), such as the potential risk of inducing genomic and/or epigenomic alterations during iPSCs reprogramming [94,95]. Nevertheless, over the past years, rapid and extensive research has been done to improve iPSCs technology to be applied in regenerative medicine, drug therapy, and disease modeling [96].

Table 1. Overview of the advantages and limitations of induced pluripotent stem cells generation and establishment from somatic cells.

Advantages	Limitations
No ethical concerns	Risk of tumor formation
Evidence on a pluripotent profile (ES-like cells)	Epigenetic and genetic alterations
Highly flexible technique	Oncogenes reactivation
Derivation from any somatic cell	Expensive and time-consuming
Patient-specific source (no immune rejection)	

The generation of iPSCs have already been done from a wide range of tissues, from adult human fibroblasts [91,97] to liver and stomach [98,99]. In 2007, Yu et al. modified the gene set used by Takahashi and Yamanaka and instead of the tumorigenic c-MYC, the authors used Lin-28 obtaining a similar population of iPSCs [100]. Moreover, Nakagawa et al. (2008) observed that supplementation with c-Myc was not crucial for iPSCs induction and although the authors reported a significantly lower reprogramming efficiency, they reduced down to zero the probability of teratoma formation after transplantation [101].

On the contrary to ESCs, the use of iPSCs as a valuable source for cell transplantation was well accepted mainly due to the absence of ethical concerns. However, iPSCs also underwent some challenges; namely by the inappropriate use of animal-derived components and the use of retroviral vectors to transfect somatic cells. Thus, novel integration-free methods and xeno-free cultures were developed as well as innovative virus-free strategies [102,103]. These latter advances prompted exponentially the therapeutic applicability of iPSCs by decreasing the risk of tumorigenicity associated with viral genomic-integration.

In 2014, Dr. Takahashi and his team (RIKEN, Kobe, Japan) submitted the first-in-human trial using iPSCs (funded by Highway Program for Realization of Regenerative Medicine and others; University Hospital Medical Information Network Clinical Trials Registry [UMIN-CTR] no. UMIN000011929). A patient with neovascular age-related macular degeneration (AMD), a degenerative retinal disease, received a transplant of a sheet of retinal pigment epithelial (RPE). The RPE cells were differentiated using autologous iPSCs from skin fibroblasts and no immunosuppressive agents were administrated to the patient. After transplantation, neither signs of immune rejection were observed nor aberrant genomic alterations, suggesting no tumorigenesis of the cell graft [104]. These positive outcomes highlight all the potentialities behind iPSC technology as a novel tool for cellular therapy and have launched the beginning of more clinical trials targeting many other conditions (see the Kavyasudha et al., 2018 review [105]).

Human iPSCs are mainly obtained from skin fibroblasts however, a skin biopsy may not be the best source due to the risk of infection and scar formation [97,106]. Thus, other less invasive somatic cell sources have been considered, such as peripheral blood due to the minimal procedures necessary to collect it. In fact, clinicians and researchers have strong expectations in peripheral blood as a gold standard clinical-grade source of iPSCs for the future [80,107].

Additionally, iPSCs technology has also been explored for disease modelling. The establishment of some disease-specific iPSCs lines have already allowed a better understanding of the mechanisms that trigger and are behind certain diseases [108]. The first successful report was based on the generation of iPSCs from a child with Spinal Muscular Atrophy (SMA) [109]. Studies on drug screening and validation have also been conducted using patient-specific cell lines, and relevant advances have already been achieved, for instance, in Rett syndrome [110], and in Fanconi anemia [111].

In conclusion, iPSCs represent a very flexible technology that opened new and challenging opportunities to develop cell-based therapies due to its ability to differentiated into any cell-type given the right culture conditions. The numerous advantages of induced stem cells, from no immune rejection to high reproducibility, prompted the field to employ them in patient-specific diseases studies, developmental studies, cell transplantation as well as in drug screening. As a consequence, we are now moving fast towards a more personalized medicine.

2.2.3. Neural Stem Cells

In the past, researchers assumed that neurons were only generated during embryogenesis, however, Altman and Das (1964) published a remarkable report describing the generation of new neurons in the hippocampal dentate gyrus of an adult rat brain [112]. The generation of new neurons from NSCs is a highly tuned process during nervous system development. Nevertheless, neurogenesis also occurs throughout adult life as an extremely limited process that attempts to sustain a proper balance between self-renewal and differentiation [113,114]. In the adult brain, the two best described niches that harbor NSCs are the subventricular zone (SVZ) and the periventricular region of the spinal cord [113,115].

Therefore, the idea of transplanting NSCs is a very promising therapeutic approach for many neurodevelopmental, neurodegenerative, and neurotraumatic diseases by replacing and reestablishing damaged neuronal circuities [114]. Thus, one of the first topics that should be discussed is how would NSCs be obtained taking in consideration both the cell source and the cell dosage required for adequate transplantation. Until this point, there are three main sources: direct isolation from primary CNS tissue (either from the fetal or adult brain); differentiation from pluripotent stem cells; and, transdifferentiation from somatic cells (Figure 5).

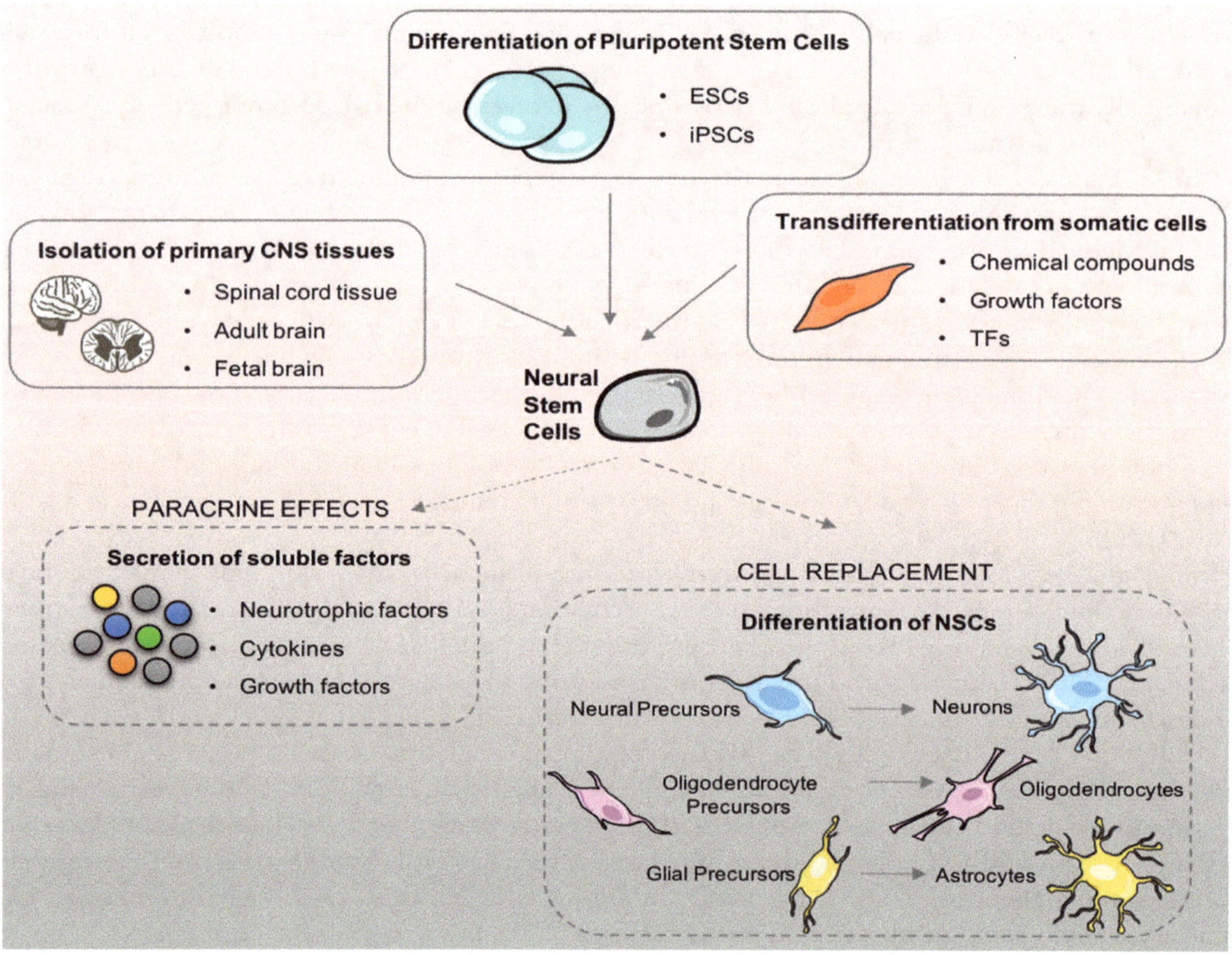

Figure 5. Neural stem cell (NSCs) sources and their therapeutic applicability after cell transplantation. There are three main sources to generate NSCs: isolation from primary central nervous system (CNS) tissue; differentiation of pluripotent stem cells, and lineage reprogramming of somatic cells. After obtaining a considerable number of cells that fulfill the needs of cell transplantation cells can be applied. Once on the injury site, NSCs can be differentiated and also secrete paracrine factors that may also support neurological repair.

NSCs from CNS primary tissues. In 1992, Reynolds and Weiss were the first to report the isolation and culture of NSCs in spherical clusters (neurospheres) from the striatal neurogenic area of an adult mouse brain [116]. Two years later, they remarkably demonstrated in vivo that the subependymal region is a viable source of NSCs in the mouse brain [117]. Concomitantly with their work, two specific mitogenic growth factors, the epidermal growth factor (EGF) and the bFGF were identified as critical factors that cooperatively induce self-renewal, proliferation, and expansion of NSCs in clonal aggregates [115,116]. Indeed, after isolation, NSCs can grow into single-cell suspensions that ultimately form regular neurospheres. These non-adherent neurospheres are particularly interesting due to their self-renewal capacity and because of their capability of establishing a favorable extracellular-matrix microenvironment that helps to maintain stemness. Moreover, neurospheres can be sub-cultured and expanded to increase the available pool of cells. Adult NSCs have, however, the disadvantage of not being able to be used as an autologous cell source.

Differentiation of NSCs from pluripotent stem cells. PSCs have been used as a very attractive alternative to primary tissue isolation. Differentiation of NSCs from ESCs and iPSCs gained a lot of attention due to their therapeutic applicability potential. As previously discussed, iPSC-derived NSCs have striking advantages over ESC-derived NSCs, namely the possibility of autologous transplantation. Regarding differentiation protocols, PSCs have been cultured either as embryoid bodies (EB) or in monolayer cultures. Considering EBs, they grow in suspension and can be differentiated into neural tube-like rosettes and, subsequently, into NPCs under specific conditions [118]. More recently, differentiation protocols of NSCs using iPSC-derived EBs have also been standardized and applied as a promising alternative for cell transplantation [119,120]. Additionally, NSCs can be generated in monolayer cultures using serum-free specific inhibitors and growth factors that contribute to neuronal specification [121,122]. Overall, when comparing both techniques there are no major differences on the typical expression markers of NSCs and morphology. Nevertheless, there are some drawbacks associated with both assays. The EBs are 3-dimensional (3-D) spheroids structures capable of spontaneous differentiation mimicking better the embryonic development by promoting a heterogeneous differentiation, which is also a synonym of low reproducibility of the technique [123,124]. On the other hand, monolayer cultures need continuous passaging to maintain self-renewal and cell potency. 2-D attachment also interferes with the shape and geometry of colonies, which might be deleterious for internal cytoskeleton shape [125,126].

Transdifferentiation of NSCs from somatic cells. Transdifferentiation is the differentiation of cells to a certain cell-type that does not follow the "normal" programmed differentiation mechanism [127]. This term was first applied by Selman and Kafatos (1974) and it is characterized by a direct reprogramming or conversion of one mature somatic cell type into another cell type without undergoing an intermediate pluripotent state [128]. Lineage reprogramming is mainly induced by the expression of endogenous lineage-specific transcription factors (TFs) [129] and by specific chemical compounds [130]. Yao et al. (2015) produced transdifferentiated induced NSCs (iNSCs) after conditionally overexpressing specific TFs (Oct4, Sox2, Klf4, c-Myc) from mouse embryonic fibroblasts. The transdifferentiated cells differentiated into mature astrocytes, neurons, and oligodendrocytes in vitro, and after being transplanted into a stroke rat model, they were able to reduce the lesion size and promote the recovery of motor and sensory function [131]. The TF-induced transdifferentiation has inherent issues associated with the use of exogenous viruses, so, chemical compounds [132] and growth factor-induced transdifferentiation [133] have been developed ensuring advantages in terms of safety. Transdifferentiation has become a powerful tool to study how cells might be manipulated for specific therapeutic purposes [134]. Nevertheless, this field is very recent and further investigation is still needed before the development of personalized regenerative therapies.

2.3. Advances on NSC-based Therapy for SCI

In 1999, McDonald et al. were the first to demonstrate the potentialities of NPCs transplantation in a SCI context. After deriving neural progenitors from mouse ESCs (mESCs) and transplanting them into a rat spinal cord 9 days post-injury they observed that grafts had the capacity to survive and differentiate into neurons, oligodendrocytes, and astrocytes, and to migrate along the rostro-caudal axis from the lesion epicenter. More importantly, the transplanted experimental group showed hind limb weight support and partial walk coordination [135]. From then on, numerous studies have been deciphering the mechanisms behind NSCs effects on SCI. However, there are still some critical questions that remain to be answered and should be addressed, such as, the optimal time-window of efficacy, the number of transplanted cells, the cellular source, safety, and administration routes.

After grafting mouse fetal striatal NS/PCs 12 wpi into a contusion T10 mice model, Kumamaru et al. (2013) observed that cells were capable of releasing multiple regenerative molecules and to differentiate into neurons/oligodendrocytes contributing for a neurogenic spinal cord environment, however, no locomotor improvements were observed [136]. Efforts were also done by Cheng et al. (2017) to explore the appropriate timing for NSCs administration. After injecting hNSCs in a contusion T10 SCI model 1 or 4 wpi, both groups showed significant functional improvement at the motor level, but the effect was more prominent in the acute 1 wpi group [137]. Using NOD/SCID mice, after a T9 injury model, hCNS-derived NSCs were immediately injected after the inflicted injury and no locomotor recovery was observed [138], on the other hand, when Salazar et al. (2010) only applied the cells 4 wpi mice displayed locomotor improvements [139]. Despite the disparities, cells differentiate into all the three CNS lineages, survived, and migrated within the injured spinal cord suggesting that hCNS-derived NSCs transplantation can be effective depending on the time-window of intervention.

Injecting the cells in an earlier phase might be more beneficial to restore the damaged neural circuits before the formation of the glial scar barrier. Nevertheless, the current number of chronic patients is highly considerable which should also stimulate the field to get novel strategies and boost cell transplantation effects in a more chronic phase. Yet, more preclinical studies are needed to better understand the best time window of NSCs transplantation. As mention above, SCI is a two-phase injury process with multiphasic cellular and molecular responses that varies along time which makes it difficult to find the best time-window of treatment [133]. To tackle such oscillations with cell transplantation between acute and chronic SCI, different protocols must be designed. For instance, in the acute phase NSCs may need to be transplanted together with some neuroprotective drug because several biological events are happening in this phase that may hamper cell survival. On the other hand, NSCs transplanted in the chronic phase may need the help of drugs that degrade the glial scar in order to better integrate in the host tissue.

The cellular source to obtain NSCs is also an important variable to be considered. First, animal studies must be carried out to better comprehend and explore the cellular viability and to decipher some potential targets of NSCs after transplantation. Further, preclinical studies are mandatory before conducting a clinical trial mainly to assess safety. Fetal brain and spinal cord are the two main sources used to generate viable NSCs. Using mouse fetal cortex, Cheng et al. (2016) injected NSCs in an acute contusion SCI mice 7 dpi and observed a reduction in M1 macrophages activation, neutrophils and iNOS^{+}/Mac-2^{+} cells at the epicenter of the injured area. Although the underlying factors remain unknown, this beneficial anti-inflammatory profile was translated into a significantly enhanced neurological function in mice [140]. Additionally, different studies have also reported some locomotor improvements after chronic transplantation of NSCs using different cellular backgrounds from the mouse striatum [141], to shrew fetal hippocampus [142], to the rat fetal brain [143].

Concerning human fetal spinal cord NSCs, positive results have also been reported regarding axonal growth at the injured site. For instance, Kadoya et al., showed that after transplantation there is an extensive regeneration of the corticospinal axons, improving synaptic connectivity and forelimb functioning [144]. Meanwhile, Robinson et al. (2017) added to E14 spinal cord-derived NPCs a 4-factor cocktail (BDNF, bFGF, VEGF, MDL) which promoted significant maintenance of grafts survival and neural differentiation, fulfilling the lesion site [145].

The capacity of pluripotent mESCs to differentiate into the neural lineage has also been explored to reestablish the damaged circuits after a SCI. In a contusive SCI model, NSCs derived from a mESC line J1 were intrathecally transplanted 3 wpi showing the ability to differentiate into spinal GABAergic neurons and to attenuate chronic neuropathic pain [146]. In a moderate compression injury of the spinal cord, Salewski et al. (2015) performed acute transplantation of mESC-derived NSCs and the treated group showed significant functional improvements 8 wpi. During the differentiation protocol used, the group described an intermediate step of LIF-dependent neurospheres formation, named as primitive NSCs (pNSCs). Interestingly, they transplanted pNSCs to assess tumorigenic potential which resulted in teratoma formation, raising the warning for tumor formation potential of mESC-derived NSCs as a real safety concern that must be explored during differentiation protocols [53].

Furthermore, preclinical studies have been conducted, approaching different cell sources, to better comprehend better the cellular response after transplantation namely immune rejection, tumor risk formation, and grafts survival. Using a human primary source of neural precursors from the fetal spinal cord (SPC-01) it was showed strong immunomodulatory properties through astroglial p65 NF-κB inhibition which significantly impacted the reduction of the glial scar and the cavity size [147]. Moreover, the well-defined human H9 ESC-derived NSC line has also been commonly addressed as a cellular source with high reproducibility. These cells are characterized by the expression of NSC-specific markers, Nestin and SOX2, and the ability to differentiate into neurons, oligodendrocytes, and astrocytes [148]. After its transplantation to immunodeficient rats, the grafts showed signs of a continuous maturation over a follow-up of 1.5 years. After 3 months, mature neuronal markers were the first to be expressed, 6 months later mature astrocytes showed up, and only 1 year after transplantation mature oligodendrocytes were detected. NSC-derived astrocytes migrated longer-distances in the lesion site when compared with other cell-types and synergistically engrafted with host astrocytes resulting in modest improvements in forelimb motor function without any critical adverse outcomes [149,150].

On the other hand, human pluripotent cells have been yielding in the generation and maintenance of NSCs. Kumamaru and coworkers demonstrated that under specific cues human ESCs (hESCs) can be derived into NSCs committed to the spinal cord improving the potential of neural cells to restore the damaged circuities. After transplantation, cellular grafts revealed to be enriched in excitatory neurons, promoting a robust corticospinal regeneration, engraftment within the host increased synaptic formation, which has culminated in hind-limb improvements [151].

The discovery of iPSCs was one of the most remarkable innovations in regenerative medicine and biological research. The concept of convert adult somatic cells, such as blood cells or skin fibroblasts, into NSCs through iPSCs incited numerous studies in the field. Promising results have been observed after iPSC-derived NSC transplantation into SCI animal models, promoting cell survival, tissue preservation, and neuronal differentiation of cells. Moreover, functional recovery was also observed through the remyelination of axons and upregulation of supportive neurotrophic factors in the spinal cord [53,152,153].

Summing up, animal studies have been very useful to evaluate and decipher novel mechanistic insights after cell transplantation, yet preclinical studies are essential to target critical questions as immune rejection and tumor formation. To circumvent ethical issues and immunosuppression, iPSCs are now the most attractive human cell source, but further studies are required to ensure efficacy, feasibility and safety.

After getting a valid cellular source other questions need to be addressed, namely, the following question raised is, how many cells are needed for a positive outcome? The optimal number of transplanted cells is still very debatable and few studies have been in order to elucidate the field. Yousefifard et al. (2016) have recently performed recently a systemic and meta-analysis to tackle some of these questions regarding NS/PCs transplantation. They reported that the median number of the cells per kilograms of animal's body weight was 4.3106 (interquartile range = 1.1106–2107), but the higher the number of transplanted cells the better was the functional recovery [154,155]. This might be related with a higher chance of cellular survival, and in addition, it was also observed that the number of transplanted cells improves hyperalgesia in the animals [155]. Therefore, it would be important to further study the optimal range of transplanted cells in order to facilitated the translation to humans.

The tumorigenicity risk associated with NSCs transplantation is also a real concern that must be addressed to ensure patients' safety. While some studies do not report any tumor formation [139,156] others documented tumorigenic risk mainly associated with pluripotent-derived NSCs [157,158]. Moreover, as the field advances, evidence has been accumulating on iPSC-derived NSCs tumorigenicity that must be addressed to ensure high clinical quality in the application of these strategies. There are two main forms of tumorigenicity, teratomas and true tumors formation [159], yet the mechanisms triggered behind each of them are not fully understood. Some studies reported the use of tumor-inducing reprogramming factors and some residual undifferentiated cells as the main causes that induce epigenetic alterations in iPSC-derived NSCs [93,94].

Teratomas development is mainly associated with an existent "epigenetic memory" and the lack of purification in the cellular sample used for transplantation [93]. Some strategies that can be undertaken are: increasing the number of passages to dissolve the "epigenetic memory"; develop purification systems with higher yield; reprogram iPSCs to drive away from the teratoma-inducing lineage; or even transplant cells in a more differentiated state.

To avoid tumor formation during iPSCs reprogramming and differentiation there are some critical steps that must be carefully performed to avoid epigenetic and genomic instability in colonies [94]. The choice of the reprogramming method is a key-step to avoid genome disturbance by choosing integration-free systems over integrative vectors [101,102]. Further, the selection of the reprogramming factors is also critical, since c-Myc from Yamanaka's factors is by itself sufficient to induce tumorigenesis [90,100]. However, it was already showed that c-Myc is not indispensable for iPSCs generation, avoiding its application [99,100,160]. Recently, based on these withdraws, Kojima et al. (2018) introduced a specific gene into a tumorigenic human iPSC-NSCs line to successfully ablate immature proliferating cells, and after transplantation, animals did not develop any tumor, moreover, this cells promoted motor recovery [156].

The route of administration is also an important topic that must be considered when addressing cell transplantation. Three main injection routes have been tested to be applied in SCI context: intraspinal, intrathecal, and intravenous. Amemori et al. (2015) studied different administration routes in an acute SCI model. NSCs were either injected intraspinally into the lesion center or intrathecally into the subarachnoid space of rats with compression lesion. Both treatments facilitated functional locomotor recovery, yet the intraspinal implantation had a higher positive effect in gray and white matter sparing and axonal sprouting, and reduced astrogliosis when compared to the intrathecal injection [152]. Nevertheless, when Cheng et al. (2012) injected hNSCs both locally at the injury site or distally no significant differences were observed in functional behavior [161].

Intraspinal injections are the most commonly used route by researchers, however, it is important to have in consideration some positive results published regarding intravenous administration [162,163]. Nishimura's et al. (2013) reported that after hNSC intravenous administration animals showed behavioral improvements, electrophysiological recovery, suppression of glial scar formation, and preservation of nerve fibers. These results suggest that cells are able to survive, proliferate, and migrate into the lesion site [163]. Moreover, Osaka et al. (2010) also support intravenous administration of cells as a minimally invasive approach with high therapeutic potential [164]. Once again, more investigation should be performed considering the ideal route of administration. Minimal invasive administration procedures avoid surgical complications to patients, however, we may also lose some therapeutic efficacy. All these factors should be well studied in the preclinical set up.

On Table 2 it is represented selected preclinical studies employing NSCs for SCI repair. Overall, from a morphological point of view, NSCs are able to differentiate into neurons, astrocytes, and oligodendrocytes promoting axonal regrowth, remyelination and regeneration of the CST [145,150,165]. In addition, NSCs grafts showed consistently the capacity of filling the lesion cavity, reducing the glial scar and a high chance of survive after transplantation [144,166]. Physiologically, Kumamaru et al. (2018)

showed that differentiated cells from NSCs form new synapses within the host spinal cord below the lesion. After assessing cell grafts, they also observed that cells present mainly an excitatory neuronal fate which promotes the host-to-graft connectivity [151]. Moreover, NSCs transplantation has consistently demonstrated to promote functional motor recovery in SCI animal models. For instance, Kadoya et al. (2016) demonstrated that transplanted rats have an improved motor function, by performing the staircase task, which is a supraspinal dependent test and requires a skilled forelimb control [144]. Lu et al. (2017) also reported that even 18 months after NSCs transplantation, cells differentiate and promote functional recovery [150]. Finally, and particularly important, the vast majority of the studies transplanted human-derived NSCs into animal models, which imposes the use of immunosuppressant drugs in combination with the cells. From the immunological point of view, several studies showed that when exogenous NSCs are combined with immunosuppressant drugs they can successfully integrate in the rat/mouse spinal cord without immune rejection [27,166,167]. However, data from clinical trials have shown that when the immunosuppressant therapy is over, patients experience complications related with immune rejection of the new tissue (please see Section 2.4) [168]. For this reason, the development of iPSCs-based therapies is very important to minimize the probabilities of immune rejection by the patient. Therefore, differentiation of NSCs from iPSCs allows to acquire a patient-specific source of suitable cells that can differentiate into neuronal lineages with the aim to replace and assist the damaged neurons.

Due to the complexity of the SCI pathophysiology, different approaches have been developed combining cell-based transplantation with other target-therapies. For instance, after combining chondroitinase ABC (ChABC) treatment with iPSC-derived NSCs mice showed improvements in the forelimb grip strength and forelimb/hindlimb locomotion. The cells were injected after injury, but the ChABC treatment was only administrated 7 wpi. Interestingly, the grafts showed improved survival and differentiation potentially promoting functional synaptic connectivity [27]. With a different strategy, Okubo et al. (2018) injected gamma-secretase inhibitor (GSI)-treated hiPSC-NS/PC into a chronic SCI model. After injection mice showed a significant increase in axonal growth, remyelination, inhibitory synapse formation within the host neural circuitry, and reticulospinal tract fiber formation. In fact, previous work from the group, demonstrated that GSI treatment inhibits Notch signaling promoting neuronal differentiation [169]. Finally, combining these favorable factors leads to motor improvements in lesioned animals [165].

Moreover, biomaterials have also been currently applied as artificial extracellular matrix with the aim to increase the survival of transplanted stem cells. Using a laminin-coated hydrogel with dual porosity, iPSC-NPs were seeded and further transplanted into a rat model of chronic SCI. The cells survived over time and promoted the growth of host axons, astrocytes, and blood vessels; however, no locomotor recovery was observed [166].

Overall, a vast number of approaches have been employed to achieve the best outcome and a significant regeneration of the damaged neurons after SCI, however, some challenges remain to be overcome. Cell-based therapy is a promising strategy since it is capable to target different events, allowing a neuroprotective environment and regenerative support in the injured spinal cord. Therefore, regeneration of the adult spinal cord cannot be thought as a one-step process, but rather as a multiple cascade-process overtime.

Table 2. Preclinical studies using neural stem cells transplantation to target spinal cord injury repair.

SCI	Animal Model	Injury	Transplanted Cells	Time	Additional Treatments	Outcomes	REF
Transection	Fischer 344 Rat C57BL/6 Mice	T3 C4	Rat E14 SC-derived NPCs Mouse E12 SC-derived cells	2 w		Cell grafts survival Full-fill of the cavitation site Axonal CST regeneration and functional synaptic formation Improved forelimb function	[144]
Contusion	C57BL/6 Mice	T9/10	Mouse Fetal Brain NSCs	1 w		Migration from the injection site toward the injury Locomotor improvement Reduction in neutrophils and $iNOS^+/Mac\text{-}2^+$ cells Downregulation of TNF-α, IL-1β, IL-6 and IL-12	[170]
Hemisection	Fischer 344 Rat	C5	Rat E14 SC-derived NPCs	2 w	4-factor cocktail	Consistent graft survival Neuronal differentiation Reduction of the lesion site	[145]
Compression	Wistar Rat	T10	Human Fetal Spinal Cord SPC-01 cell line	1 w		Downregulation of TNF-α Inhibition of p65 NF-κB Reduction of glial scar and cavity size Gray matter preservation	[147]
Compression	C57BL/6 Mice	T6	ES-dNSC	1 w		Enhancement of spared neural tissue Differentiation into oligodendrocytes Motor improvement	[171]
Hemisection	Nude Rat	C5	H9 ESC-derived NSCs	2 w		Graft size stable over time Differentiation into mature neurons and glia Long axonal regrowth Glial migration to host white matter	[150]
Contusion	NOD-scid Mice	T9	hCNS-derived NSCs	0		Astroglial differentiation of donor cells in the lesion site No locomotor recovery	[138]
Transection	Nude Rat	C4	hPSC-derived Spinal Cord NSCs	2 w		NSCs committed to a spinal cord phenotype Differentiation into excitatory neurons Regeneration of the CST Host-to-graft synaptic connectivity	[151]
Compression	WT Mouse C3Fe.SWV-Mbpshi/J Mice	T6	iPS-derived NSCs	1 w		Integration within the lesion site Differentiation to oligodendrocytes *wt*-iPS-dNSCs promote remyelination and axonal function Motor Improvements	[53]

Table 2. *Cont.*

SCI	Animal Model	Injury	Transplanted Cells	Time	Additional Treatments	Outcomes	REF
Compression	Wistar Rat	T8	iPS-derived NPs	1 w		Intraspinal implantation promote: > gray and white matter sparing > axonal sprouting > astrogliosis reduction Moderate functional recovery	[152]
Compression	Wistar Rat	T8/T9	hiPSC-derived NPs	1 w		Cell survival and tissue preservation Differentiation into the three germ layers Motor improvement Increased expression of NFs Neuronal regeneration	[153]
Contusion	C57BL/6 Mice	T10	iPSC-derived NPCs	1 w		Neuronal lineage differentiation No tumor formation No locomotor recovery	[167]
Contusion	Long-Evans hooded Rat	T10	Human Fetal Brain NSCs	4 w		Trophic effect in the CSF Motor improvement	[140]
Contusion	C57BL/6 Mice	T9	Mouse Striatal NS/PCs	7–10 d	Treadmill Training	Differentiation into neurons, oligodendrocytes, and astrocytes Electrophysiologic recovery Locomotor improvements	[141]
Contusion	Rat	T10	Rat Spinal Cord NSCs	13 w	Ch combined with NFs	60% of survival < 40% of the lesion site covered Improvement in bladder function	[172]
Hemisection	Tree Shrew	T10	Shrew Fetal NSCs	9 d		Self-renewal potential Differentiation into neurons and astrocytes Production of NFs (CNTF, TGF-β1, GDNF, NGF, BDNF and IGF)	[142]
Contusion	Wistar Rat	C6/C7	Rat Fetal Brain NSCs	10 d		Long-term survival Differentiation along the oligodendroglial lineage Reduction in M1 macrophages Lower density of iNOS Functional recovery Reduction in apoptosis	[143]
Contusion	Sprague–Dawley Rat	T12	mESC-derived NPCs	3 w		In vitro differentiation into a spinal GABAergic phenotype Attenuation of chronic neuropathic pain	[146]
Hemisection	Nude Rat	C5	Human H9 ESC-derived NSCs	2 w		No cellular migration Improvement in skilled forelimb motor function	[149]

Table 2. *Cont.*

SCI	Animal Model	Injury	Transplanted Cells	Time	Additional Treatments	Outcomes	REF
Contusion	C57BL/6 Mice	C6/C7	iPS-derived NSCs	8 w	Intrathecal ChABC	Cell survival Remyelination and synaptic formation Behavioral recovery of the forelimb grip strength and locomotion	[27]
Contusion	NOD-SCID Mice	T10	hiPSC-derived NS/PCs	6 w	GSI	Axonal regrowth and remyelination Reticulo-spinal tract fiber formation Motor functional recovery	[165]
Compression	Wistar Rat	T8/T8	hiPSC-derived NS/PCs	5 w	Laminin-coated pHEMA-MOETACl hydrogel	Survival and integration within the lesion spinal cord Reduction in cavity depth and axonal growth Increased number of astrocytes, blood vessels, and TH^+ fibers No locomotor recovery	[166]

Abbreviations: w weeks; d days; wt wild-type; ChABC chondroitinase ABC; NTFs neurotrophic factors; GSI gamma-secretase inhibitor; CST corticospinal tract; BDNF brain-derived neurotrophic Factor; bFGF basic-fibroblastic growth Factor; VEGF vascular endothelial growth factor; NSC neural stem cell; NPC neural progenitor cell; iPSC-derived NSC induced pluripotent stem cell-derived NSCs; mESC-derived NPCs mouse embryonic stem cell–derived NPCs; hiPSC-derived NS/PCs human induced pluripotent stem cell-derived NS/PCs; ES-dNSC embryonic stem-definitive NSCs; hCNS-derived NSCs human central nervous system-derived NSCs.

2.4. SCI Clinical Trials Based on NSCs

Translational medicine has been one of the biggest challenges in science and medicine. Interestingly, the European Society for Translational Medicine (EUSTM) defined it as *an interdisciplinary branch of the biomedical field supported by three main pillars: benchside, bedside, and community* [173]. Promising studies have been developed concerning NSCs transplantation to different SCI models, inciting now an important and necessary transition from the *benchside*-to-*bedside*. Although the encouraging results reported in preclinical studies, translation into the clinical set is still very challenging [174], being the main limitations: anatomical differences between experimental animal models and human SCI [175]; inconsistency observed in the therapeutic efficacy; variability in NSCs generation; number of transplanted cells; logistics to obtain donor cells that can be reliable and safely stored for clinical use; ethical concerns; sample size and subject selection criteria; absence of standardization in the post-assessment tests; and extensive costs of running clinical trials.

To date, a low number of clinical trials have been conducted for SCI patients using NSCs, nevertheless, some have already been concluded and others are still ongoing (Table 3).

The first clinical trial using NSCs was approved in 2005 by the Yonsei University Health System, Severance Hospital, Republic of Korea (Clinical Research Information Service (CRIS), Registration Number: KCT0000879). The phase I/ II clinical trial was based on the transplantation of NSC-derived from brain fetal tissue. Human NSCs neurospheres between P10–P20 were carefully selected and prepared for transplantation into 19 patients which were subdivided into four groups according to the time window between the injury onset and transplantation: acute (<1 week), early subacute (1–8 weeks), late subacute (9 weeks–6 months), and chronic (>6 months). A control group was also addressed to the clinical trial of 15 patients with traumatic cervical SCI. After 1 year, the study concluded that hNSCs transplantation is safe and well-tolerable by patients since no adverse evidence was observed. The patients did not exhibit evidence of cord damage, syrinx or tumor formation, neither neurological deterioration nor exacerbating neuropathic pain and spasticity. Regarding neurological outcomes, based on the American Spinal Injury Association Impairment Scale (AIS) grade, 5 out of 19 transplanted patients showed beneficial alterations, including recovery at the motor level and increased motor scores, whereas only 1 patient in the control group showed improvement [176].

Table 3. Spinal Cord Injury Clinical Trials using NSC-based therapies.

Start Year	Sponsor	Country	NTC/I.D.	Clinical Phase	SCI Cohort	Cell-Type	Cell Source	Safety	Improvements	Others	REF
2005	Yonsei University Health System, Severance Hospital	KR	KCT0000879	Phase I/II	Cervical	hNSPCs	Fetal brain	Safe and well-tolerable	Partial sensorimotor function	No cord damage, syrinx or tumor formation No neurological deterioration, and exacerbating neuropathic pain or spasticity Incomplete sensory recovery	[176]
2011	StemCells, Inc.	CAN CH	NCT01321333	Phase I/II	T2-T11	HuCNS-SCs	Fetal brain	Safe and well-tolerable	Segmental sensory	Decline in sensory gains lost after withdrawal of the immunosuppressive	[168]
2012	StemCells, Inc.	CH	NCT01725880	Phase I/II	T2-T11	HuCNS-SCs	Fetal brain	Study terminated based on a business decision			[177]
2013	Neuralstem Inc.	US	NCT01772810	Phase I	T2-T12	NSI-566 cell line	Fetal spinal cord (cervical and upper thoracic regions)	Safe and no side effects 18–27 months after cell delivery		Low sample size (n = 4) Still Recruiting	[178]
2014	StemCells, Inc.	US CAN	NCT02163876	Phase I/II	C5-C7	HuCNS-SCs	Fetal brain	Slight motor strength but the study was terminated based on a business decision			[179]
2017	University of Zurich	CH	NCT03069404	Phase I/II	T2-T11	HuCNS-SCs	Fetal brain	No data			[180]
2014	Federal Research Clinical Center of Federal Medical & Biological Agency	RU	NCT02326662	Phase I/II	Neck, thoracic or lumbar	drNSCs	BMCs	Safe with any complications	Neurologic state		[181]
2016	Chinese Academy of Sciences	CN	NCT02688049	Phase I/II	C5-T12	NSCs		No data Still recruiting			[182]
2010	Asterias Biotherapeutics	US	NCT01217008	Phase I	Neurologically Complete, Subacute	GRNOPC1	hESCs	The study was terminated based on financial issues			[183]
2015	Asterias Biotherapeutics	US	NCT02302157	Phase I/II	C4-C7	AST-OPC1	hESCs	Favorable safety profile	Some hand functions		[184]

Abbreviations: T thoracic; US United States; CAN Canada; CH Switzerland; CN China; RU Russian Federation; KR Republic of Korea; NSCs neural stem cells; hESCs human embryonic stem cells; BMCs bone marrow cells; HuCNS-SCs human central nervous system stem cells; NSI-566 cell line human spinal-cord-derived NSC; drNSC directly reprogrammed autologous NSCs; AST-OPC1 AST-oligodendrocyte progenitor cells; GRNOPC1 human embryonic stem cell-derived OPCs.

Neuralstem Inc. (Germantown, MD, USA) began a phase I safety trial (clinicaltrials.gov identifier: NCT01772810) at the University of California San Diego to intramedullary injected an FDA-approved NSI-566RSC cell line into thoracic (T2-T12) SCI subjects. NSI-566RSC line is derived from the cervical and upper thoracic regions of the spinal cord from an 8 gestational weeks human fetus. The first report was published by Curtis et al. (2018) showing that NSI-566 grafts are safe and have no detectable side effects after 18–27 months of cell transplantation [178]. However, the small sample size (n = 4) is a major drawback in the assessment of this one-open-arm study. Nevertheless, future studies are needed and justified due to the positive results regarding the safety and tolerability of NSI-566RSC cells in subjects.

As mentioned before, Asterias Biotherapeutics Inc. (Fremont, CA, USA) has also begun a safety trial in the implementation of human ESC-derived oligodendrocyte progenitors (GRNOPC1 cells) [78] in patients with neurologically complete subacute SCI (clinicaltrials.gov identifier no. NCT01217008). Although some financial problems delay the initial study, a second clinical trial was initiated as a phase I/IIa dose-escalation study using the same embryonic-derived OPCs (NCT02302157). Preliminary results suggest improvements in motor function, but further data still needed [80].

In 2014, a different clinical trial was also initiated to evaluate the safety and the potential of directly reprogrammed autologous NSCs (drNSCs) in subacute and chronic SCI subjects (Federal Research Clinical Center of Federal Medical & Biological Agency, Russia, NCT02326662). Directly reprogrammed NSCs were generated from patients' bone marrow cells (BMCs) using a patented reprogramming xeno-free cocktail. The grafts were directly injected into the white and grey matter of the spinal cord adjacent to the lesion after the implantation of a regeneration matrix (RMx). Although the sample size presented by the study is extremely limited (n = 5), after 6–9 months of follow-up there was no complications or side effects associated with the intervention, and all patients showed improvements in the neurologic state.

Many different reports have already described the benefits of research cell lines transplantation into rodent models of thoracic contusion SCI [185–188]. Concomitantly to these results, Stemcells, Inc. led a phase II clinical trial in thoracic SCI patients using the HuCNS-SCs cell line (NCT02163876). The main aim was to escalate the dose safety and efficacy, 4 months after injury, of intramedullary injections rostral and caudally to C5-C7 injury. An optimistic press release of interim 6-month data (November 18, 2015) reported improvements in motor strength in 4 out of 5 subjects. Using the same HuCNS-SCs, Anderson et al. (2017) inject them in an in vivo preclinical study to validate locomotor and sensory recovery, cell engraftment, migration, and neural lineage fate of cells [48]. Yet, no evidence of HuCNS-SCs efficacy was observed raising awareness for the necessity of validation of cell lines and/or in cell manufacture/processing, to diminish possible variations and ensure consistency along preclinical studies to clinical trials. Nevertheless, after one-year post-transplantation, no evidence of additional spinal cord damage, new lesions, or syrinx formation was observed in patients. An efficacy threshold was previously set by the sponsor to further support the study and by citing a lack of significant improvements and trend for improvements over time, StemCells Inc. actually terminated the study [189].

In 2011, a new phase I/II clinical trial (NCT01321333) was sponsored by Stem Cells Inc. and managed at the University Hospital Balgrist (Zurich, Switzerland). Based on previous preclinical studies, the main focus was to assess the safety and preliminary efficacy of human CNS stem cells (HuCNS-SC) transplantation. The trial included 12 thoracic (T2-T11) SCI patients who sustained an injury within 3–12 months prior to cell transplantation. At the injection time, patients received approximately a total of 20 million cells directly into the spinal cord, 2 injections rostral and 2 caudally to the injury site. After 12-months o, HuCNS-SC showed to be safe and feasible concerning the surgery and the cellular transplant. More interestingly, 7 out of the 12 patients experienced sensory improvements after neurological stability [178].

Following these positive results, a second clinical trial was approved (NCT01725880) to perform a long-term follow-up of the transplanted HuCNS-SC subjects. However, some obstacles appeared that should be carefully considered. After 9 months of immunosuppression, the agents were removed and the sensory gains were lost. It seems that the immune system was rejecting the transplanted cells which culminate with the ceasing of the long-term follow up. Although the result observed in SCI patients was not expected, this warned the field for a real problem in transplant non-patient cells that might be challenging the host immune system. Consequently, the cell source used for clinical cell transplantation must be rethought being NSCs-derived from iPSCs one of the most attractive alternatives.

Okano's team in Japan is proposing the launch of the human clinical study using allogenic iPSC-derived NSCs for subacute SCI patients. The costs associated with quality testing, safety concerns and time-consuming for autologous transplants have led the team to an increased interest in an allogeneic alternative. Therefore, the Center for iPS Cell Research and Application (CiRA) at Kyoto University will donate "iPSCs of human leucocyte antigen (HLA) super-donors" for cell transplant intervention, which are clinical-grade allogenic immunologically match clones and no adverse outcomes are expected. Thus, the conduction of this clinical trial intends firstly to address safety and tumorigenesis issues associated with the transplantation of these clones into humans as a future viable therapeutic intervention [190,191].

Overall, clinical trials have been showing some modest improvements to the SCI patients. More important, these trials have not shown major safety problems, however the clinical trial perform by University Hospital Balgrist shown that after stopping immunosuppression complications may arise. For these reasons, autologous iPSC-derived NSCs are the most promising cell source to repair the injured spinal cord. This section was only based on the NSCs-based, however, several different therapeutic agents were or are being testing in clinical settings with the aim to promote SCI repair. For more information about clinical trials in a SCI context please read the following reviews [192–195].

3. Future Perspectives

NSCs are a promising therapeutic approach for SCI repair. NSCs can differentiate and replace the lost neural tissue as well as secrete neurotrophic factors that can protect or regenerate the tissue. Nevertheless, further studies are necessary to confirm neurological and functional benefits, safety, adjusting doses and administrations periods, and to select the most promising cellular sources to obtain NSCs. Despite all the efforts and progress, the match between preclinical models and human SCI is still poorly established but several ongoing clinical can provide an important avenue for future cell transplantation research. It is also important to highlight that cellular transplantation alone may not be a sufficient approach to completely treat the injured spinal cord, therefore, combinatory therapies may be necessary for the treatment of this devastating injury.

Author Contributions: I.M.P.: Conception and design, manuscript writing; A.M.: Manuscript writing; A.J.S.: manuscript writing; and N.A.S.: Conception and design, manuscript writing, final approval of manuscript.

References

1. James, S.L.; Theadom, A.; Ellenbogen, R.G.; Bannick, M.S.; Montjoy-Venning, W.; Lucchesi, L.R.; Abbasi, N.; Abdulkader, R.; Abraha, H.N.; Adsuar, J.C.; et al. Global, regional, and national burden of traumatic brain injury and spinal cord injury, 1990–2016: A systematic analysis for the Global Burden of Disease Study 2016. *Lancet Neurol.* **2019**, *18*, 56–87. [CrossRef]
2. Karunakaran, K.D.; He, J.; Zhao, J.; Cui, J.-L.; Zang, Y.-F.; Zhang, Z.; Biswal, B.B. Differences in Cortical Gray Matter Atrophy of Paraplegia and Tetraplegia after Complete Spinal Cord Injury. *J. Neurotrauma* **2019**. (In press) [CrossRef]
3. McDonald, J.W.; Sadowsky, C. Spinal-cord injury. *Lancet* **2002**, *359*, 417–425. [CrossRef]
4. Tator, C.H. Update on the Pathophysiology and Pathology of Acute Spinal Cord Injury. *Brain Pathol.* **1995**, *5*, 407–413. [CrossRef]
5. Allen, A.R. Surgery of experimental lesion of spinal cord equivalent to crush injury of fracture dislocation of spinal column: A preliminary report. *J. Am. Med. Assoc.* **1911**, *LVII*, 878. [CrossRef]

6. Hagen, E.M. Acute complications of spinal cord injuries. *World J. Orthop.* **2015**, *6*, 17. [CrossRef] [PubMed]
7. Benton, R.L.; Hagg, T. Vascular Pathology as a Potential Therapeutic Target in SCI. *Transl. Stroke Res.* **2011**, *2*, 556–574. [CrossRef]
8. Li, X.-Q.; Fang, B.; Tan, W.-F.; Wang, Z.-L.; Sun, X.-J.; Zhang, Z.-L.; Ma, H. miR-320a affects spinal cord edema through negatively regulating aquaporin-1 of blood–spinal cord barrier during bimodal stage after ischemia reperfusion injury in rats. *BMC Neurosci.* **2016**, *17*, 10. [CrossRef]
9. Phillips, A.A.; Krassioukov, A.V. Contemporary Cardiovascular Concerns after Spinal Cord Injury: Mechanisms, Maladaptations, and Management. *J. Neurotrauma* **2015**, *32*, 1927–1942. [CrossRef]
10. Visavadiya, N.P.; Patel, S.P.; VanRooyen, J.L.; Sullivan, P.G.; Rabchevsky, A.G. Cellular and subcellular oxidative stress parameters following severe spinal cord injury. *Redox Biol.* **2016**, *8*, 59–67. [CrossRef] [PubMed]
11. Gwak, Y.S.; Hulsebosch, C.E. GABA and central neuropathic pain following spinal cord injury. *Neuropharmacology* **2011**, *60*, 799–808. [CrossRef]
12. Park, E.; Velumian, A.A.; Fehlings, M.G. The Role of Excitotoxicity in Secondary Mechanisms of Spinal Cord Injury: A Review with an Emphasis on the Implications for White Matter Degeneration. *J. Neurotrauma* **2004**, *21*, 754–774. [CrossRef] [PubMed]
13. David, S.; Kroner, A.; Greenhalgh, A.D.; Zarruk, J.G.; López-Vales, R. Myeloid cell responses after spinal cord injury. *J. Neuroimmunol.* **2018**, *321*, 97–108. [CrossRef] [PubMed]
14. Gensel, J.C.; Zhang, B. Macrophage activation and its role in repair and pathology after spinal cord injury. *Brain Res.* **2015**, *1619*, 1–11. [CrossRef] [PubMed]
15. Monteiro, S.; Salgado, A.; Silva, N. Immunomodulation as a neuroprotective strategy after spinal cord injury. *Neural Regen. Res.* **2018**, *13*, 423. [PubMed]
16. Lim, S.-W.; Shiue, Y.-L.; Ho, C.-H.; Yu, S.-C.; Kao, P.-H.; Wang, J.-J.; Kuo, J.-R. Anxiety and Depression in Patients with Traumatic Spinal Cord Injury: A Nationwide Population-Based Cohort Study. *PLoS ONE* **2017**, *12*, e0169623. [CrossRef] [PubMed]
17. Maldonado-Bouchard, S.; Peters, K.; Woller, S.A.; Madahian, B.; Faghihi, U.; Patel, S.; Bake, S.; Hook, M.A. Inflammation is increased with anxiety- and depression-like signs in a rat model of spinal cord injury. *Brain Behav. Immun.* **2016**, *51*, 176–195. [CrossRef] [PubMed]
18. Anderson, M.A.; Burda, J.E.; Ren, Y.; Ao, Y.; O'Shea, T.M.; Kawaguchi, R.; Coppola, G.; Khakh, B.S.; Deming, T.J.; Sofroniew, M.V. Astrocyte scar formation aids central nervous system axon regeneration. *Nature* **2016**, *532*, 195–200. [CrossRef]
19. Dias, D.O.; Kim, H.; Holl, D.; Werne Solnestam, B.; Lundeberg, J.; Carlén, M.; Göritz, C.; Frisén, J. Reducing Pericyte-Derived Scarring Promotes Recovery after Spinal Cord Injury. *Cell* **2018**, *173*, 153–165. [CrossRef] [PubMed]
20. Gallo, V.; Bertolotto, A.; Levi, G. The proteoglycan chondroitin sulfate is present in a subpopulation of cultured astrocytes and in their precursors. *Dev. Biol.* **1987**, *123*, 282–285. [CrossRef]
21. Hackett, A.R.; Lee, J.K. Understanding the NG2 Glial Scar after Spinal Cord Injury. *Front. Neurol.* **2016**, *7*, 199. [CrossRef]
22. Feng, N.; Hao, G.; Yang, F.; Qu, F.; Zheng, H.; Liang, S.; Jin, Y. Transplantation of mesenchymal stem cells promotes the functional recovery of the central nervous system following cerebral ischemia by inhibiting myelin-associated inhibitor expression and neural apoptosis. *Exp. Ther. Med.* **2016**, *11*, 1595–1600. [CrossRef]
23. Kucher, K.; Johns, D.; Maier, D.; Abel, R.; Badke, A.; Baron, H.; Thietje, R.; Casha, S.; Meindl, R.; Gomez-Mancilla, B.; et al. First-in-Man Intrathecal Application of Neurite Growth-Promoting Anti-Nogo-A Antibodies in Acute Spinal Cord Injury. *Neurorehabil. Neural Repair* **2018**, *32*, 578–589. [CrossRef]
24. Dyck, S.M.; Karimi-Abdolrezaee, S. Chondroitin sulfate proteoglycans: Key modulators in the developing and pathologic central nervous system. *Exp. Neurol.* **2015**, *269*, 169–187. [CrossRef]
25. Andrews, P.W. From teratocarcinomas to embryonic stem cells. *Philos. Trans. R. Soc. Lond. B. Biol. Sci.* **2002**, *357*, 405–417. [CrossRef]
26. Lang, B.T.; Cregg, J.M.; DePaul, M.A.; Tran, A.P.; Xu, K.; Dyck, S.M.; Madalena, K.M.; Brown, B.P.; Weng, Y.-L.; Li, S.; et al. Modulation of the proteoglycan receptor PTPσ promotes recovery after spinal cord injury. *Nature* **2015**, *518*, 404–408. [CrossRef]

27. Suzuki, H.; Ahuja, C.S.; Salewski, R.P.; Li, L.; Satkunendrarajah, K.; Nagoshi, N.; Shibata, S.; Fehlings, M.G. Neural stem cell mediated recovery is enhanced by Chondroitinase ABC pretreatment in chronic cervical spinal cord injury. *PLoS ONE* **2017**, *12*, e0182339. [CrossRef]
28. Oni-Orisan, A.; Kaushal, M.; Li, W.; Leschke, J.; Ward, B.D.; Vedantam, A.; Kalinosky, B.; Budde, M.D.; Schmit, B.D.; Li, S.-J.; et al. Alterations in Cortical Sensorimotor Connectivity following Complete Cervical Spinal Cord Injury: A Prospective Resting-State fMRI Study. *PLoS ONE* **2016**, *11*, e0150351. [CrossRef]
29. Theodore, N.; Hadley, M.N.; Aarabi, B.; Dhall, S.S.; Gelb, D.E.; Hurlbert, R.J.; Rozzelle, C.J.; Ryken, T.C.; Walters, B.C. Prehospital Cervical Spinal Immobilization After Trauma. *Neurosurgery* **2013**, *72*, 22–34. [CrossRef]
30. Li, Y.; Walker, C.L.; Zhang, Y.P.; Shields, C.B.; Xu, X.-M. Surgical decompression in acute spinal cord injury: A review of clinical evidence, animal model studies, and potential future directions of investigation. *Front. Biol.* **2014**, *9*, 127–136. [CrossRef]
31. Bartholdi, D.; Schwab, M.E. Methylprednisolone inhibits early inflammatory processes but not ischemic cell death after experimental spinal cord lesion in the rat. *Brain Res.* **1995**, *672*, 177–186. [CrossRef]
32. Ahuja, C.S.; Schroeder, G.D.; Vaccaro, A.R.; Fehlings, M.G. Spinal Cord Injury—What Are the Controversies? *J. Orthop. Trauma* **2017**, *31*, S7–S13. [CrossRef] [PubMed]
33. Caruso, M.C.; Daugherty, M.C.; Moody, S.M.; Falcone, R.A.; Bierbrauer, K.S.; Geis, G.L. Lessons learned from administration of high-dose methylprednisolone sodium succinate for acute pediatric spinal cord injuries. *J. Neurosurg. Pediatr.* **2017**, *20*, 567–574. [CrossRef]
34. Shultz, R.; Zhong, Y. Minocycline targets multiple secondary injury mechanisms in traumatic spinal cord injury. *Neural Regen. Res.* **2017**, *12*, 702. [PubMed]
35. Casha, S.; Zygun, D.; McGowan, M.D.; Bains, I.; Yong, V.W.; John Hurlbert, R. Results of a phase II placebo-controlled randomized trial of minocycline in acute spinal cord injury. *Brain* **2012**, *135*, 1224–1236. [CrossRef] [PubMed]
36. Nagoshi, N.; Nakashima, H.; Fehlings, M. Riluzole as a Neuroprotective Drug for Spinal Cord Injury: From Bench to Bedside. *Molecules* **2015**, *20*, 7775–7789. [CrossRef]
37. Vasconcelos, N.L.; Gomes, E.D.; Oliveira, E.P.; Silva, C.J.; Lima, R.; Sousa, N.; Salgado, A.J.; Silva, N.A. Combining neuroprotective agents: Effect of riluzole and magnesium in a rat model of thoracic spinal cord injury. *Spine J.* **2016**, *16*, 1015–1024. [CrossRef]
38. Chow, D.S.L.; Teng, Y.; Toups, E.G.; Aarabi, B.; Harrop, J.S.; Shaffrey, C.I.; Johnson, M.M.; Boakye, M.; Frankowski, R.F.; Fehlings, M.G.; et al. Pharmacology of riluzole in acute spinal cord injury. *J. Neurosurg. Spine* **2012**, *17*, 129–140. [CrossRef]
39. Fehlings, M.G.; Nakashima, H.; Nagoshi, N.; Chow, D.S.L.; Grossman, R.G.; Kopjar, B. Rationale, design and critical end points for the Riluzole in Acute Spinal Cord Injury Study (RISCIS): A randomized, double-blinded, placebo-controlled parallel multi-center trial. *Spinal Cord* **2016**, *54*, 8–15. [CrossRef]
40. Zhou, Y.; Wang, Z.; Li, J.; Li, X.; Xiao, J. Fibroblast growth factors in the management of spinal cord injury. *J. Cell. Mol. Med.* **2018**, *22*, 25–37. [CrossRef]
41. Nordblom, J.; Persson, J.K.E.; Brismar, H.; Sjodahl, J.; Josephson, A.; Frostell, A.; Thams, S.; Brundin, L.; Svensson, M.; Mattsson, P. FGF1 containing biodegradable device with peripheral nerve grafts induces corticospinal tract regeneration and motor evoked potentials after spinal cord resection. *Restor. Neurol. Neurosci.* **2012**, *30*, 91–102.
42. Nishio, Y.; Koda, M.; Kamada, T.; Someya, Y.; Kadota, R.; Mannoji, C.; Miyashita, T.; Okada, S.; Okawa, A.; Moriya, H.; et al. Granulocyte Colony-Stimulating Factor Attenuates Neuronal Death and Promotes Functional Recovery After Spinal Cord Injury in Mice. *J. Neuropathol. Exp. Neurol.* **2007**, *66*, 724–731. [CrossRef]
43. Kamiya, K.; Koda, M.; Furuya, T.; Kato, K.; Takahashi, H.; Sakuma, T.; Inada, T.; Ota, M.; Maki, S.; Okawa, A.; et al. Neuroprotective therapy with granulocyte colony-stimulating factor in acute spinal cord injury: A comparison with high-dose methylprednisolone as a historical control. *Eur. Spine J.* **2015**, *24*, 963–967. [CrossRef] [PubMed]
44. Takahashi, H.; Yamazaki, M.; Okawa, A.; Sakuma, T.; Kato, K.; Hashimoto, M.; Hayashi, K.; Furuya, T.; Fujiyoshi, T.; Kawabe, J.; et al. Neuroprotective therapy using granulocyte colony-stimulating factor for acute spinal cord injury: A phase I/IIa clinical trial. *Eur. Spine J.* **2012**, *21*, 2580–2587. [CrossRef] [PubMed]

45. Kigerl, K.A.; Gensel, J.C.; Ankeny, D.P.; Alexander, J.K.; Donnelly, D.J.; Popovich, P.G. Identification of two distinct macrophage subsets with divergent effects causing either neurotoxicity or regeneration in the injured mouse spinal cord. *J. Neurosci. Off. J. Soc. Neurosci.* **2009**, *29*, 13435–13444. [CrossRef] [PubMed]
46. Francos-Quijorna, I.; Amo-Aparicio, J.; Martinez-Muriana, A.; López-Vales, R. IL-4 drives microglia and macrophages toward a phenotype conducive for tissue repair and functional recovery after spinal cord injury. *Glia* **2016**, *64*, 2079–2092. [CrossRef] [PubMed]
47. Lima, R.; Monteiro, S.; Lopes, J.; Barradas, P.; Vasconcelos, N.; Gomes, E.; Assunção-Silva, R.; Teixeira, F.; Morais, M.; Sousa, N.; et al. Systemic Interleukin-4 Administration after Spinal Cord Injury Modulates Inflammation and Promotes Neuroprotection. *Pharmaceuticals* **2017**, *10*, 83. [CrossRef]
48. Anderson, K.D.; Guest, J.D.; Dietrich, W.D.; Bartlett Bunge, M.; Curiel, R.; Dididze, M.; Green, B.A.; Khan, A.; Pearse, D.D.; Saraf-Lavi, E.; et al. Safety of Autologous Human Schwann Cell Transplantation in Subacute Thoracic Spinal Cord Injury. *J. Neurotrauma* **2017**, *34*, 2950–2963. [CrossRef]
49. Gomes, E.D.; Mendes, S.S.; Assunção-Silva, R.C.; Teixeira, F.G.; Pires, A.O.; Anjo, S.I.; Manadas, B.; Leite-Almeida, H.; Gimble, J.M.; Sousa, N.; et al. Co-Transplantation of Adipose Tissue-Derived Stromal Cells and Olfactory Ensheathing Cells for Spinal Cord Injury Repair: Co-transplantation of ASCs and OECs for SCI Repair. *Stem Cells* **2018**, *36*, 696–708. [CrossRef]
50. May, Z.; Kumar, R.; Fuehrmann, T.; Tam, R.; Vulic, K.; Forero, J.; Osma, A.L.; Fenrich, K.; Assinck, P.; Lee, M.J.; et al. Adult skin-derived precursor Schwann cell grafts form growths in the injured spinal cord of Fischer rats. *Biomed. Mater.* **2018**, *13*, 034101. [CrossRef]
51. Gomes, E.D.; Mendes, S.S.; Leite-Almeida, H.; Gimble, J.M.; Tam, R.Y.; Shoichet, M.S.; Sousa, N.; Silva, N.A.; Salgado, A.J. Combination of a peptide-modified gellan gum hydrogel with cell therapy in a lumbar spinal cord injury animal model. *Biomaterials* **2016**, *105*, 38–51. [CrossRef]
52. Kawabata, S.; Takano, M.; Numasawa-Kuroiwa, Y.; Itakura, G.; Kobayashi, Y.; Nishiyama, Y.; Sugai, K.; Nishimura, S.; Iwai, H.; Isoda, M.; et al. Grafted Human iPS Cell-Derived Oligodendrocyte Precursor Cells Contribute to Robust Remyelination of Demyelinated Axons after Spinal Cord Injury. *Stem Cell Rep.* **2016**, *6*, 1–8. [CrossRef]
53. Salewski, R.P.; Mitchell, R.A.; Li, L.; Shen, C.; Milekovskaia, M.; Nagy, A.; Fehlings, M.G. Transplantation of Induced Pluripotent Stem Cell-Derived Neural Stem Cells Mediate Functional Recovery Following Thoracic Spinal Cord Injury Through Remyelination of Axons: Myelination Following SCI With iPS-dNSC Treatment. *Stem Cell. Transl. Med.* **2015**, *4*, 743–754. [CrossRef]
54. Tam, P.P.L.; Rossant, J. Mouse embryonic chimeras: Tools for studying mammalian development. *Development* **2003**, *130*, 6155–6163. [CrossRef]
55. Arkell Ruth, M.; Tam Patrick, P.L. Initiating head development in mouse embryos: Integrating signalling and transcriptional activity. *Open Biol.* **2012**, *2*, 120030. [CrossRef]
56. Takata, N.; Sakakura, E.; Eiraku, M.; Kasukawa, T.; Sasai, Y. Self-patterning of rostral-caudal neuroectoderm requires dual role of Fgf signaling for localized Wnt antagonism. *Nat. Commun.* **2017**, *8*, 1339. [CrossRef]
57. Purves, D.; Augustine, G.J.; Fitzpatrick, D.; Katz, L.C.; LaMantia, A.-S.; McNamara, J.O.; Williams, S.M. *The Initial Formation of the Nervous System: Gastrulation and Neurulation*, 2nd ed.; Sinauer Associates: Sunderland, MA, USA, 2001.
58. Gouti, M.; Tsakiridis, A.; Wymeersch, F.J.; Huang, Y.; Kleinjung, J.; Wilson, V.; Briscoe, J. In Vitro Generation of Neuromesodermal Progenitors Reveals Distinct Roles for Wnt Signalling in the Specification of Spinal Cord and Paraxial Mesoderm Identity. *PLoS Biol.* **2014**, *12*, e1001937. [CrossRef]
59. Henrique, D.; Abranches, E.; Verrier, L.; Storey, K.G. Neuromesodermal progenitors and the making of the spinal cord. *Development* **2015**, *142*, 2864–2875. [CrossRef]
60. Javali, A.; Misra, A.; Leonavicius, K.; Acharyya, D.; Vyas, B.; Sambasivan, R. Co-expression of Tbx6 and Sox2 identifies a novel transient neuromesoderm progenitor cell state. *Dev. Camb. Engl.* **2017**, *144*, 4522–4529. [CrossRef]
61. Lippmann, E.S.; Williams, C.E.; Ruhl, D.A.; Estevez-Silva, M.C.; Chapman, E.R.; Coon, J.J.; Ashton, R.S. Deterministic HOX Patterning in Human Pluripotent Stem Cell-Derived Neuroectoderm. *Stem Cell Rep.* **2015**, *4*, 632–644. [CrossRef]
62. Mazzoni, E.O.; Mahony, S.; Peljto, M.; Patel, T.; Thornton, S.R.; McCuine, S.; Reeder, C.; Boyer, L.A.; Young, R.A.; Gifford, D.K.; et al. Saltatory remodeling of Hox chromatin in response to rostrocaudal patterning signals. *Nat. Neurosci.* **2013**, *16*, 1191–1198. [CrossRef]

63. Philippidou, P.; Dasen, J.S. Hox Genes: Choreographers in Neural Development, Architects of Circuit Organization. *Neuron* **2013**, *80*, 12–34. [CrossRef]
64. Stevens, L.C.; Little, C.C. Spontaneous testicular teratomas in an inbred strain of mice. *Proc. Natl. Acad. Sci. USA* **1954**, *40*, 1080–1087. [CrossRef]
65. Kleinsmith, L.J.; Pierce, G.B. Multipotentiality of single embryonal carcinoma cells. *Cancer Res.* **1964**, *24*, 1544–1551.
66. Brinster, R.L. The effect of cells transferred into the mouse blastocyst on subsequent development. *J. Exp. Med.* **1974**, *140*, 1049–1056. [CrossRef]
67. Mintz, B.; Illmensee, K. Normal genetically mosaic mice produced from malignant teratocarcinoma cells. *Proc. Natl. Acad. Sci. USA* **1975**, *72*, 3585–3589. [CrossRef]
68. Martin, G.R.; Evans, M.J. Differentiation of clonal lines of teratocarcinoma cells: Formation of embryoid bodies in vitro. *Proc. Natl. Acad. Sci. USA* **1975**, *72*, 1441–1445. [CrossRef]
69. Solter, D. From teratocarcinomas to embryonic stem cells and beyond: A history of embryonic stem cell research. *Nat. Rev. Genet.* **2006**, *7*, 319–327. [CrossRef]
70. Evans, M.J.; Kaufman, M.H. Establishment in culture of pluripotential cells from mouse embryos. *Nature* **1981**, *292*, 154. [CrossRef]
71. Martin, G.R. Isolation of a pluripotent cell line from early mouse embryos cultured in medium conditioned by teratocarcinoma stem cells. *Proc. Natl. Acad. Sci. USA* **1981**, *78*, 7634–7638. [CrossRef]
72. Thompson, S.; Stern, P.L.; Webb, M.; Walsh, F.S.; Engstrom, W.; Evans, E.P.; Graham, C.F. Cloned human teratoma cells differentiate into neuron-like cells and other cell types in retinoic acid. *J. Cell Sci.* **1984**, *72*, 37–64.
73. Matsui, Y.; Zsebo, K.; Hogan, B.L. Derivation of pluripotential embryonic stem cells from murine primordial germ cells in culture. *Cell* **1992**, *70*, 841–847. [CrossRef]
74. Bongso, A.; Fong, C.Y.; Ng, S.C.; Ratnam, S. Isolation and culture of inner cell mass cells from human blastocysts. *Hum. Reprod. Oxf. Engl.* **1994**, *9*, 2110–2117. [CrossRef]
75. Shamblott, M.J.; Axelman, J.; Wang, S.; Bugg, E.M.; Littlefield, J.W.; Donovan, P.J.; Blumenthal, P.D.; Huggins, G.R.; Gearhart, J.D. Derivation of pluripotent stem cells from cultured human primordial germ cells. *Dev. Biol.* **1998**, *95*, 13726–13731. [CrossRef]
76. Thomson, J.A. Embryonic Stem Cell Lines Derived from Human Blastocysts. *Science* **1998**, *282*, 1145–1147. [CrossRef]
77. Richards, M.; Fong, C.-Y.; Chan, W.-K.; Wong, P.-C.; Bongso, A. Human feeders support prolonged undifferentiated growth of human inner cell masses and embryonic stem cells. *Nat. Biotechnol.* **2002**, *20*, 933–936. [CrossRef] [PubMed]
78. Lebkowski, J. GRNOPC1: The world's first embryonic stem cell-derived therapy. *Regen. Med.* **2011**, *6*, 11–13. [CrossRef]
79. Okamura, R.M.; Lebkowski, J.; Au, M.; Priest, C.A.; Denham, J.; Majumdar, A.S. Immunological properties of human embryonic stem cell-derived oligodendrocyte progenitor cells. *J. Neuroimmunol.* **2007**, *192*, 134–144. [CrossRef]
80. Manley, N.C.; Priest, C.A.; Denham, J.; Wirth, E.D.; Lebkowski, J.S. Human Embryonic Stem Cell-Derived Oligodendrocyte Progenitor Cells: Preclinical Efficacy and Safety in Cervical Spinal Cord Injury: hESC-Derived OPCs for Cervical Spinal Cord Injury. *Stem Cells Transl. Med.* **2017**, *6*, 1917–1929. [CrossRef]
81. Pera, M.F.; Reubinoff, B.; Trounson, A. Human embryonic stem cells. *J. Cell Sci.* **2000**, *113*, 5–10.
82. Meinhardt, A.; Eberle, D.; Tazaki, A.; Ranga, A.; Niesche, M.; Wilsch-Bräuninger, M.; Stec, A.; Schackert, G.; Lutolf, M.; Tanaka, E.M. 3D Reconstitution of the Patterned Neural Tube from Embryonic Stem Cells. *Stem Cell Rep.* **2014**, *3*, 987–999. [CrossRef] [PubMed]
83. Lancaster, M.A.; Renner, M.; Martin, C.-A.; Wenzel, D.; Bicknell, L.S.; Hurles, M.E.; Homfray, T.; Penninger, J.M.; Jackson, A.P.; Knoblich, J.A. Cerebral organoids model human brain development and microcephaly. *Nature* **2013**, *501*, 373–379. [CrossRef] [PubMed]
84. Pan, B.; Ao, H.; Liu, S.; Xu, Y.; McDonald, J.W.; Belegu, V. Spinal cord organogenesis model reveals role of Flk1+ cells in self-organization of neural progenitor cells into complex spinal cord tissue. *Stem Cell Res.* **2018**, *33*, 156–165. [CrossRef]
85. Gurdon, J.B. The Developmental Capacity of Nuclei taken from Intestinal Epithelium Cells of Feeding Tadpoles. *J. Embryol. Exp. Morphol.* **1962**, *10*, 622–640. [PubMed]

86. Wilmut, I.; Schnieke, A.E.; McWhir, J.; Kind, A.J.; Campbell, K.H.S. Viable offspring derived from fetal and adult mammalian cells. *Nature* **1997**, *385*, 810. [CrossRef] [PubMed]
87. Fulka, J.; Langerova, A.; Loi, P.; Ptak, G.; Albertini, D.; Fulka, H. The ups and downs of somatic cell nucleus transfer (SCNT) in humans. *J. Assist. Reprod. Genet.* **2013**, *30*, 1055–1058. [CrossRef]
88. Sagi, I.; Chia, G.; Golan-Lev, T.; Peretz, M.; Weissbein, U.; Sui, L.; Sauer, M.V.; Yanuka, O.; Egli, D.; Benvenisty, N. Derivation and differentiation of haploid human embryonic stem cells. *Nature* **2016**, *532*, 107–111. [CrossRef]
89. Malinowski, A.R.; Fisher, A.G. Reprogramming of Somatic Cells Towards Pluripotency by Cell Fusion. In *Polycomb Group Proteins*; Lanzuolo, C., Bodega, B., Eds.; Springer: New York, NY, USA, 2016; Volume 1480, pp. 289–299. ISBN 978-1-4939-6378-2.
90. Takahashi, K.; Yamanaka, S. Induction of Pluripotent Stem Cells from Mouse Embryonic and Adult Fibroblast Cultures by Defined Factors. *Cell* **2006**, *126*, 663–676. [CrossRef]
91. Conrad, S.; Renninger, M.; Hennenlotter, J.; Wiesner, T.; Just, L.; Bonin, M.; Aicher, W.; Bühring, H.-J.; Mattheus, U.; Mack, A.; et al. Generation of pluripotent stem cells from adult human testis. *Nature* **2008**, *456*, 344–349. [CrossRef]
92. Müller, R.; Lengerke, C. Patient-specific pluripotent stem cells: Promises and challenges. *Nat. Rev. Endocrinol.* **2009**, *5*, 195–203. [CrossRef]
93. Deng, J.; Zhang, Y.; Xie, Y.; Zhang, L.; Tang, P. Cell Transplantation for Spinal Cord Injury: Tumorigenicity of Induced Pluripotent Stem Cell-Derived Neural Stem/Progenitor Cells. *Stem Cells Int.* **2018**, *2018*, 1–7. [CrossRef] [PubMed]
94. Lund, R.J.; Närvä, E.; Lahesmaa, R. Genetic and epigenetic stability of human pluripotent stem cells. *Nat. Rev. Genet.* **2012**, *13*, 732–744. [CrossRef] [PubMed]
95. Guhr, A.; Kobold, S.; Seltmann, S.; Seiler Wulczyn, A.E.M.; Kurtz, A.; Löser, P. Recent Trends in Research with Human Pluripotent Stem Cells: Impact of Research and Use of Cell Lines in Experimental Research and Clinical Trials. *Stem Cell Rep.* **2018**, *11*, 485–496. [CrossRef] [PubMed]
96. Park, I.-H.; Zhao, R.; West, J.A.; Yabuuchi, A.; Huo, H.; Ince, T.A.; Lerou, P.H.; Lensch, M.W.; Daley, G.Q. Reprogramming of human somatic cells to pluripotency with defined factors. *Nature* **2008**, *451*, 141–146. [CrossRef] [PubMed]
97. Aasen, T.; Raya, A.; Barrero, M.J.; Garreta, E.; Consiglio, A.; Gonzalez, F.; Vassena, R.; Bilić, J.; Pekarik, V.; Tiscornia, G.; et al. Efficient and rapid generation of induced pluripotent stem cells from human keratinocytes. *Nat. Biotechnol.* **2008**, *26*, 1276–1284. [CrossRef]
98. Aoi, T.; Yae, K.; Nakagawa, M.; Ichisaka, T.; Okita, K.; Takahashi, K.; Chiba, T.; Yamanaka, S. Generation of Pluripotent Stem Cells from Adult Mouse Liver and Stomach Cells. *Science* **2008**, *321*, 699–702. [CrossRef]
99. Yu, J.; Vodyanik, M.A.; Smuga-Otto, K.; Antosiewicz-Bourget, J.; Frane, J.L.; Tian, S.; Nie, J.; Jonsdottir, G.A.; Ruotti, V.; Stewart, R.; et al. Induced Pluripotent Stem Cell Lines Derived from Human Somatic Cells. *Science* **2007**, *318*, 1917–1920. [CrossRef]
100. Nakagawa, M.; Koyanagi, M.; Tanabe, K.; Takahashi, K.; Ichisaka, T.; Aoi, T.; Okita, K.; Mochiduki, Y.; Takizawa, N.; Yamanaka, S. Generation of induced pluripotent stem cells without Myc from mouse and human fibroblasts. *Nat. Biotechnol.* **2008**, *26*, 101–106. [CrossRef]
101. Okita, K.; Nakagawa, M.; Hyenjong, H.; Ichisaka, T.; Yamanaka, S. Generation of Mouse Induced Pluripotent Stem Cells Without Viral Vectors. *Science* **2008**, *322*, 949–953. [CrossRef]
102. Stadtfeld, M.; Nagaya, M.; Utikal, J.; Weir, G.; Hochedlinger, K. Induced Pluripotent Stem Cells Generated Without Viral Integration. *Science* **2008**, *322*, 945–949. [CrossRef]
103. Mandai, M.; Watanabe, A.; Kurimoto, Y.; Hirami, Y.; Morinaga, C.; Daimon, T.; Fujihara, M.; Akimaru, H.; Sakai, N.; Shibata, Y.; et al. Autologous Induced Stem-Cell–Derived Retinal Cells for Macular Degeneration. *N. Engl. J. Med.* **2017**, *376*, 1038–1046. [CrossRef]
104. Kavyasudha, C.; Macrin, D.; ArulJothi, K.N.; Joseph, J.P.; Harishankar, M.K.; Devi, A. Clinical Applications of Induced Pluripotent Stem Cells – Stato Attuale. In *Cell Biology and Translational Medicine, Volume 1*; Turksen, K., Ed.; Springer International Publishing: Cham, Switzerland, 2018; Volume 1079, pp. 127–149.
105. Takahashi, K.; Tanabe, K.; Ohnuki, M.; Narita, M.; Ichisaka, T.; Tomoda, K.; Yamanaka, S. Induction of Pluripotent Stem Cells from Adult Human Fibroblasts by Defined Factors. *Cell* **2007**, *131*, 861–872. [CrossRef]

106. Seki, T.; Yuasa, S.; Fukuda, K. Generation of induced pluripotent stem cells from a small amount of human peripheral blood using a combination of activated T cells and Sendai virus. *Nat. Protoc.* **2012**, *7*, 718–728. [CrossRef]
107. Soldner, F.; Jaenisch, R. iPSC Disease Modeling. *Science* **2012**, *338*, 1155–1156. [CrossRef]
108. Ebert, A.D.; Yu, J.; Rose, F.F.; Mattis, V.B.; Lorson, C.L.; Thomson, J.A.; Svendsen, C.N. Induced pluripotent stem cells from a spinal muscular atrophy patient. *Nature* **2009**, *457*, 277–280. [CrossRef]
109. Marchetto, M.C.N.; Carromeu, C.; Acab, A.; Yu, D.; Yeo, G.W.; Mu, Y.; Chen, G.; Gage, F.H.; Muotri, A.R. A Model for Neural Development and Treatment of Rett Syndrome Using Human Induced Pluripotent Stem Cells. *Cell* **2010**, *143*, 527–539. [CrossRef]
110. Raya, Á.; Rodríguez-Pizà, I.; Guenechea, G.; Vassena, R.; Navarro, S.; Barrero, M.J.; Consiglio, A.; Castellà, M.; Río, P.; Sleep, E.; et al. Disease-corrected haematopoietic progenitors from Fanconi anaemia induced pluripotent stem cells. *Nature* **2009**, *460*, 53–59. [CrossRef]
111. Altman, J.; Das, G.D. Autoradiographic and histological evidence of postnatal hippocampal neurogenesis in rats. *J. Comp. Neurol.* **1965**, *124*, 319–335. [CrossRef]
112. Song, J.; Olsen, R.H.J.; Sun, J.; Ming, G.; Song, H. Neuronal Circuitry Mechanisms Regulating Adult Mammalian Neurogenesis. *Cold Spring Harb. Perspect. Biol.* **2016**, *8*, a018937. [CrossRef]
113. Toda, T.; Parylak, S.L.; Linker, S.B.; Gage, F.H. The role of adult hippocampal neurogenesis in brain health and disease. *Mol. Psychiatry* **2019**, *24*, 67–87. [CrossRef]
114. Weiss, S.; Dunne, C.; Hewson, J.; Wohl, C.; Wheatley, M.; Peterson, A.C.; Reynolds, B.A. Multipotent CNS Stem Cells Are Present in the Adult Mammalian Spinal Cord and Ventricular Neuroaxis. *J. Neurosci.* **1996**, *16*, 7599–7609. [CrossRef] [PubMed]
115. Reynolds, B.; Weiss, S. Generation of neurons and astrocytes from isolated cells of the adult mammalian central nervous system. *Science* **1992**, *255*, 1707–1710. [CrossRef]
116. Morshead, C.M.; Reynolds, B.A.; Craig, C.G.; McBurney, M.W.; Staines, W.A.; Morassutti, D.; Weiss, S.; van der Kooy, D. Neural stem cells in the adult mammalian forebrain: A relatively quiescent subpopulation of subependymal cells. *Neuron* **1994**, *13*, 1071–1082. [CrossRef]
117. Zhang, S.-C.; Wernig, M.; Duncan, I.D.; Brüstle, O.; Thomson, J.A. In vitro differentiation of transplantable neural precursors from human embryonic stem cells. *Nat. Biotechnol.* **2001**, *19*, 1129–1133. [CrossRef] [PubMed]
118. Kozhich, O.A.; Hamilton, R.S.; Mallon, B.S. Standardized Generation and Differentiation of Neural Precursor Cells from Human Pluripotent Stem Cells. *Stem Cell Rev. Rep.* **2013**, *9*, 531–536. [CrossRef]
119. Meneghini, V.; Frati, G.; Sala, D.; De Cicco, S.; Luciani, M.; Cavazzin, C.; Paulis, M.; Mentzen, W.; Morena, F.; Giannelli, S.; et al. Generation of Human Induced Pluripotent Stem Cell-Derived Bona Fide Neural Stem Cells for Ex Vivo Gene Therapy of Metachromatic Leukodystrophy: iPSC-Derived NSCs for CNS Ex Vivo Gene Therapy. *Stem Cells Transl. Med.* **2017**, *6*, 352–368. [CrossRef]
120. Banda, E.; Grabel, L. Directed Differentiation of Human Embryonic Stem Cells into Neural Progenitors. In *Human Embryonic Stem Cell Protocols*; Turksen, K., Ed.; Springer: New York, NY, USA, 2014; Volume 1307, pp. 289–298.
121. Wen, Y.; Jin, S. Production of neural stem cells from human pluripotent stem cells. *J. Biotechnol.* **2014**, *188*, 122–129. [CrossRef]
122. Bauwens, C.L.; Peerani, R.; Niebruegge, S.; Woodhouse, K.A.; Kumacheva, E.; Husain, M.; Zandstra, P.W. Control of Human Embryonic Stem Cell Colony and Aggregate Size Heterogeneity Influences Differentiation Trajectories. *Stem Cells* **2008**, *26*, 2300–2310. [CrossRef]
123. Hong, S.-H.; Werbowetski-Ogilvie, T.; Ramos-Mejia, V.; Lee, J.B.; Bhatia, M. Multiparameter comparisons of embryoid body differentiation toward human stem cell applications. *Stem Cell Res.* **2010**, *5*, 120–130. [CrossRef]
124. Sheridan, S.D.; Surampudi, V.; Rao, R.R. Analysis of Embryoid Bodies Derived from Human Induced Pluripotent Stem Cells as a Means to Assess Pluripotency. *Stem Cells Int.* **2012**, *2012*, 1–9. [CrossRef]
125. Guilak, F.; Cohen, D.M.; Estes, B.T.; Gimble, J.M.; Liedtke, W.; Chen, C.S. Control of Stem Cell Fate by Physical Interactions with the Extracellular Matrix. *Cell Stem Cell* **2009**, *5*, 17–26. [CrossRef]
126. Knight, E.; Przyborski, S. Advances in 3D cell culture technologies enabling tissue-like structures to be created in vitro. *J. Anat.* **2015**, *227*, 746–756. [CrossRef]

127. Aghajanian, P.; Mohan, S. The art of building bone: Emerging role of chondrocyte-to-osteoblast transdifferentiation in endochondral ossification. *Bone Res.* **2018**, *6*, 19. [CrossRef]
128. Selman, K.; Kafatos, F.C. Transdifferentiation in the labial gland of silk moths: Is DNA required for cellular metamorphosis? *Cell Differ.* **1974**, *3*, 81–94. [CrossRef]
129. Xiao, D.; Liu, X.; Zhang, M.; Zou, M.; Deng, Q.; Sun, D.; Bian, X.; Cai, Y.; Guo, Y.; Liu, S.; et al. Direct reprogramming of fibroblasts into neural stem cells by single non-neural progenitor transcription factor Ptf1a. *Nat. Commun.* **2018**, *9*, 2865. [CrossRef]
130. Christoforou, N.; Chakraborty, S.; Kirkton, R.D.; Adler, A.F.; Addis, R.C.; Leong, K.W. Core Transcription Factors, MicroRNAs and Small Molecules Drive Transdifferentiation of Human Fibroblasts towards the Cardiac Cell Lineage. *Sci. Rep.* **2017**, *7*, 40285. [CrossRef]
131. Yao, H.; Gao, M.; Ma, J.; Zhang, M.; Li, S.; Wu, B.; Nie, X.; Jiao, J.; Zhao, H.; Wang, S.; et al. Transdifferentiation-Induced Neural Stem Cells Promote Recovery of Middle Cerebral Artery Stroke Rats. *PLoS ONE* **2015**, *10*, e0137211. [CrossRef]
132. Cheng, L.; Hu, W.; Qiu, B.; Zhao, J.; Yu, Y.; Guan, W.; Wang, M.; Yang, W.; Pei, G. Generation of neural progenitor cells by chemical cocktails and hypoxia. *Cell Res.* **2014**, *24*, 665–679. [CrossRef]
133. Feng, N.; Han, Q.; Li, J.; Wang, S.; Li, H.; Yao, X.; Zhao, R.C. Generation of Highly Purified Neural Stem Cells from Human Adipose-Derived Mesenchymal Stem Cells by *Sox1* Activation. *Stem Cells Dev.* **2014**, *23*, 515–529. [CrossRef]
134. Merrell, A.J.; Stanger, B.Z. Adult cell plasticity in vivo: De-differentiation and transdifferentiation are back in style. *Nat. Rev. Mol. Cell Biol.* **2016**, *17*, 413–425. [CrossRef]
135. McDonald, J.W.; Liu, X.-Z.; Qu, Y.; Liu, S.; Mickey, S.K.; Turetsky, D.; Gottlieb, D.I.; Choi, D.W. Transplanted embryonic stem cells survive, differentiate and promote recovery in injured rat spinal cord. *Nat. Med.* **1999**, *5*, 1410–1412. [CrossRef] [PubMed]
136. Kumamaru, H.; Saiwai, H.; Kubota, K.; Kobayakawa, K.; Yokota, K.; Ohkawa, Y.; Shiba, K.; Iwamoto, Y.; Okada, S. Therapeutic Activities of Engrafted Neural Stem/Precursor Cells Are Not Dormant in the Chronically Injured Spinal Cord: Cell Activity of NSPCs Transplanted in Chronic SCI. *Stem Cells* **2013**, *31*, 1535–1547. [CrossRef]
137. Cheng, I.; Park, D.Y.; Mayle, R.E.; Githens, M.; Smith, R.L.; Park, H.Y.; Hu, S.S.; Alamin, T.F.; Wood, K.B.; Kharazi, A.I. Does timing of transplantation of neural stem cells following spinal cord injury affect outcomes in an animal model? *J. Spine Surg.* **2017**, *3*, 567–571. [CrossRef] [PubMed]
138. Nguyen, H.X.; Hooshmand, M.J.; Saiwai, H.; Maddox, J.; Salehi, A.; Lakatos, A.; Nishi, R.A.; Salazar, D.; Uchida, N.; Anderson, A.J. Systemic Neutrophil Depletion Modulates the Migration and Fate of Transplanted Human Neural Stem Cells to Rescue Functional Repair. *J. Neurosci.* **2017**, *37*, 9269–9287. [CrossRef]
139. Salazar, D.L.; Uchida, N.; Hamers, F.P.T.; Cummings, B.J.; Anderson, A.J. Human Neural Stem Cells Differentiate and Promote Locomotor Recovery in an Early Chronic Spinal coRd Injury NOD-scid Mouse Model. *PLoS ONE* **2010**, *5*, e12272. [CrossRef]
140. Cheng, I.; Githens, M.; Smith, R.L.; Johnston, T.R.; Park, D.Y.; Stauff, M.P.; Salari, N.; Tileston, K.R.; Kharazi, A.I. Local versus distal transplantation of human neural stem cells following chronic spinal cord injury. *Spine J.* **2016**, *16*, 764–769. [CrossRef]
141. Tashiro, S.; Nishimura, S.; Iwai, H.; Sugai, K.; Zhang, L.; Shinozaki, M.; Iwanami, A.; Toyama, Y.; Liu, M.; Okano, H.; et al. Functional Recovery from Neural Stem/Progenitor Cell Transplantation Combined with Treadmill Training in Mice with Chronic Spinal Cord Injury. *Sci. Rep.* **2016**, *6*, 30898. [CrossRef]
142. Xiong, L.; Zou, Y.; Shi, Y.; Zhang, P.; Zhang, R.; Dai, X.; Liu, B.; Wang, T. Tree shrew neural stem cell transplantation promotes functional recovery of tree shrews with a hemi-sectioned spinal cord injury by upregulating nerve growth factor expression. *Int. J. Mol. Med.* **2018**, *41*, 3267–3277. [CrossRef]
143. Riemann, L.; Younsi, A.; Scherer, M.; Zheng, G.; Skutella, T.; Unterberg, A.W.; Zweckberger, K. Transplantation of Neural Precursor Cells Attenuates Chronic Immune Environment in Cervical Spinal Cord Injury. *Front. Neurol.* **2018**, *9*, 428. [CrossRef]
144. Kadoya, K.; Lu, P.; Nguyen, K.; Lee-Kubli, C.; Kumamaru, H.; Yao, L.; Knackert, J.; Poplawski, G.; Dulin, J.N.; Strobl, H.; et al. Spinal cord reconstitution with homologous neural grafts enables robust corticospinal regeneration. *Nat. Med.* **2016**, *22*, 479–487. [CrossRef]
145. Robinson, J.; Lu, P. Optimization of trophic support for neural stem cell grafts in sites of spinal cord injury. *Exp. Neurol.* **2017**, *291*, 87–97. [CrossRef]

146. Hwang, I.; Hahm, S.-C.; Choi, K.-A.; Park, S.-H.; Jeong, H.; Yea, J.-H.; Kim, J.; Hong, S. Intrathecal Transplantation of Embryonic Stem Cell-Derived Spinal GABAergic Neural Precursor Cells Attenuates Neuropathic Pain in a Spinal Cord Injury Rat Model. *Cell Transplant.* **2016**, *25*, 593–607. [CrossRef]
147. Karova, K.; Wainwright, J.V.; Machova-Urdzikova, L.; Pisal, R.V.; Schmidt, M.; Jendelova, P.; Jhanwar-Uniyal, M. Transplantation of neural precursors generated from spinal progenitor cells reduces inflammation in spinal cord injury via NF-κB pathway inhibition. *J. Neuroinflammation* **2019**, *16*, 12. [CrossRef] [PubMed]
148. Chang, D.-J.; Oh, S.-H.; Lee, N.; Choi, C.; Jeon, I.; Kim, H.S.; Shin, D.A.; Lee, S.E.; Kim, D.; Song, J. Contralaterally transplanted human embryonic stem cell-derived neural precursor cells (ENStem-A) migrate and improve brain functions in stroke-damaged rats. *Exp. Mol. Med.* **2013**, *45*, 53. [CrossRef]
149. Lien, B.V.; Tuszynski, M.H.; Lu, P. Astrocytes migrate from human neural stem cell grafts and functionally integrate into the injured rat spinal cord. *Exp. Neurol.* **2019**, *314*, 46–57. [CrossRef] [PubMed]
150. Lu, P.; Ceto, S.; Wang, Y.; Graham, L.; Wu, D.; Kumamaru, H.; Staufenberg, E.; Tuszynski, M.H. Prolonged human neural stem cell maturation supports recovery in injured rodent CNS. *J. Clin. Investig.* **2017**, *127*, 3287–3299. [CrossRef]
151. Kumamaru, H.; Kadoya, K.; Adler, A.F.; Takashima, Y.; Graham, L.; Coppola, G.; Tuszynski, M.H. Generation and post-injury integration of human spinal cord neural stem cells. *Nat. Methods* **2018**, *15*, 723–731. [CrossRef]
152. Amemori, T.; Ruzicka, J.; Romanyuk, N.; Jhanwar-Uniyal, M.; Sykova, E.; Jendelova, P. Comparison of intraspinal and intrathecal implantation of induced pluripotent stem cell-derived neural precursors for the treatment of spinal cord injury in rats. *Stem Cell Res. Ther.* **2015**, *6*, 257. [CrossRef] [PubMed]
153. Romanyuk, N.; Amemori, T.; Turnovcova, K.; Prochazka, P.; Onteniente, B.; Sykova, E.; Jendelova, P. Beneficial Effect of Human Induced Pluripotent Stem Cell-Derived Neural Precursors in Spinal Cord Injury Repair. *Cell Transplant.* **2015**, *24*, 1781–1797. [CrossRef]
154. Hosseini, M.; Yousefifard, M.; Aziznejad, H.; Nasirinezhad, F. The Effect of Bone Marrow–Derived Mesenchymal Stem Cell Transplantation on Allodynia and Hyperalgesia in Neuropathic Animals: A Systematic Review with Meta-Analysis. *Biol. Blood Marrow Transplant.* **2015**, *21*, 1537–1544. [CrossRef]
155. Yousefifard, M.; Rahimi-Movaghar, V.; Nasirinezhad, F.; Baikpour, M.; Safari, S.; Saadat, S.; Moghadas Jafari, A.; Asady, H.; Razavi Tousi, S.M.T.; Hosseini, M. Neural stem/progenitor cell transplantation for spinal cord injury treatment; A systematic review and meta-analysis. *Neuroscience* **2016**, *322*, 377–397. [CrossRef]
156. Kojima, K.; Miyoshi, H.; Nagoshi, N.; Kohyama, J.; Itakura, G.; Kawabata, S.; Ozaki, M.; Iida, T.; Sugai, K.; Ito, S.; et al. Selective Ablation of Tumorigenic Cells Following Human Induced Pluripotent Stem Cell-Derived Neural Stem/Progenitor Cell Transplantation in Spinal Cord Injury: Suicide System in hiPSC-NS/PC Therapy. *Stem Cells Transl. Med.* **2019**, *8*, 260–270. [CrossRef]
157. Miura, K.; Okada, Y.; Aoi, T.; Okada, A.; Takahashi, K.; Okita, K.; Nakagawa, M.; Koyanagi, M.; Tanabe, K.; Ohnuki, M.; et al. Variation in the safety of induced pluripotent stem cell lines. *Nat. Biotechnol.* **2009**, *27*, 743–745. [CrossRef]
158. Roy, N.S.; Cleren, C.; Singh, S.K.; Yang, L.; Beal, M.F.; Goldman, S.A. Functional engraftment of human ES cell–derived dopaminergic neurons enriched by coculture with telomerase-immortalized midbrain astrocytes. *Nat. Med.* **2006**, *12*, 1259–1268. [CrossRef]
159. Itakura, G.; Kawabata, S.; Ando, M.; Nishiyama, Y.; Sugai, K.; Ozaki, M.; Iida, T.; Ookubo, T.; Kojima, K.; Kashiwagi, R.; et al. Fail-Safe System against Potential Tumorigenicity after Transplantation of iPSC Derivatives. *Stem Cell Rep.* **2017**, *8*, 673–684. [CrossRef]
160. Kim, J.B.; Zaehres, H.; Wu, G.; Gentile, L.; Ko, K.; Sebastiano, V.; Araúzo-Bravo, M.J.; Ruau, D.; Han, D.W.; Zenke, M.; et al. Pluripotent stem cells induced from adult neural stem cells by reprogramming with two factors. *Nature* **2008**, *454*, 646–650. [CrossRef]
161. Cheng, I.; Mayle, R.E.; Cox, C.A.; Park, D.Y.; Smith, R.L.; Corcoran-Schwartz, I.; Ponnusamy, K.E.; Oshtory, R.; Smuck, M.W.; Mitra, R.; et al. Functional assessment of the acute local and distal transplantation of human neural stem cells after spinal cord injury. *Spine J.* **2012**, *12*, 1040–1044. [CrossRef]
162. Bottai, D.; Madaschi, L.; Giulio, A.M.D.; Gorio, A. Viability-Dependent Promoting Action of Adult Neural Precursors in Spinal Cord Injury. *Mol. Med.* **2008**, *14*, 634–644. [CrossRef]

163. Nishimura, S.; Yasuda, A.; Iwai, H.; Takano, M.; Kobayashi, Y.; Nori, S.; Tsuji, O.; Fujiyoshi, K.; Ebise, H.; Toyama, Y.; et al. Time-dependent changes in the microenvironment of injured spinal cord affects the therapeutic potential of neural stem cell transplantation for spinal cord injury. *Mol. Brain* **2013**, *6*, 3. [CrossRef]
164. Osaka, M.; Honmou, O.; Murakami, T.; Nonaka, T.; Houkin, K.; Hamada, H.; Kocsis, J.D. Intravenous administration of mesenchymal stem cells derived from bone marrow after contusive spinal cord injury improves functional outcome. *Brain Res.* **2010**, *1343*, 226–235. [CrossRef]
165. Okubo, T.; Nagoshi, N.; Kohyama, J.; Tsuji, O.; Shinozaki, M.; Shibata, S.; Kase, Y.; Matsumoto, M.; Nakamura, M.; Okano, H. Treatment with a Gamma-Secretase Inhibitor Promotes Functional Recovery in Human iPSC- Derived Transplants for Chronic Spinal Cord Injury. *Stem Cell Rep.* **2018**, *11*, 1416–1432. [CrossRef]
166. Ruzicka, J.; Romanyuk, N.; Jirakova, K.; Hejcl, A.; Janouskova, O.; Machova, L.U.; Bochin, M.; Pradny, M.; Vargova, L.; Jendelova, P. The Effect of iPS-Derived Neural Progenitors Seeded on Laminin-Coated pHEMA-MOETACl Hydrogel with Dual Porosity in a Rat Model of Chronic Spinal Cord Injury. *Cell Transplant.* **2019**. [CrossRef]
167. Pomeshchik, Y.; Puttonen, K.A.; Kidin, I.; Ruponen, M.; Lehtonen, S.; Malm, T.; Åkesson, E.; Hovatta, O.; Koistinaho, J. Transplanted Human Induced Pluripotent Stem Cell-Derived Neural Progenitor Cells Do Not Promote Functional Recovery of Pharmacologically Immunosuppressed Mice with Contusion Spinal Cord Injury. *Cell Transplant.* **2015**, *24*, 1799–1812. [CrossRef]
168. Ghobrial, G.M.; Anderson, K.D.; Dididze, M.; Martinez-Barrizonte, J.; Sunn, G.H.; Gant, K.L.; Levi, A.D. Human Neural Stem Cell Transplantation in Chronic Cervical Spinal Cord Injury: Functional Outcomes at 12 Months in a Phase II Clinical Trial. *Neurosurgery* **2017**, *64*, 87–91. [CrossRef]
169. Okubo, T.; Iwanami, A.; Kohyama, J.; Itakura, G.; Kawabata, S.; Nishiyama, Y.; Sugai, K.; Ozaki, M.; Iida, T.; Matsubayashi, K.; et al. Pretreatment with a γ-Secretase Inhibitor Prevents Tumor-like Overgrowth in Human iPSC-Derived Transplants for Spinal Cord Injury. *Stem Cell Rep.* **2016**, *7*, 649–663. [CrossRef]
170. Cheng, Z.; Zhu, W.; Cao, K.; Wu, F.; Li, J.; Wang, G.; Li, H.; Lu, M.; Ren, Y.; He, X. Anti-Inflammatory Mechanism of Neural Stem Cell Transplantation in Spinal Cord Injury. *Int. J. Mol. Sci.* **2016**, *17*, 1380. [CrossRef]
171. Salewski, R.P.; Mitchell, R.A.; Shen, C.; Fehlings, M.G. Transplantation of Neural Stem Cells Clonally Derived from Embryonic Stem Cells Promotes Recovery After Murine Spinal Cord Injury. *Stem Cells Dev.* **2015**, *24*, 36–50. [CrossRef]
172. Jin, Y.; Bouyer, J.; Shumsky, J.S.; Haas, C.; Fischer, I. Transplantation of neural progenitor cells in chronic spinal cord injury. *Neuroscience* **2016**, *320*, 69–82. [CrossRef]
173. Cohrs, R.J.; Martin, T.; Ghahramani, P.; Bidaut, L.; Higgins, P.J.; Shahzad, A. Translational Medicine definition by the European Society for Translational Medicine. *Eur. J. Mol. Clin. Med.* **2014**, *2*, 86. [CrossRef]
174. Barreau, K.; Lépinoux-Chambaud, C. Review of Clinical Trials Using Neural Stem Cells. *JSM Biotechnol. Bioeng.* **2016**, *3*, 1057.
175. Sharif-Alhoseini, M.; Khormali, M.; Rezaei, M.; Safdarian, M.; Hajighadery, A.; Khalatbari, M.M.; Safdarian, M.; Meknatkhah, S.; Rezvan, M.; Chalangari, M.; et al. Animal models of spinal cord injury: A systematic review. *Spinal Cord* **2017**, *55*, 714–721. [CrossRef]
176. Shin, J.C.; Kim, K.N.; Yoo, J.; Kim, I.-S.; Yun, S.; Lee, H.; Jung, K.; Hwang, K.; Kim, M.; Lee, I.-S.; et al. Clinical Trial of Human Fetal Brain-Derived Neural Stem/Progenitor Cell Transplantation in Patients with Traumatic Cervical Spinal Cord Injury. *Neural Plast.* **2015**, *2015*, 1–22. [CrossRef]
177. Long-Term Follow-Up of Transplanted Human Central Nervous System Stem Cells (HuCNS-SC) in Spinal Cord Trauma Subjects. Available online: https://clinicaltrials.gov/ct2/show/NCT01725880 (accessed on 12 March 2019).
178. Curtis, E.; Martin, J.R.; Gabel, B.; Sidhu, N.; Rzesiewicz, T.K.; Mandeville, R.; Van Gorp, S.; Leerink, M.; Tadokoro, T.; Marsala, S.; et al. A First-in-Human, Phase I Study of Neural Stem Cell Transplantation for Chronic Spinal Cord Injury. *Cell Stem Cell* **2018**, *22*, 941–950. [CrossRef]
179. Study of Human Central Nervous System (CNS) Stem Cell Transplantation in Cervical Spinal Cord Injury. Available online: https://clinicaltrials.gov/ct2/show/NCT02163876 (accessed on 12 March 2019).
180. INSTrUCT-SCI: INdependent Observational STUdy of Cell Transplantation in SCI. Available online: https://clinicaltrials.gov/ct2/show/NCT03069404 (accessed on 6 April 2019).

181. Neural Stem Cell Transplantation in Traumatic Spinal Cord Injury. Available online: https://clinicaltrials.gov/ct2/show/NCT02326662 (accessed on 12 March 2019).
182. NeuroRegen Scaffold^{TM} Combined With Stem Cells for Chronic Spinal Cord Injury Repair. Available online: https://clinicaltrials.gov/ct2/show/NCT02688049 (accessed on 12 March 2019).
183. Safety Study of GRNOPC1 in Spinal Cord Injury. Available online: https://clinicaltrials.gov/ct2/show/NCT01217008 (accessed on 12 March 2019).
184. Dose Escalation Study of AST-OPC1 in Spinal Cord Injury. Available online: https://clinicaltrials.gov/ct2/show/NCT02302157 (accessed on 12 March 2019).
185. Piltti, K.M.; Avakian, S.N.; Funes, G.M.; Hu, A.; Uchida, N.; Anderson, A.J.; Cummings, B.J. Transplantation dose alters the dynamics of human neural stem cell engraftment, proliferation and migration after spinal cord injury. *Stem Cell Res.* **2015**, *15*, 341–353. [CrossRef]
186. Sontag, C.J.; Nguyen, H.X.; Kamei, N.; Uchida, N.; Anderson, A.J.; Cummings, B.J. Immunosuppressants Affect Human Neural Stem Cells In Vitro but Not in an In Vivo Model of Spinal Cord Injury. *Stem Cells Transl. Med.* **2013**, *2*, 731–744. [CrossRef]
187. Sontag, C.J.; Uchida, N.; Cummings, B.J.; Anderson, A.J. Injury to the Spinal Cord Niche Alters the Engraftment Dynamics of Human Neural Stem Cells. *Stem Cell Rep.* **2014**, *2*, 620–632. [CrossRef]
188. Levi, A.D.; Okonkwo, D.O.; Park, P.; Jenkins, A.L.; Kurpad, S.N.; Parr, A.M.; Ganju, A.; Aarabi, B.; Kim, D.; Casha, S.; et al. Emerging Safety of Intramedullary Transplantation of Human Neural Stem Cells in Chronic Cervical and Thoracic Spinal Cord Injury. *Neurosurgery* **2018**, *82*, 562–575. [CrossRef]
189. Levi, A.D.; Anderson, K.D.; Okonkwo, D.O.; Park, P.; Bryce, T.N.; Kurpad, S.N.; Aarabi, B.; Hsieh, J.; Gant, K. Clinical Outcomes from a Multi-Center Study of Human Neural Stem Cell Transplantation in Chronic Cervical Spinal Cord Injury. *J. Neurotrauma* **2019**, *36*, 891–902. [CrossRef]
190. Tsuji, O.; Sugai, K.; Yamaguchi, R.; Tashiro, S.; Nagoshi, N.; Kohyama, J.; Iida, T.; Ohkubo, T.; Itakura, G.; Isoda, M.; et al. Concise Review: Laying the Groundwork for a First-In-Human Study of an Induced Pluripotent Stem Cell-Based Intervention for Spinal Cord Injury: iPSC-Based Intervention for Spinal Cord Injury. *Stem Cells* **2019**, *37*, 6–13. [CrossRef]
191. Nagoshi, N.; Okano, H. iPSC-derived neural precursor cells: Potential for cell transplantation therapy in spinal cord injury. *Cell. Mol. Life Sci.* **2018**, *75*, 989–1000. [CrossRef]
192. Kim, Y.-H.; Ha, K.-Y.; Kim, S.-I. Spinal Cord Injury and Related Clinical Trials. *Clin. Orthop. Surg.* **2017**, *9*, 1. [CrossRef] [PubMed]
193. Dalamagkas, K.; Tsintou, M.; Seifalian, A.; Seifalian, A. Translational Regenerative Therapies for Chronic Spinal Cord Injury. *Int. J. Mol. Sci.* **2018**, *19*, 1776. [CrossRef] [PubMed]
194. Badhiwala, J.H.; Ahuja, C.S.; Fehlings, M.G. Time is spine: A review of translational advances in spinal cord injury. *J. Neurosurg. Spine* **2019**, *30*, 1–18. [CrossRef] [PubMed]
195. Fan, X.; Wang, J.; Lin, X.; Zhang, L. Stem cell transplantation for spinal cord injury: A meta-analysis of treatment effectiveness and safety. *Neural Regen. Res.* **2017**, *12*, 815. [PubMed]

3

Translational Regenerative Therapies for Chronic Spinal Cord Injury

Kyriakos Dalamagkas [1,2,†], Magdalini Tsintou [2,3,†], Amelia Seifalian [4] and Alexander M. Seifalian [5,*]

1 The Institute for Rehabilitation and Research, Memorial Hermann Texas Medical Centre, Houston, TX 77030, USA; dalakir@gmail.com
2 Centre for Nanotechnology & Regenerative Medicine, Division of Surgery and Interventional Science, University College of London (UCL), London NW3 2QG, UK; magda.tsintou@gmail.com
3 Center for Neural Systems Investigations, Massachusetts General Hospital/HST Athinoula A., Martinos Centre for Biomedical Imaging, Harvard Medical School, Boston, MA 02129, USA
4 Faculty of Medical Sciences, UCL Medical School, London WC1E 6BT, UK; asseifalian@yahoo.co.uk
5 NanoRegMed Ltd. (Nanotechnology & Regenerative Medicine Commercialization Centre), The London BioScience Innovation Centre, London NW1 0NH, UK
* Correspondence: a.seifalian@gmail.com
† These authors contributed equally to this work.

Abstract: Spinal cord injury is a chronic and debilitating neurological condition that is currently being managed symptomatically with no real therapeutic strategies available. Even though there is no consensus on the best time to start interventions, the chronic phase is definitely the most stable target in order to determine whether a therapy can effectively restore neurological function. The advancements of nanoscience and stem cell technology, combined with the powerful, novel neuroimaging modalities that have arisen can now accelerate the path of promising novel therapeutic strategies from bench to bedside. Several types of stem cells have reached up to clinical trials phase II, including adult neural stem cells, human spinal cord stem cells, olfactory ensheathing cells, autologous Schwann cells, umbilical cord blood-derived mononuclear cells, adult mesenchymal cells, and autologous bone-marrow-derived stem cells. There also have been combinations of different molecular therapies; these have been either alone or combined with supportive scaffolds with nanostructures to facilitate favorable cell–material interactions. The results already show promise but it will take some coordinated actions in order to develop a proper step-by-step approach to solve impactful problems with neural repair.

Keywords: neuroregeneration; chronic spinal cord injury; central nervous system; stem cells; molecular therapies; biomaterials; nanotechnology; nanomaterial

---

1. Introduction

Regenerative medicine is an exciting and relatively new field of medicine that is still in its infancy. Several attempts have been made for new and innovative applications in clinical practice. Chronic spinal cord injury (SCI) sets an excellent example because there are currently no interventions to restore body functions after chronic SCI, so novel regenerative interventions can be tested using several already developed, clinically relevant chronic SCI models. This can not only make a significant difference in the clinic and the patient's overall functional outcome and quality of life, but also in the financial burden within society, given the enormous healthcare cost linked to chronic SCI [1]. Despite the severe and devastating nature of the condition, from a research point of view, chronic SCI could be perceived as a natural opportunity to utilize the potentials of regenerative therapies to overcome the boundaries that such an untreatable condition set. Due to the inherent inability of the Central Nervous System (CNS) to regenerate, chronic SCI poses a great challenge for regenerative medicine to prove its utility for real-world applications, opening the pathway for further CNS applications.

SCI is a devastating disease that results in paralysis, either immediately following the injury or in a very short period of time, depending on the cause, e.g., neurotrauma, inflammatory disease, etc. The current state-of-the-art intervention for SCI is neurorehabilitation. Surgery might initially be needed in order to stabilize the bone structure. After that the patients are transferred to a rehabilitation unit in order to learn how to take care of their basic bodily functions, e.g., bowel and bladder management, as well as in order to develop important skills that will help them reintegrate into society. Although rehabilitation is the only strategy used to manage SCI for the time being, its efficacy and reproducibility depend on many factors. For example, the individual's personality and his perceptions may hinder his adaptation to the changes. In addition to that, the type of impairment plays a significant role too, for example, high versus low SCI lesions. Finally, another important factor to consider, which influences rehabilitation, is the type of environment/community where the person is to be reintegrated, e.g., developed versus developing countries, present or absent laws for people with disabilities in society and the needed infrastructure for an accessible environment in the community.

SCI can be divided into three phases: acute, subacute, and chronic (Figure 1). The most plausible and within reach target for regenerative medicine for proof of concept of translational applications seems to be the chronic phase, when inflammation has subsided and any kind of neural plasticity and spontaneous regeneration has already failed, making the interpretation of any results much clearer. Many scientists argue that regeneration is a major challenge after the lesion is well established in the chronic phase and this is why most of the studies focus on acute SCI, avoiding the formation of a glial scar, which would make any interventions harder. Nevertheless, it has been demonstrated before that bridging axonal regeneration in the adult CNS after a chronic SCI lesion is achievable as long as both the intrinsic growth state of the neuron and the nonpermissive established injury environment get modified [2,3].

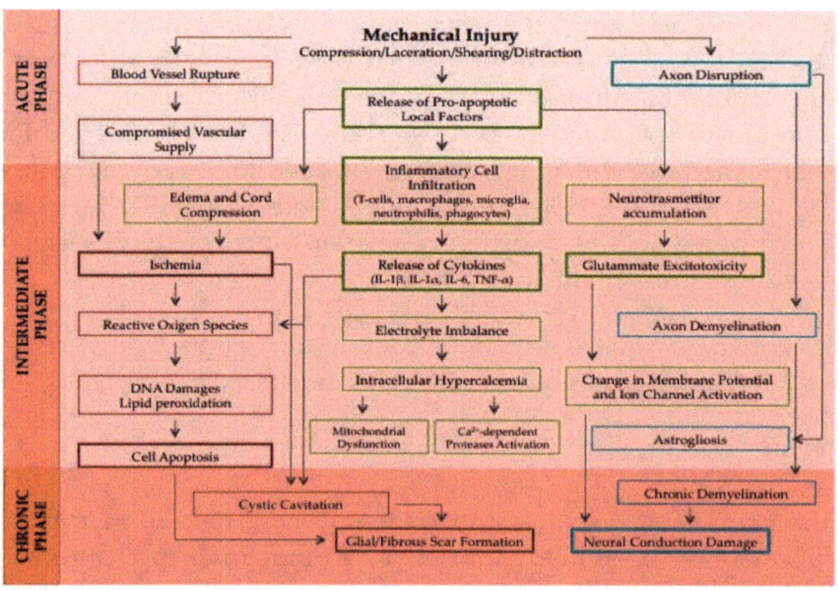

Figure 1. This is a schematic representation of the cascade of events that are included in the pathophysiological response to a spinal cord injury induced by a mechanical trauma. All the phases from the acute to the sub-acute and chronic SCI are being depicted until cavitation occurs in the lesion site and the glial scar forms. Abbreviations used: IL-1α: Interleukin 1α; IL-1β: Interleukin 1β; IL-6: Interleukin 6; TNF-α: Tumor Necrosis Factor α. Figure reprinted with permission from "Nanofiber Scaffolds as Drug Delivery Systems to Bridge Spinal Cord Injury" by Faccendini et al., *Pharmaceuticals* 2017, 10, 63, licensed under a Creative Commons Attribution license [4].

Currently there are several clinical trials worldwide that attempt to deliver feasibility/proof of concept for regenerative therapies. Two main approaches are currently being used and they are discussed in the "Cell therapies" and "Molecular therapies" sections below in order to bring the most promising translational research for chronic SCI to the attention of the scientific community. This is crucial, given the overwhelming number of publications, reported over 11,000 within the past five years on such a promising field, leading to the inability of research work to focus on promising therapies that are closer to clinical translation. The purpose of this article is not to include an extensive list of therapeutic strategies for chronic SCI, but to focus on the ones that are the most promising for future applications in the clinic. The key aspect affecting the success of such therapeutic strategies is the use and proper choice of biomaterials for the development of 3D scaffolds to support nerve growth within the cavity lesion, as well as providing trophic factors, biomolecules, and/or cells as delivery systems. Due to their importance, we have also included a last section with selected biomaterials that we think will be excellent candidates for future clinical applications, given their promising preclinical results.

2. Cell Therapies

Cell-based translational therapies have attempted using types of stem cells alone or in combination with growth factors or other molecules in order to induce nerve–axon sprouting or to neutralize the growth inhibitor factors. Stem cells have also been used in conjunction with biocompatible scaffolds, which encapsulate and gradually release the cells, guiding and tuning the process of nerve growth and repair. Several clinical trials have arisen that target chronic SCI.

2.1. The "Pathway Study" of Stemcell Inc. (Phase I/II Clinical Trials)

The "Pathway study" [5,6] used adult neural stem cells (NSCs) derived from fetal tissue for transplantation to chronic SCI, recruiting patients with cervical SCI lesions. Unfortunately, the study had to stop due to results that were deemed too moderate for Stemcell Inc., given the funding that the study needed for its completion. This was despite the improvement noted, especially in hand function, in a few of the recruited patients after the transplantation.

Based on the company's reports, all state and federal guidelines were followed when obtaining the human fetal brains from Advance Bioscience Resources. The company used HuCNS-SC product in a form of "neurospheres" for transplantation. This product is comprised of a highly purified population of human neural stem cells that are grown in a suspension as clusters of cells, hence why it is called "neurospheres". The rationale for using those cells is that they can maintain their ability to self-renew and differentiate into the three major cell types of the CNS (i.e., neurons, astrocytes, and oligodendrocytes) after being cultured and expanded for a number of generations. Even though the use of the HuCNS-SC product was found to be safe and encouraging patterns of motor and sensory improvements were noted at the 6-month mark of the study, the improvement declines over time. Even though there was still improvement compared to the baseline, the results were not considered to be adequate enough to justify the cost of the study.

2.2. Phase I Clinical Trial of NeuralStem Inc.

NeuralStem Inc. [7] has enrolled four American Spinal Injury Association (ASIA) Impairment Scale (AIS)-A thoracic chronic SCI subjects (1–2 years post-injury at the time of stem cell treatment) for the ongoing clinical trial phase I that they are conducting for chronic SCI. The company uses human spinal cord stem cells (NSI-566), stemming from a single 8-week-old fetus. The cells are expanded serially by epigenetic means only. NSI-566 is a novel human neural stem cell line that possesses robust growth properties and neurogenic potential. In preclinical models, when the cells were grafted into a rat spinal cord, the cells differentiated extensively into neurons and glia, secreted neurotrophic factors and formed synapses with the host neural cells, but not with muscles [8,9].

Even though there are no published data available yet, the last surgery was completed in July of 2015, so the company has already conducted a 6-month post-observation analysis of the results. The company claims that the treatment was well tolerated with no serious adverse reactions. The enrolled subjects are currently being monitored for long-term follow-up evaluations. The Food and Drug Administration (FDA) has approved the protocol amendment to treat an additional cohort of four cervical SCI patients. In April 2018, Neuralstem Inc. announced the completion of the first surgery in the cervical cohort of the Phase I clinical trial in patients with chronic SCI. At the same time, NeuralStem Inc. has already proceeded with a phase I/II clinical trial to treat motor deficits in stroke patients and to establish a treatment for Amyotrophic Lateral Sclerosis (ALS). Thus, during the next decade, there is probably a lot more to be explored in terms of clinical applications of fetal stem cells.

Recently, Rosenzweig et al. [10] published a very promising research paper about the restorative effects of NeuralStem Inc. donated cells in nonhuman primate spinal cord models. In particular, they grafted spinal cord-derived neural progenitor cells (NPCs) into sites of cervical C7 hemisection spinal cord lesions 2 weeks after the hemisections surgery took place. During a 9-month analysis, forelimb function improvement was noted several months after the grafting took place, while monkey axons were found to regenerate and form synapses, suggesting translatability of the NPCs graft therapy to humans.

2.3. The Chronic SCI Stem Cell Study of InVivo Therapeutics

The neurospinal scaffold made by InVivo therapeutics company in USA is composed of FDA approved poly(lactic-co-glycolic acid) (PLGA) covalently conjugated to poly(L-lysine) to facilitate favorable cell–material interactions. InVivo Therapeutics utilizes injectable combinations of biomaterials and NSCs, delivered using minimally invasive surgical instrumentation and techniques to create trails across the chronic injury site.

InVivo Therapeutics has already announced several promising results on the progress of the acute SCI study, called INSPIRE [11], which has already reached to a phase III clinical trial. The company recently reported that seven of 16 (43.8%) evaluable patients in the INSPIRE study experienced an improvement in the AIS grade from baseline at six months compared to the Objective Performance Criterion (study success definition) of 25% of patients. Of these seven patients, three of five individuals who had converted from AIS A SCI (complete) to AIS B SCI (sensory incomplete) in the first six-month period of follow-up subsequently further improved to AIS C SCI (motor incomplete) within 12 to 24 months, including a recent patient who converted from AIS B to AIS C at the 12-month exam in January 2018.

Unfortunately, three deaths were witnessed during the INSPIRE study that were considered to be unrelated to the Neuro-Spinal Scaffold used and the implantation technique. Nevertheless, the company has elected, based in part on discussions with the company's independent Data Safety Monitoring Board, to implement a temporary halt to enrolment as it engages with the FDA to determine whether any changes to patient enrolment criteria related to patients who may have a higher mortality risk or other study modifications are deemed necessary.

As a result of the temporary enrolment halt, the company anticipated completing INSPIRE enrolment in the first half of 2018 and submitting a Humanitarian Device Exemption (HDE) application in the second half of 2018. As per a recent press release of the company in March 2018, the company has received supplemental Investigational Device Exemption (IDE) approval from the US FDA for a second pivotal clinical study of the company's Neuro-Spinal Scaffold in patients with acute SCI.

In the meantime, InVivo therapeutics took the decision to focus only on the INSPIRE study for the time being, so they announced the temporary suspension of the chronic SCI stem cell study.

2.4. "Walk Again Project"

Raisman and co-workers in London, who pioneered the "Walk Again Project" [12]. Unfortunately, he passed away but his work is being continued by Tabakow and co-workers in Poland, the leading neurosurgeon involved in Raisman's project. The project focuses on the use of Olfactory Ensheathing Cells (OECs) in order to accomplish functional improvement after SCI. Even though there are many unidentified mechanisms involved, OECs have been used for years in clinical trials for CNS repair and one of their functions is thought to be helping the local propriospinal interneurons to create new circuits for bypassing the lesion. The first clinical trials of OECs have already taken place in China, Australia, and Spain in 2003, 2005, and 2006, respectively [13–15]. Ever since, significant progress has been accomplished and the safety of OECs transplantation in humans has been established through several phase I clinical trials [16]. Nevertheless, the need for robust, well-designed phase II clinical trials is still unmet in order to measure the efficacy of that technique. Through such future clinical trials, the technique can be optimized in order to accomplish the optimal harvesting methodology and maximize the viability of the cells after transplantation [17].

Despite all the current limitations regarding the OECs transplantation technique, Geoffrey Raisman's team in UCL reported very promising results, from an injured patient, in 2014 (Figure 2). As per the report, the recipient of the transplanted OECs demonstrated significant functional recovery below the level of SCI, favoring the use of OECs as an efficient treatment of SCI [12]. It is remarkable that the patient went from complete paraplegia to incomplete (ASIA A to ASIA C) and has regained considerable functions. Nevertheless, expectations from this study have to be tempered since we are now talking about a single patient. Chronic SCI patients are still (since March 2016) being recruited for a new clinical trial taking place in Poland (Tabakow and colleagues). As far as we know, the clinical trial follows the same protocol as the one that was applied to the first patient, i.e., extraction of olfactory cells from the olfactory bulb in the patient's brain, transplantation into the spinal cord and a peripheral nerve graft. Only patients with a transected/severed spinal cord can apply for the trial and not patients with contused spinal cord.

2.5. "Miami Project" Phase I Clinical Trial

Schwan cells (SCs) are supporting cells surrounding the peripheral nerves. In the peripheral nervous system (PNS) they are thought to provide guidance to the axons for regeneration to take place [18]. The idea of using SCs after chronic SCI stems from the observation that SCs have been found around the lesion site after SCI [19,20], demonstrating beneficial effects. Nevertheless, it has been shown that apoptosis is a big obstacle, given the hostile CNS environment that does not favor the survival of those cells [21,22]. Despite the challenges, SCs are being used, for years now, in clinical trials targeting CNS lesions. Their safety has already been demonstrated in two already completed clinical trials involving SCs transplantation in human spinal cords. Currently, two more clinical trials phase I are in progress in Miami, Florida, USA, both studying sub-acute and chronic SCI subjects, in order to establish the safety of SCs before proceeding.

The "Miami Project" is a Phase I clinical trial for chronic SCI patients, it is currently recruiting patients and is expected to be completed by January 2019. Trial enrolment will target 2 cohorts. The study uses autologous Schwann cells harvested from the sural nerve of the participant, those cells are being transplanted into the epicenter of the participant's SCI. The first cohort is announced to be thoracic (T) level 2–12 AIS grade A, B, or C (n = up to 4) and the second one to be cervical (C) level 5 through T1 AIS A, B, or C (n = up to 6).

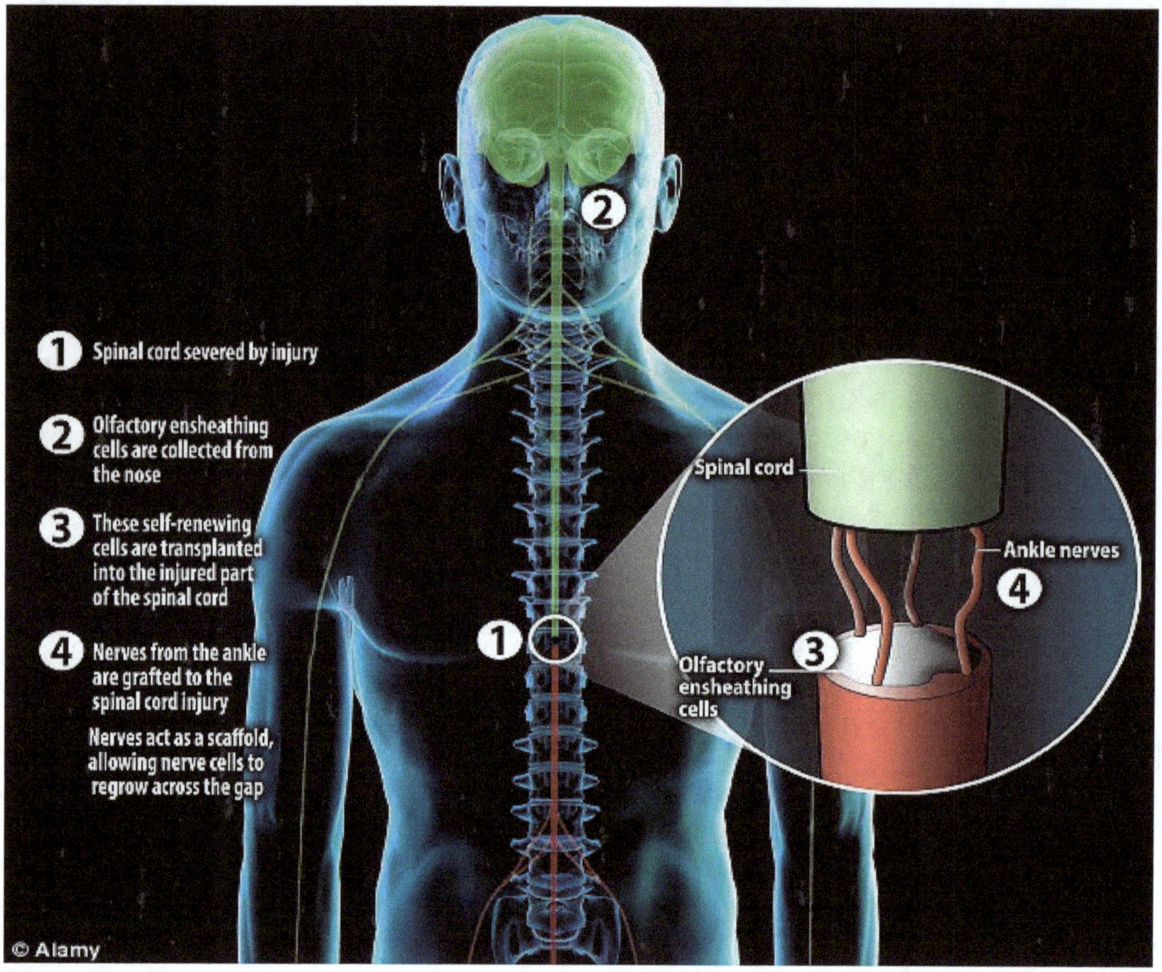

Figure 2. Schematic diagram shows steps of the treatment of Spinal Cord Injury (SCI) in a male patient who was paralyzed due to knife injury in 2010. He was treated with Olfactory Ensheathing Cells (OECs), a type of cell which is produced at the base of brain and through which human beings get their sense of smell. The surgeon extracted OECs from the nasal cavity and cultured those in the lab. Then nerve grafts were extracted from the ankle of the patient to support the regeneration of severed spinal cord nerve fibers to fill the spinal cavity. Both nerve grafts and stem cells were injected into the spinal cord injured site of the patient. This figure is also available online: http://www.dailymail.co.uk/sciencetech/article-2800988/world-man-spinal-cord-severed-walks-paralysed-fireman-recovers-thanks-uk-research.html.

2.6. Umbilical Cord Blood & Lithium ChinaSCINet Phase II Clinical Trial

In the fall of 2014, Wise Young, from Rutgers University and SCINetChina (available online: http://www.chinascinet.org), presented some preliminary information from the Umbilical Cord Blood & Lithium Phase II clinical trial that had taken place in China. In this trial [23], umbilical cord blood mononuclear cells (UCB-MNC) and lithium are used as a combinatorial therapy. The rationale for using lithium is that, apart from the low cost and availability in the clinic, it is known to stimulate UCB-MNC cells to secrete Nerve Growth Factor (NGF), Neurotrophin-3 (NT-3), and Glial cell line-derived Neurotrophic Factor (GDNF). In terms of the selection of UCB-MNCs, the aim is to improve recovery after chronic SCI. Several mechanisms have been proposed for the UCB-MNCs to improve recovery after CNS injury, involving secretion of anti-inflammatory cytokines [24–26], growth factors release [27–29], matrix metalloproteinase upregulation [25], tissue plasminogen activator downregulation [26], apoptosis prevention [24], mediation in myelination process [30,31], decreased gliosis [32], and increased angiogenesis [33].

Several groups have been known to attempt UCB-MNCs transplantation in patients with SCI with favorable outcomes. In the ChinaSCINet Phase I and II clinical trials [23], the patients were treated in Hong Kong (HK) and Kunming (KM) to assess the safety and efficacy of transplanting escalating doses of human leukocyte antigen (HLA)-matched UCB-MNCs into the spinal cords of people with chronic (1–19 years after) complete SCI. Wise Young explained in his presentation on the preliminary findings of the clinical trials that although none of the chronic ASIA A participants had improved motor scores, 15 out of the 20 patients were able to take steps with the aid of a walker whilst in rehabilitation.

Even though the motor scores of the chronic ASIA A patients did not improve, "functional recovery" was noted, which has raised some concerns. The main limitation is the absence of appropriate controls to assess the real effect of the UCB-MNCs transplantation. The fact that the intensive physiotherapy program was followed in combination with the stem cell transplant made it difficult to assess the real source of the improvements noted and would require further assessment. There is a possibility for the conduction of a phase IIb similar clinical trial in United States, aiming at proving the efficacy of the treatment. The structure of that new study is meant to be as follows: three groups of nine ASIA A, C5-T10 patients. The first group will get UCB-MNCs injections plus six weeks of oral lithium plus intensive rehabilitation. The second group will get UCB-MNCs plus intensive rehabilitation. Group three will get intensive rehabilitation only. This new study's structure would certainly overcome the limitations of the previous study conducted in HK and KM.

2.7. The Puerta de Hierro Phase I/II Clinical Trial

In the Puerta de Hierro Phase I/II clinical trials [34], autologous bone marrow adult mesenchymal stem cells (MSCs) were used for the studies, establishing the safety of the technique. MSCs have already been correlated with beneficial outcomes when being transplanted in CNS lesions in small and big preclinical animal models, paving the way towards clinical translation. Even though MSCs were traditionally known to be able to selfrenew and differentiate into cells of mesodermal origin, they have also been found to differentiate into tissue of nonmesoderm origin (i.e., nerve tissue) and they have the potential to modulate the inflammatory response [35,36]. In that trial, the MSCs were administered by intrathecal injection (subarachnoid and intramedullary). Improvement was noted even in the patients with the longest chronicity, while the team studied both complete and incomplete chronic SCI.

In the complete chronic SCI study, the recovery noted was considered to be a result of cytokine release by the transplanted MSCs, activating preserved but nonfunctional circuits, rather than inducing nerve regeneration. This is because the recovery of infralesional sensitivity and vegetative functions (e.g., bladder, bowel, and sexual functions) occurred soon after surgery. In addition, a dose-dependent beneficial effect of the MSCs transplantation was suggested because the improvement noted in the scaled used (e.g., ASIA, International Association of Neurorestoratology Spinal Cord Injury Functional Rating Scale (IANR-SCIFRS) and neurogenic bowel dysfunction (NBD)) was more significant for higher numbers of transplanted cells.

In the incomplete chronic SCI study, the repeated subarachnoid administrations of autologous MSCs supported in autologous plasma at months 1, 4, 7, and 10 of the study improved the patients' quality of life. Nevertheless, objective neuroimaging findings that would suggest morphological changes in the lesion site after the repeated subarachnoid administration of MSCs were absent. Therefore, the improvements were considered to be a result of the release of neurotrophic factors. It is in fact thought that the potential of MSCs transplantation for CNS regeneration relies on the ability of the MSCs to modulate the environment through their secretome. Classic growth factors and cytokines packed and secreted by the MSCs [37] are now thought to play a significant role for SCI repair, possibly by decreasing the levels of proinflammatory cytokines like Interleukine-2 (IL-2), Interleukine-6 (IL-6), and Tumor Necrosis Factor α (TNFα), among other mechanisms. This is demonstrated in a recent paper of Cizkova et al., where the molecular cocktail found in the MSCs after the MSCs transplantation in the rat SCI model was thought to be responsible for the observed motor function recovery, the attenuated inflammatory response and for the spared spinal cord tissue [38].

The Puerta de Hierro clinical trial phase II has been completed but an announcement on future trials is still pending.

2.8. *"Neurocell" Pre-Clinical Study of Neuroplast (Phase I Clinical Trial in Preparation)*

A preclinical study of Neuroplast, a company based in the Netherlands, showed that NEUROCELL (Neuroplast proprietary cells that are autologous bone-marrow-derived stem cells) significantly improved both locomotor functions and survival in those spinal cord-lesioned rats as compared to rats treated with a placebo. It is thought that autologous bone-marrow-derived stem cells can lead to functional improvement after CNS injuries by contributing towards the neuroplasticity and/or by exerting a paracrine effect. Neuroplast is currently preparing a Phase I clinical trial for chronic SCI patients. The trial will involve the transplantation of Neurocells and is expected to take place in Europe. The Neurocells are meant to have a positive effect, both in terms of neuroprotection and neuroplasticity, and thus contribute to a level of functional return in the case of both chronic and acute SCI. The first chronic SCI patients are expected to be recruited during 2018.

2.9. *Less Strictly Regulated Clinical Trials*

It should be noted that further trials in SCI patients are being conducted all over the world, but they are not performed under strict regulatory environments so caution is advised when assessing the results of such studies until further work is done in order to confirm findings in a better regulated setting [39–45].

3. Molecular Therapies

A summary of the various molecular therapies in the nanoscale projects is included in Table 1.

Table 1. Summary of the various molecular therapies in the nanoscale projects that show promise for the treatment of SCI. Keys: CNS: Central Nervous System; SCI: spinal cord injury; Ch'ase: Chondroitinase.

Project Name	Mechanism	Current Progress	Future Outlook	Ref.
Nogo Trap of ReNetX Bio	A decoy receptor that binds growth inhibitors, allowing for the nerve fibers to grow naturally and directly.	Nogo Trap has demonstrated improved neurologic function following CNS damage in several animal models.	Planning phase Ib–IIa clinical trials to test safety and efficacy for patients with a chronic cervical incomplete SCI.	[46]
CHASE-IT Preclinical Initiative of the International Spinal Research Trust (ISRT)	The application of the biological enzyme Ch'ase in animal models is reported to have degraded scar tissue, promoted growth and improved activity.	Ch'ase has proven to be effective in rats, delivered to both thoracic and cervical contusion injury sites. Latest animal studies took place in 2016 and proved that longer-term application of the enzyme led to more significant motor control improvement.	Promising outcome, but one should bear in mind that data is based on rodent in vivo models; will this translate to humans?	[47]
Intracellular sigma peptide (ISP), Ch'ase and combinations preclinical projects	Using the biological enzyme Ch'ase in combinations with intracellular sigma peptide in order to restore breathing after long chronic C2 hemisection injury.	These projects are at a single center led by Jerry Silver. Currently these applications are at a pre-clinical stage.	Development of the product and preparation for clinical trials.	[48]

3.1. *Nogo Trap of ReNetX Bio (Formerly Known as Axerion Therapeutics)*

Nogo Trap is a decoy receptor developed by the ReNetX Bio company. The decoy receptor is meant to modify the hostile CNS environment by binding to the growth inhibitors within the CNS. This allows new nerve fiber growth, targeting restoration across all facets of growth: axonal regeneration (long distance), axonal sprouting (medium distance), and synaptic plasticity. The main difference to the widely-known "Anti-NoGo" technology, as per the ReNetX representatives, is that the Nogo Trap is able to bind and neutralize three types of inhibitors and is not limited to the NoGo-inhibitor alone.

Nogo Trap has demonstrated improved neurologic function following CNS damage in several animal models. Based on these promising results, the company thought that Nogo Trap should be evaluated in chronic SCI patients. ReNetX Bio is planning a phase Ib–IIa clinical trial in order to test the safety and efficacy of the treatment for patients with chronic cervical incomplete SCI.

3.2. CHASE-IT Preclinical Initiative of the International Spinal Research Trust (ISRT)

Chondroitinase, or Ch'ase [49], is a bacterial enzyme that has attracted the attention of neuroscientists because of its ability to degrade the glial scar tissue that develops in chronic SCI. Apart from that, it has also repeatedly been proven to promote growth and to improve recovery in preclinical animal experiments. Therefore, Ch'ase is able to modify the scar tissue that develops after SCI and promote rewiring of the nervous system. This was only made possible by the molecular re-engineering of Ch'ase, developed by Muir and colleagues [50] at the University of Cambridge, who created a version of Ch'ase that could be expressed by human cells.

Gene therapy using a modified Chondroitinase ABC (ChABC) gene compatible with expression and secretion by mammalian host cells confers sustained and long-term delivery of ChABC to the injured spinal cord. It has been shown to be effective in rats to promote functional recovery in both thoracic and cervical contusion injury paradigms [51].

Several milestones have been reached since the CHASE-IT Initiative started in 2014. In particular: (1) The gene for Ch'ase can now be expressed in an active form in human cells; (2) expression of Ch'ase in the spinal cord can now be controlled, switching it on and off using an inducible switch responsive to the antibiotic doxycycline; and (3) treatment gives rise to improved walking and unprecedented upper limb function in clinically-relevant SCI models.

4. Selected Biomaterials That Hold Promise for Future Clinical Trials on Chronic Sci

The application of biomaterials in SCI is divided into two strategies. The first strategy involves the application of biomaterials as a scaffold for the neuronal cells or the encapsulation of certain cells for delivery. The second strategy is using biomaterials that mimic the soft tissue mechanical properties and the high conductivity required for electrical transmission in the native spinal cord for nerve tissue regeneration.

The use of biomaterials is of great importance for CNS regeneration and repair. It was soon observed that the use of potent stem cells alone could be dangerous, given the possibility of tumor formation. It has been demonstrated that the use of certain injectable hydrogels loaded with pluripotent stem cells can promote cell survival, integration, and differentiation, thereby reducing the risk of tumorigenicity that has been linked with the use of such cell lines [52,53].

The careful choice of the appropriate biomaterial for that specific application could not only guide the process with different topographical cues, but it could also provide the necessary structural support to build a temporary bridge within the cavity that is formed in chronic SCI lesions until nerve sprouting occurs.

The use of biomaterials for CNS regeneration purposes can also use nanotechnology in order to encapsulate the cells within nanoparticle-based hydrogels and develop a sustained release system that would allow a prolonged, tuned effect to accomplish the desired outcome. Trophic factors (e.g., growth factors) can also be incorporated in a scaffold made from the appropriate biomaterial in order to support the transplanted cells to live longer or even trigger endogenous regeneration through stem cell niches.

Several biomaterials have been used for supportive scaffold formation in order to accomplish CNS regeneration after chronic SCI lesions, but so far, only limited biomaterials have made it towards clinical trials as mentioned above (e.g., PLGA). There is an overwhelming amount of different combinations of biomaterials used in chronic SCI in terms of basic science experimentation, but this would be beyond the focus of the current review. Below, we will only mention a couple of selected biomaterials that we consider to be very promising in terms of future clinical applications.

Graphene Oxide (GO) 3D nano-structured scaffolds, considered "wonder biomaterials" with extraordinary potentials in the next few years based on preclinical results:

Studies have shown graphene to have great potential as a bioscaffold at the site of the lesion in chronic SCI allowing for neuronal regeneration [4,54–60]. GO nanocomposite is considered to be a favorable material for use in treatment because of its unique electro-physico-chemical properties and it is conductivity. GO has the ability to stimulate neuronal differentiation and axonal alignment at sites of SCI by providing a space for the growth, attachment, and survival of neural tissue at the lesion. Toxicity and biocompatibility of reduced graphene oxide is a debatable obstacle facing use of the material, with intravenous studies in mice showing dose-dependent toxicity and pathological damage present at lower doses [61,62]. Other routes of administration, however, such as oral [63], intravitreal [64], intraperitoneal [63], and subcutaneous [65], have proven the material to be nontoxic. The conductive properties of GO make it a viable product to use in the healing of SCI. The benefit of using GO is that the inflammatory response seen with other biomaterials is reduced and not as damaging at the site of the SCI.

GO combined with hydrogel has been used to fill the hemispinal cord transection lesion that was made in twenty rats [66]. After three months, histologic evaluation of the lesion in the spinal cords of the rats showed graphene nanoscaffolds adhering to the spinal cord tissue and an ingrowth of connective tissue elements, blood vessels, neurofilaments, and Schwann cells around the area of the graphene nanoscaffolds. A control study was carried out whereby similar rats with hemispinal cord transections had a hydrogel-only matrix injected into the lesion at site of injury. Three months later, histological evaluation showed pseudocyst cavities where the hydrogel matrix had been injected and the site of the lesion devoid of any tissue or substantial regrowth of neural cells. Even though this was a study on acute SCI, this in vivo preclinical study brings promise that the graphene nanoscaffolds material has potential to be used for stimulation of axonal regeneration into the lesion.

Another aspect stressing the significance and potential of Graphene, in terms of future clinical SCI repair-related applications, is the fact that Graphene has been chosen as the key biomaterial to be used as part of the project "Neurofibers" (Biofunctionalised Electroconducting Microfibers for the Treatment of Spinal Cord Injury). The project has recently started and it was selected by the European Commission in the framework of the Horizon 2020 (H2020) program in the area of emerging technologies (FET Proactive—Boosting emerging technologies) (for more information from the European Commission's website: https://cordis.europa.eu/project/rcn/206185_en.html).

4.1. Fibrin-Based Scaffolds and Hydrogels Have Shown Impressive Results in Terms of Supporting CNS Regeneration in SCI Lesions in the Right Settings

The Fibrin glue has been approved by FDA and it is used successfully in clinically repairing cranial nerves and other tissues [67,68]. The Fibrin sealant (like the commercially available TISSEEL® (Baxter) product) has been used for years by neurosurgeons as a hemostatic agent and in order to control cerebrospinal fluid (CSF) leaks. This is of particular importance for spinal surgeries given the CSF leakage that can occur after the durotomy. In human patients, Fibrin has also been combined with FGF and the mixture was applied to the injured spinal segment of patients in order to prevent postoperative CSF leakage. The application of the FGF-containing Fibrin matrices resulted in significant motor and sensory improvements in the patients [69]. In terms of CNS repair and regenerative medicine, Fibrin could act as a carrier for therapeutic agents, such as neurotrophic factors and stem cells [70–72].

Fibrin matrices have been tested for supporting stem cells, specially embedded NSCs in fibrin matrices in order to increase the cells' viability, when transplanted after SCI [73]. Even though the increase in NSCs viability was significant compared to the initial poor survival of the cells without the fibrin matrices, the results were even more remarkable when growth factor cocktails were added in the NSCs-containing fibrin matrices. This way the combination of NSCs with fibrin matrices and growth factors accomplished enhanced cells survival with the cells filling large lesion cavities and being differentiated into neurons and glia after spinal cord transection [2,73,74]. In a very recent paper, Rosenzweig et al. [10] used a similar methodology in nonhuman primate models, proving for one more time that testing a promising treatment in nonhuman primates is crucial for the successful translation to humans. After several modifications to the rodent grafting technique (e.g., grafting matrix modifications, CSF drainage, more extensive immunosuppression), successful engraftment was achieved, paving the path towards clinical translation of the proposed therapy. The same group of researchers had accomplished before that the longest axonal sprouting, to the best of our knowledge, using a cocktail of growth factors and fibrin matrices. Ten growth factors were embedded in a fibrin gel to support rat or human neural stem cells grafted to the completely transected spinal cord of adult rats, accomplishing axons extending at least 25 mm in each direction in all subjects [75].

Further combinatorial approaches have been attempted using Fibrin with certain growth factors and grafts to enhance the restorative results with very promising results.

The FGF/Fibrin mixture along with human Schwann-cell grafts has been engrafted to transected rat spinal cords, stimulating fiber regeneration throughout the implant [76]. This also has been coupled with an autologous peripheral intercostal nerve segment to bridge a 5 mm gap within the transected rat spinal cords [77]. Even though this is only a small part of the literature supporting the use of Fibrin for CNS repair, it is evident that this biomaterial is also a very good candidate for future clinical applications in terms of regenerative therapeutic strategies in chronic SCI.

4.2. Collagen/Heparin Sulfate Scaffolds Fabricated by a 3D Bioprinter

One promising, new approach is the use of a 3D bioprinter in producing collagen and heparin sulfate based bioscaffolds for the treatment of SCI [78]. The use of a 3D bioprinter, in order to produce the bioscaffold, is thought to have significantly amplified the mechanical properties of the mixture when compared to methods of production without the use of a 3D printer therefore methods using a 3D bioprinter will be discussed here. The current priorities when producing a bioscaffold for SCI is the biocompatibility of the scaffold, that it is made of a porous material in order to allow for neural regeneration and for it to have great strength. The team working on the 3D bioprinted collagen/heparin sulfate scaffolds believes it will be the answer to treating and stimulating neural regeneration in patients with SCI.

Locomotor recovery is the most important outcome to assess during preclinical and clinical studies and was seen in rats with SCI that had had the collagen/heparin sulfate bioscaffold implanted at the site of the lesion, during preclinical in vivo studies. The improved locomotor function after implantation and biodegradable and biocompatible properties of the collagen/heparin sulfate mixture gives promise for the use of such a bioscaffold in clinical practice to help improve the outcome of patients suffering with SCI.

4.3. Peripheral Nerve Grafts Combined with Chitosan-Laminin Scaffold

Chitosan is a suitable biomaterial for use in neuronal repair due to its biocompatible and biodegradable properties [79]. It has been considered as a suitable material for many biomedical and industrial applications, such as drug delivery, due to its nontoxicity and biodegradability. Laminin is a glycoprotein that acts as a neurite outgrowth-promoting factor and so is suitable for combination in the bioscaffold. The combination of chitosan and laminin provide a promising biomaterial for use as a scaffold in promoting axonal growth and preventing neural degeneration.

Studies have shown that the use of chitosan channels containing nerve grafts promote axonal regeneration when applied to chronic SCI lesions [80]. Preclinical studies have shown that the use of chitosan-laminin scaffolds combined with peripheral nerve grafts supported axonal regeneration and positive outcomes include motor function improvement, as well as functional sensory improvement when the bioscaffolds were implanted in chronic nerve lesions [40]. Further investigation of this biomaterial would be recommended as it proves to be a promising option in the field of treatment of chronic SCI.

5. Conclusions and Future Perspectives

In conclusion, it is evident that more promising therapies will come up in the future regarding chronic SCI. We anticipate that the management of chronic SCI will change during the next few decades due to the fast pace of advances in the field of nanotechnology/smart materials and regenerative medicine. A combinatorial approach using cells and/or growth factors or other molecules along with biocompatible nanostructured scaffolds, that would allow fine-tuning of the release of the incorporated factors and would guide nerve growth in the CNS environment, would most probably be the key for success in such a complex tissue.

One significant component seems to be the ability to catalyze the translation of all the promising new therapies into clinical practice. This refers to imaging technology, and more specifically, Magnetic Resonance Imaging (MRI) sequences that can help assess and objectively quantify the biological response of the CNS to the tested intervention, solving a known issue of reproducibility and quantification in the application of all the new therapies. MRI could assess the biological significance, detecting tissue-related changes, while techniques like surface electromyography could assess the functional outcomes in a more objective way, leading together to the development of the much needed objective clinical scales that would take into consideration the statistical, biological and clinical significance associated with the tested therapeutic strategy or management plan. In addition, the combination of imaging technology along with the implementation of new, clinically relevant models, like the nonhuman primate model of SCI developed for evaluating pharmacologic treatments, and could open the pathway to safer and more efficient clinical application to patients in the future [81]. Nevertheless, we do anticipate that the use of bioengineered models on-a-chip and further advancements in nanomedicine might revolutionize the field and change the translational pathway in the future, accelerating the drug approval process and the implementation of new treatments in the clinic.

From the practical standpoint, there are several obstacles that need to be tackled, like the lack of published data from companies that have done significant work on SCI regeneration and repair through clinical trials. The inclusion of controls is crucial for obtaining reliable outcomes and yet certain clinical trials either fail to implement controls in their study plan or they avoid reporting the outcomes in a timely manner, hindering the progress in the field. In addition to that, researchers mainly use less clinically relevant SCI models like hemisections/transection models. There is a significant need for inclusion of contusion SCI models that are more similar to the lesions usually managed in the clinic. Last but not least, it should be stressed that acute SCI models are mainly used for research purposes aiming to address the problem soon after the injury in the clinic and to avoid complications (e.g., formation of glial scar that would hinder neuroregeneration). The inclusion of more chronic SCI models in research might seem to be a challenging task, but it is very important for the reliable assessment of the therapeutic interventions in order to solve significant questions on CNS regeneration, ensuring the safe application of future treatments to any SCI patient.

Author Contributions: A.M.S. proposed the review article and M.T., K.D., and A.S. worked on data gathering and drafting the review. All four authors critically analyzed and reviewed the topic and completed the review with future direction of the research.

Acknowledgments: M.T. was supported by Onassis Foundation during that study.

References

1. National Spinal Cord Injury Statistical Center. *Spinal Cord Injury (SCI) Facts and Figures at a Glance*; National Spinal Cord Injury Statistical Center: Birmingham, AL, USA, 2017.
2. Kadoya, K.; Tsukada, S.; Lu, P.; Coppola, G.; Geschwind, D.; Filbin, M.; Blesch, A.; Tuszynski, M.H. Combined Intrinsic and Extrinsic Neuronal Mechanisms Facilitate Bridging Axonal Regeneration One Year After Spinal Cord Injury. *Neuron* **2009**, *64*, 165–172. [CrossRef] [PubMed]

3. Gelain, F.; Panseri, S.; Antonini, S.; Cunha, C.; Donega, M.; Lowery, J.; Taraballi, F.; Cerri, G.; Montagna, M.; Baldissera, F.; et al. Transplantation of Nanostructured Composite Scaffolds Results in the Regeneration of Chronically Injured Spinal Cords. *ACS Nano* **2011**, *5*, 227–236. [CrossRef] [PubMed]
4. Faccendini, A.; Vigani, B.; Rossi, S.; Sandri, G.; Bonferoni, M.C.; Caramella, C.M.; Ferrari, F. Nanofiber Scaffolds as Drug Delivery Systems to Bridge Spinal Cord Injury. *Pharmaceuticals* **2017**, *10*, 63. [CrossRef] [PubMed]
5. StemCells Inc. *Pathway Study*; StemCells Inc.: Newark, CA, USA, 2015.
6. StemCells Inc. *Phase II Trial in Cervical Spinal Cord Injury (SCI)*; StemCells Inc.: Newark, CA, USA, 2015.
7. NeuralStem Inc. *Neuralstem Reports Third Quarter 2015 Financial Results—Nov 9, 2015*; NeuralStem Inc.: Rockville, MD, USA, 2015.
8. Yan, J.; Xu, L.; Welsh, A.M.; Hatfield, G.; Hazel, T.; Johe, K.; Koliatsos, V.E. Extensive neuronal differentiation of human neural stem cell grafts in adult rat spinal cord. *PLoS Med.* **2007**, *4*, e39. [CrossRef] [PubMed]
9. Xu, L.; Yan, J.; Chen, D.; Welsh, A.M.; Hazel, T.; Johe, K.; Hatfield, G.; Koliatsos, V.E. Human neural stem cell grafts ameliorate motor neuron disease in SOD-1 transgenic rats. *Transplantation* **2006**, *82*, 865–875. [CrossRef] [PubMed]
10. Rosenzweig, E.S.; Brock, J.H.; Lu, P.; Kumamaru, H.; Salegio, E.A.; Kadoya, K.; Weber, J.L.; Liang, J.J.; Moseanko, R.; Hawbecker, S.; et al. Restorative effects of human neural stem cell grafts on the primate spinal cord. *Nat. Med.* **2018**, *24*, 484–490. [CrossRef] [PubMed]
11. Theodore, N.; Hlubek, R.; Danielson, J.; Neff, K.; Vaickus, L.; Ulich, T.R.; Ropper, A.E. First Human Implantation of a Bioresorbable Polymer Scaffold for Acute Traumatic Spinal Cord Injury: A Clinical Pilot Study for Safety and Feasibility. *Neurosurgery* **2016**, *79*, E305–E312. [CrossRef] [PubMed]
12. Tabakow, P.; Raisman, G.; Fortuna, W.; Czyz, M.; Huber, J.; Li, D.; Szewczyk, P.; Okurowski, S.; Miedzybrodzki, R.; Czapiga, B.; et al. Functional regeneration of supraspinal connections in a patient with transected spinal cord following transplantation of bulbar olfactory ensheathing cells with peripheral nerve bridging. *Cell Transpl.* **2014**, *23*, 1631–1655. [CrossRef] [PubMed]
13. Huang, H.; Chen, L.; Wang, H.; Xiu, B.; Li, B.; Wang, R.; Zhang, J.; Zhang, F.; Gu, Z.; Li, Y.; et al. Influence of patients' age on functional recovery after transplantation of olfactory ensheathing cells into injured spinal cord injury. *Chin. Med. J.* **2003**, *116*, 1488–1491. [PubMed]
14. Féron, F.; Perry, C.; Cochrane, J.; Licina, P.; Nowitzke, A.; Urquhart, S.; Geraghty, T.; Mackay-Sim, A. Autologous olfactory ensheathing cell transplantation in human spinal cord injury. *Brain* **2005**, *128*, 2951–2960. [CrossRef] [PubMed]
15. Lima, C.; Pratas-Vital, J.; Escada, P.; Hasse-Ferreira, A.; Capucho, C.; Peduzzi, J.D. Olfactory Mucosa Autografts in Human Spinal Cord Injury: A Pilot Clinical Study. *J. Spinal Cord Med.* **2006**, *29*, 191–203. [CrossRef] [PubMed]
16. Li, L.; Adnan, H.; Xu, B.; Wang, J.; Wang, C.; Li, F.; Tang, K. Effects of transplantation of olfactory ensheathing cells in chronic spinal cord injury: A systematic review and meta-analysis. *Eur. Spine J.* **2015**, *24*, 919–930. [CrossRef] [PubMed]
17. Choi, D.; Gladwin, K. Olfactory Ensheathing Cells: Part II—Source of Cells and Application to Patients. *World Neurosurg.* **2015**, *83*, 251–256. [CrossRef] [PubMed]
18. Son, Y.-J.; Thompson, W.J. Schwann cell processes guide regeneration of peripheral axons. *Neuron* **1995**, *14*, 125–132. [CrossRef]
19. Bruce, J.H.; Norenberg, M.D.; Kraydieh, S.; Puckett, W.; Marcillo, A.; Dietrich, D. Schwannosis: Role of gliosis and proteoglycan in human spinal cord injury. *J. Neurotrauma* **2000**, *17*, 781–788. [CrossRef] [PubMed]
20. Guest, J.D.; Hiester, E.D.; Bunge, R.P. Demyelination and Schwann cell responses adjacent to injury epicenter cavities following chronic human spinal cord injury. *Exp. Neurol.* **2005**, *192*, 384–393. [CrossRef] [PubMed]
21. Bunge, M.B.; Wood, P.M. Realizing the maximum potential of Schwann cells to promote recovery from spinal cord injury. *Handb. Clin. Neurol.* **2012**, *109*, 523–540. [CrossRef] [PubMed]
22. Wiliams, R.R.; Bunge, M.B. Schwann cell transplantation: A repair strategy for spinal cord injury? *Prog. Brain Res.* **2012**, *201*, 295–312. [CrossRef] [PubMed]
23. Zhu, H.; Poon, W.; Liu, Y.; Leung, G.K.-K.; Wong, Y.; Feng, Y.; Ng, S.C.P.; Tsang, K.S.; Sun, D.T.F.; Yeung, D.K.; et al. Phase I–II Clinical Trial Assessing Safety and Efficacy of Umbilical Cord Blood Mononuclear Cell Transplant Therapy of Chronic Complete Spinal Cord Injury. *Cell Transpl.* **2016**, *25*, 1925–1943. [CrossRef] [PubMed]

24. Dasari, V.R.; Veeravalli, K.K.; Tsung, A.J.; Gondi, C.S.; Gujrati, M.; Dinh, D.H.; Rao, J.S. Neuronal Apoptosis Is Inhibited by Cord Blood Stem Cells after Spinal Cord Injury. *J. Neurotrauma* **2009**, *26*, 2057–2069. [CrossRef] [PubMed]
25. Veeravalli, K.K.; Dasari, V.R.; Tsung, A.J.; Dinh, D.H.; Gujrati, M.; Fassett, D.; Rao, J.S. Human umbilical cord blood stem cells upregulate matrix metalloproteinase-2 in rats after spinal cord injury. *Neurobiol. Dis.* **2009**, *36*, 200–212. [CrossRef] [PubMed]
26. Veeravalli, K.K.; Dasari, V.R.; Tsung, A.J.; Dinh, D.H.; Gujrati, M.; Fassett, D.; Rao, J.S. Stem Cells Downregulate the Elevated Levels of Tissue Plasminogen Activator in Rats After Spinal Cord Injury. *Neurochem. Res.* **2009**, *34*, 1183–1194. [CrossRef] [PubMed]
27. Kao, C.-H.; Chen, S.-H.; Chio, C.-C.; Lin, M.-T. Human Umbilical Cord Blood-derived CD34+ cells may attenuate spinal cord injury by stimulating vascular endothelial and neurotrophic factors. *Shock* **2008**, *29*, 49–55. [CrossRef] [PubMed]
28. Chua, S.J.; Bielecki, R.; Yamanaka, N.; Fehlings, M.G.; Rogers, I.M.; Casper, R.F. The Effect of Umbilical Cord Blood Cells on Outcomes After Experimental Traumatic Spinal Cord Injury. *Spine* **2010**, *35*, 1520–1526. [CrossRef] [PubMed]
29. Chung, H.; Chung, W.; Lee, J.-H.; Chung, D.-J.; Yang, W.-J.; Lee, A.-J.; Choi, C.-B.; Chang, H.-S.; Kim, D.-H.; Suh, H.J.; et al. Expression of neurotrophic factors in injured spinal cord after transplantation of human-umbilical cord blood stem cells in rats. *J. Vet. Sci.* **2016**, *17*, 97–102. [CrossRef] [PubMed]
30. Dasari, V.R.; Spomar, D.G.; Gondi, C.S.; Sloffer, C.A.; Saving, K.L.; Gujrati, M.; Rao, J.S.; Dinh, D.H. Axonal Remyelination by Cord Blood Stem Cells after Spinal Cord Injury. *J. Neurotrauma* **2007**, *24*, 391–410. [CrossRef] [PubMed]
31. Cho, S.-R.; Yang, M.S.; Yim, S.H.; Park, J.H.; Lee, J.E.; Eom, Y.; Jang, I.K.; Kim, H.E.; Park, J.S.; Kim, H.O.; et al. Neurally induced umbilical cord blood cells modestly repair injured spinal cords. *NeuroReport* **2008**, *19*, 1259–1263. [CrossRef] [PubMed]
32. Ryu, H.-H.; Byeon, Y.-E.; Park, S.-S.; Kang, B.-J.; Seo, M.-S.; Park, S.-B.; Kim, W.H.; Kang, K.-S.; Kweon, O.-K. Immunohistomorphometric Analysis of Transplanted Umbilical Cord Blood-Derived Mesenchymal Stem Cells and The Resulting Anti-Inflammatory Effects on Nerve Regeneration of Injured Canine Spinal Cord. *Tissue Eng. Regen. Med.* **2011**, *8*, 173–182.
33. Ning, G.; Tang, L.; Wu, Q.; Li, Y.; Li, Y.; Zhang, C.; Feng, S. Human umbilical cord blood stem cells for spinal cord injury: Early transplantation results in better local angiogenesis. *Regen. Med.* **2013**, *8*, 271–281. [CrossRef] [PubMed]
34. Vaquero, J.; Zurita, M.; Rico, M.A.; Bonilla, C.; Aguayo, C.; Montilla, J.; Bustamante, S.; Carballido, J.; Marin, E.; Martinez, F.; et al. An approach to personalized cell therapy in chronic complete paraplegia: The Puerta de Hierro phase I/II clinical trial. *Cytotherapy* **2016**, *18*, 1025–1036. [CrossRef] [PubMed]
35. Deans, R.J.; Moseley, A.B. Mesenchymal stem cells. *Exp. Hematol.* **2000**, *28*, 875–884. [CrossRef]
36. Kopen, G.C.; Prockop, D.J.; Phinney, D.G. Marrow stromal cells migrate throughout forebrain and cerebellum, and they differentiate into astrocytes after injection into neonatal mouse brains. *Proc. Natl. Acad. Sci. USA* **1999**, *96*, 10711–10716. [CrossRef] [PubMed]
37. Hofer, H.R.; Tuan, R.S. Secreted trophic factors of mesenchymal stem cells support neurovascular and musculoskeletal therapies. *Stem Cell Res. Ther.* **2016**, *7*, 131. [CrossRef] [PubMed]
38. Cizkova, D.; Cubinkova, V.; Smolek, T.; Murgoci, A.-N.; Danko, J.; Vdoviakova, K.; Humenik, F.; Cizek, M.; Quanico, J.; Fournier, I.; et al. Localized Intrathecal Delivery of Mesenchymal Stromal Cells Conditioned Medium Improves Functional Recovery in a Rat Model of Spinal Cord Injury. *Int. J. Mol. Sci.* **2018**, *19*, 870. [CrossRef] [PubMed]
39. Bansal, H.; Verma, P.; Agrawal, A.; Leon, J.; Sundell, I.B.; Koka, P.S. Autologous Bone Marrow-Derived Stem Cells in Spinal Cord Injury. *J. Stem Cells* **2016**, *11*, 51–61. [PubMed]
40. Amr, S.M.; Gouda, A.; Koptan, W.T.; Galal, A.A.; Abdel-Fattah, D.S.; Rashed, L.A.; Atta, H.M.; Abdel-Aziz, M.T. Bridging defects in chronic spinal cord injury using peripheral nerve grafts combined with a chitosan-laminin scaffold and enhancing regeneration through them by co-transplantation with bone-marrow-derived mesenchymal stem cells: Case series of 14 patients. *J. Spinal Cord Med.* **2014**, *37*, 54–71. [CrossRef] [PubMed]

41. Frolov, A.A.; Bryukhovetskiy, A.S. Effects of hematopoietic autologous stem cell transplantation to the chronically injured human spinal cord evaluated by motor and somatosensory evoked potentials methods. *Cell Transpl.* **2012**, *21* (Suppl. 1), S49–S55. [CrossRef] [PubMed]
42. El-Kheir, W.A.; Gabr, H.; Awad, M.R.; Ghannam, O.; Barakat, Y.; Farghali, H.A.M.A.; El Maadawi, Z.M.; Ewes, I.; Sabaawy, H.E. Autologous bone marrow-derived cell therapy combined with physical therapy induces functional improvement in chronic spinal cord injury patients. *Cell Transpl.* **2014**, *23*, 729–745. [CrossRef] [PubMed]
43. Wong, Y.W.; Tam, S.; So, K.F.; Chen, J.Y.H.; Cheng, W.S.; Luk, K.D.K.; Tang, S.W.; Young, W. A three-month, open-label, single-arm trial evaluating the safety and pharmacokinetics of oral lithium in patients with chronic spinal cord injury. *Spinal Cord* **2011**, *49*, 94–98. [CrossRef] [PubMed]
44. Cristante, A.F.; Barros-Filho, T.E.P.; Tatsui, N.; Mendrone, A.; Caldas, J.G.; Camargo, A.; Alexandre, A.; Teixeira, W.G.J.; Oliveira, R.P.; Marcon, R.M. Stem cells in the treatment of chronic spinal cord injury: Evaluation of somatosensitive evoked potentials in 39 patients. *Spinal Cord* **2009**, *47*, 733–738. [CrossRef] [PubMed]
45. Moviglia, G.A.; Fernandez Viña, R.; Brizuela, J.A.; Saslavsky, J.; Vrsalovic, F.; Varela, G.; Bastos, F.; Farina, P.; Etchegaray, G.; Barbieri, M.; et al. Combined protocol of cell therapy for chronic spinal cord injury. Report on the electrical and functional recovery of two patients. *Cytotherapy* **2006**, *8*, 202–209. [CrossRef] [PubMed]
46. ReNetX. ReNetX Bio Launched to Advance Innovative Neuro-Regenerative Technology Developed at Yale University. Available online: http://globenewswire.com/news-release/2017/07/24/1056062/0/en/ReNetX-Bio-Launched-to-Advance-Innovative-Neuro-Regenerative-Technology-Developed-at-Yale-University.html (accessed on 20 April 2018).
47. CHASE IT. Available online: https://www.spinal-research.org/chase-it (accessed on 20 April 2018).
48. Tran, A.P.; Sundar, S.; Yu, M.; Lang, B.T.; Silver, J. Modulation of receptor protein tyrosine phosphatase sigma increases chondroitin sulfate proteoglycan degradation through Cathepsin B secretion to enhance axon outgrowth. *J. Neurosci.* **2018**, 3214–3217. [CrossRef] [PubMed]
49. Bartus, K.; James, N.D.; Didangelos, A.; Bosch, K.D.; Verhaagen, J.; Yáñez-Muñoz, R.J.; Rogers, J.H.; Schneider, B.L.; Muir, E.M.; Bradbury, E.J. Large-scale chondroitin sulfate proteoglycan digestion with chondroitinase gene therapy leads to reduced pathology and modulates macrophage phenotype following spinal cord contusion injury. *J. Neurosci.* **2014**, *34*, 4822–4836. [CrossRef] [PubMed]
50. Muir, E.; Raza, M.; Ellis, C.; Burnside, E.; Love, F.; Heller, S.; Elliot, M.; Daniell, E.; Dasgupta, D.; Alves, N.; et al. Trafficking and processing of bacterial proteins by mammalian cells: Insights from chondroitinase ABC. *PLoS ONE* **2017**, *12*, e0186759. [CrossRef] [PubMed]
51. James, N.D.; Shea, J.; Muir, E.M.; Verhaagen, J.; Schneider, B.L.; Bradbury, E.J. Chondroitinase gene therapy improves upper limb function following cervical contusion injury. *Exp. Neurol.* **2015**, *271*, 131–135. [CrossRef] [PubMed]
52. Oliveira, J.M.; Carvalho, L.; Silva-Correia, J.; Vieira, S.; Majchrzak, M.; Lukomska, B.; Stanaszek, L.; Strymecka, P.; Malysz-Cymborska, I.; Golubczyk, D.; et al. Hydrogel-based scaffolds to support intrathecal stem cell transplantation as a gateway to the spinal cord: Clinical needs, biomaterials, and imaging technologies. *NPJ Regen. Med.* **2018**, *3*, 8. [CrossRef] [PubMed]
53. Führmann, T.; Tam, R.Y.; Ballarin, B.; Coles, B.; Elliott Donaghue, I.; van der Kooy, D.; Nagy, A.; Tator, C.H.; Morshead, C.M.; Shoichet, M.S. Injectable hydrogel promotes early survival of induced pluripotent stem cell-derived oligodendrocytes and attenuates longterm teratoma formation in a spinal cord injury model. *Biomaterials* **2016**, *83*, 23–36. [CrossRef] [PubMed]
54. López-Dolado, E.; González-Mayorga, A.; Gutiérrez, M.C.; Serrano, M.C. Immunomodulatory and angiogenic responses induced by graphene oxide scaffolds in chronic spinal hemisected rats. *Biomaterials* **2016**, *99*, 72–81. [CrossRef] [PubMed]
55. Mattei, T.A. How graphene is expected to impact neurotherapeutics in the near future. *Expert Rev. Neurother.* **2014**, *14*, 845–847. [CrossRef] [PubMed]
56. Domínguez-Bajo, A.; González-Mayorga, A.; López-Dolado, E.; Serrano, M.C. Graphene-Derived Materials Interfacing the Spinal Cord: Outstanding in Vitro and in Vivo Findings. *Front. Syst. Neurosci.* **2017**, *11*, 71. [CrossRef] [PubMed]

57. Zhou, K.; Motamed, S.; Thouas, G.A.; Bernard, C.C.; Li, D.; Parkington, H.C.; Coleman, H.A.; Finkelstein, D.I.; Forsythe, J.S. Graphene Functionalized Scaffolds Reduce the Inflammatory Response and Supports Endogenous Neuroblast Migration when Implanted in the Adult Brain. *PLoS ONE* **2016**, *11*, e0151589. [CrossRef] [PubMed]
58. González-Mayorga, A.; López-Dolado, E.; Gutiérrez, M.C.; Collazos-Castro, J.E.; Ferrer, M.L.; del Monte, F.; Serrano, M.C. Favorable Biological Responses of Neural Cells and Tissue Interacting with Graphene Oxide Microfibers. *ACS Omega* **2017**, *2*, 8253–8263. [CrossRef]
59. Singh, Z. Applications and Toxicity of Graphene Family Nanomaterials and Their Composites. Available online: https://www.dovepress.com/applications-and-toxicity-of-graphene-family-nanomaterials-and-their-c-peer-reviewed-fulltext-article-NSA (accessed on 19 April 2018).
60. Kim, C.-Y.; Sikkema, W.K.A.; Hwang, I.-K.; Oh, H.; Kim, U.J.; Lee, B.H.; Tour, J.M. Spinal cord fusion with PEG-GNRs (TexasPEG): Neurophysiological recovery in 24 hours in rats. *Surg. Neurol. Int.* **2016**, *7*, S632–S636. [CrossRef] [PubMed]
61. Mendonça, M.C.P.; Soares, E.S.; de Jesus, M.B.; Ceragioli, H.J.; Batista, Â.G.; Nyúl-Tóth, Á.; Molnár, J.; Wilhelm, I.; Maróstica, M.R.; Krizbai, I.; et al. PEGylation of Reduced Graphene Oxide Induces Toxicity in Cells of the Blood-Brain Barrier: An in Vitro and in Vivo Study. *Mol. Pharm.* **2016**, *13*, 3913–3924. [CrossRef] [PubMed]
62. Zhang, X.; Yin, J.; Peng, C.; Hu, W.; Zhu, Z.; Li, W.; Fan, C.; Huang, Q. Distribution and biocompatibility studies of graphene oxide in mice after intravenous administration. *Carbon* **2011**, *49*, 986–995. [CrossRef]
63. Yang, K.; Gong, H.; Shi, X.; Wan, J.; Zhang, Y.; Liu, Z. In vivo biodistribution and toxicology of functionalized nano-graphene oxide in mice after oral and intraperitoneal administration. *Biomaterials* **2013**, *34*, 2787–2795. [CrossRef] [PubMed]
64. Yan, L.; Wang, Y.; Xu, X.; Zeng, C.; Hou, J.; Lin, M.; Xu, J.; Sun, F.; Huang, X.; Dai, L.; et al. Can Graphene Oxide Cause Damage to Eyesight? *Chem. Res. Toxicol.* **2012**, *25*, 1265–1270. [CrossRef] [PubMed]
65. Sahu, A.; Il Choi, W.; Tae, G. A stimuli-sensitive injectable graphene oxide composite hydrogel. *Chem. Commun.* **2012**, *48*, 5820–5822. [CrossRef] [PubMed]
66. Palejwala, A.H.; Fridley, J.S.; Mata, J.A.; Samuel, E.L.G.; Luerssen, T.G.; Perlaky, L.; Kent, T.A.; Tour, J.M.; Jea, A. Biocompatibility of reduced graphene oxide nanoscaffolds following acute spinal cord injury in rats. *Surg. Neurol. Int.* **2016**, *7*, 75. [CrossRef] [PubMed]
67. Wieken, K.; Angioi-Duprez, K.; Lim, A.; Marchal, L.; Merle, M. Nerve anastomosis with glue: Comparative histologic study of fibrin and cyanoacrylate glue. *J. Reconstr. Microsurg.* **2003**, *19*, 17–20. [CrossRef] [PubMed]
68. Brodbaker, E.; Bahar, I.; Slomovic, A.R. Novel use of fibrin glue in the treatment of conjunctivochalasis. *Cornea* **2008**, *27*, 950–952. [CrossRef] [PubMed]
69. Wu, J.-C.; Huang, W.-C.; Chen, Y.-C.; Tu, T.-H.; Tsai, Y.-A.; Huang, S.-F.; Huang, H.-C.; Cheng, H. Acidic fibroblast growth factor for repair of human spinal cord injury: A clinical trial. *J. Neurosurg. Spine* **2011**, *15*, 216–227. [CrossRef] [PubMed]
70. Iwakawa, M.; Mizoi, K.; Tessler, A.; Itoh, Y. Intraspinal implants of fibrin glue containing glial cell line-derived neurotrophic factor promote dorsal root regeneration into spinal cord. *Neurorehabil. Neural Repair* **2001**, *15*, 173–182. [CrossRef] [PubMed]
71. Cheng, H.; Huang, S.S.; Lin, S.M.; Lin, M.J.; Chu, Y.C.; Chih, C.L.; Tsai, M.J.; Lin, H.C.; Huang, W.C.; Tsai, S.K. The neuroprotective effect of glial cell line-derived neurotrophic factor in fibrin glue against chronic focal cerebral ischemia in conscious rats. *Brain Res.* **2005**, *1033*, 28–33. [CrossRef] [PubMed]
72. Petter-Puchner, A.H.; Froetscher, W.; Krametter-Froetscher, R.; Lorinson, D.; Redl, H.; van Griensven, M. The long-term neurocompatibility of human fibrin sealant and equine collagen as biomatrices in experimental spinal cord injury. *Exp. Toxicol. Pathol.* **2007**, *58*, 237–245. [CrossRef] [PubMed]
73. Lu, P.; Graham, L.; Wang, Y.; Wu, D.; Tuszynski, M. Promotion of Survival and Differentiation of Neural Stem Cells with Fibrin and Growth Factor Cocktails after Severe Spinal Cord Injury. *J. Vis. Exp.* **2014**. [CrossRef] [PubMed]
74. Willerth, S.M.; Faxel, T.E.; Gottlieb, D.I.; Sakiyama-Elbert, S.E. The Effects of Soluble Growth Factors on Embryonic Stem Cell Differentiation Inside of Fibrin Scaffolds. *Stem Cells* **2007**, *25*, 2235–2244. [CrossRef] [PubMed]

75. Lu, P.; Wang, Y.; Graham, L.; McHale, K.; Gao, M.; Wu, D.; Brock, J.; Blesch, A.; Rosenzweig, E.S.; Havton, L.A.; et al. Long-Distance Growth and Connectivity of Neural Stem Cells after Severe Spinal Cord Injury. *Cell* **2012**, *150*, 1264–1273. [CrossRef] [PubMed]
76. Guest, J.D.; Hesse, D.; Schnell, L.; Schwab, M.E.; Bunge, M.B.; Bunge, R.P. Influence of IN-1 antibody and acidic FGF-fibrin glue on the response of injured corticospinal tract axons to human Schwann cell grafts. *J. Neurosci. Res.* **1997**, *50*, 888–905. [CrossRef]
77. Kuo, H.-S.; Tsai, M.-J.; Huang, M.-C.; Chiu, C.-W.; Tsai, C.-Y.; Lee, M.-J.; Huang, W.-C.; Lin, Y.-L.; Kuo, W.-C.; Cheng, H. Acid fibroblast growth factor and peripheral nerve grafts regulate Th2 cytokine expression, macrophage activation, polyamine synthesis, and neurotrophin expression in transected rat spinal cords. *J. Neurosci.* **2011**, *31*, 4137–4147. [CrossRef] [PubMed]
78. Zhang, R.; Tu, Y.; Zhao, M.; Chen, C.; Liang, H.; Wang, J.; Zhang, S.; Li, X. Preparation of Bionic Collagen-Heparin Sulfate Spinal Cord Scaffold with Three-dimentional print technology. *Zhongguo Xiu Fu Chong Jian Wai Ke Za Zhi* **2015**, *29*, 1022–1027. [PubMed]
79. Chen, B.; Bohnert, D.; Borgens, R.B.; Cho, Y. Pushing the science forward: Chitosan nanoparticles and functional repair of CNS tissue after spinal cord injury. *J. Biol. Eng.* **2013**, *7*, 15. [CrossRef] [PubMed]
80. Nomura, H.; Baladie, B.; Katayama, Y.; Morshead, C.M.; Shoichet, M.S.; Tator, C.H. Delayed implantation of intramedullary chitosan channels containing nerve grafts promotes extensive axonal regeneration after spinal cord injury. *Neurosurgery* **2008**, *63*, 127–141, discussion 141–143. [CrossRef] [PubMed]
81. Seth, N.; Simmons, H.A.; Masood, F.; Graham, W.A.; Rosene, D.L.; Westmoreland, S.V.; Cummings, S.M.; Gwardjan, B.; Sejdic, E.; Hoggatt, A.F.; et al. Model of Traumatic Spinal Cord Injury for Evaluating Pharmacologic Treatments in Cynomolgus Macaques (*Macaca fasicularis*). *Comp. Med.* **2018**, *68*, 63–73. [PubMed]

4

Modified Methacrylate Hydrogels Improve Tissue Repair after Spinal Cord Injury

Aleš Hejčl [1,2,*], Jiří Růžička [1], Kristýna Kekulová [1], Barbora Svobodová [1], Vladimír Proks [3], Hana Macková [3], Kateřina Jiránková [4], Kristýna Kárová [1,5], Lucia Machová Urdziková [1], Šárka Kubinová [1], Jiří Cihlář [6], Daniel Horák [3] and Pavla Jendelová [1,5]

1 Institute of Experimental Medicine, Academy of Sciences of the Czech Republic, Vídeňská 1083, 142 20 Prague, Czech Republic; stoupa-ruza@seznam.cz (J.R.); kristyna.kekulova@iem.cas.cz (K.K.); barbora.svobodova@iem.cas.cz (B.S.); kristyna.karova@iem.cas.cz (K.K.); urdzikl@saske.sk (L.M.U.); sarka.kubinova@iem.cas.cz (S.K.); pavla.jendelova@iem.cas.cz (P.J.)

2 Department of Neurosurgery, J. E. Purkinje University, Masaryk Hospital, Sociální Péče 12A, 401 13 Ústí nad Labem, Czech Republic

3 Institute of Macromolecular Chemistry, Academy of Sciences of the Czech Republic, Heyrovského nám.2, 162 06 Praha, Czech Republic; proks@imc.cas.cz (V.P.); mackova@imc.cas.cz (H.M.); horak@imc.cas.cz (D.H.)

4 Second Faculty of Medicine, Charles University, V Úvalu 84, 150 06 Prague, Czech Republic; jirankova.katerina@seznam.cz

5 Department of Neuroscience, 2nd Faculty of Medicine, Charles University, V Úvalu 84, 150 06 Prague, Czech Republic

6 Department of Mathematics, Faculty of Science, J. E. Purkyně University, České Mládeže 8, 400 96 Ústí nad Labem, Czech Republic; jiri.cihlar@ujep.cz

* Correspondence: ales.hejcl@gmail.com

Abstract: Methacrylate hydrogels have been extensively used as bridging scaffolds in experimental spinal cord injury (SCI) research. As synthetic materials, they can be modified, which leads to improved bridging of the lesion. Fibronectin, a glycoprotein of the extracellular matrix produced by reactive astrocytes after SCI, is known to promote cell adhesion. We implanted 3 methacrylate hydrogels: a scaffold based on hydroxypropylmethacrylamid (HPMA), 2-hydroxyethylmethacrylate (HEMA) and a HEMA hydrogel with an attached fibronectin (HEMA-Fn) in an experimental model of acute SCI in rats. The animals underwent functional evaluation once a week and the spinal cords were histologically assessed 3 months after hydrogel implantation. We found that both the HPMA and the HEMA-Fn hydrogel scaffolds lead to partial sensory improvement compared to control animals and animals treated with plain HEMA scaffold. The HPMA scaffold showed an increased connective tissue infiltration compared to plain HEMA hydrogels. There was a tendency towards connective tissue infiltration and higher blood vessel ingrowth in the HEMA-Fn scaffold. HPMA hydrogels showed a significantly increased axonal ingrowth compared to HEMA-Fn and plain HEMA; while there were some neurofilaments in the peripheral as well as the central region of the HEMA-Fn scaffold, no neurofilaments were found in plain HEMA hydrogels. In conclusion, HPMA hydrogel as well as the HEMA-Fn scaffold showed better bridging qualities compared to the plain HEMA hydrogel, which resulted in very limited partial sensory improvement.

Keywords: spinal cord injury; hydrogel; connective tissue; neurofilaments; locomotor test; plantar test

1. Introduction

Functional deficits of spinal cord injury (SCI) are the result of subsequent temporal events: the primary insult leads to ischemia, followed by neuronal cell death, axon damage, and demyelination. Subsequently, glial activation, the release of inflammatory factors and cytokines, and the scar formation that prevents axons to regenerate leads to progression of the lesion. Post-traumatic syringomyelia usually develops in the chronic phase after SCI as a result of hemorrhage and tissue necrosis. The cavity is filled with tissue debris and later mostly with CSF and is surrounded by glial and mesenchymal scarring forming a barrier for tissue regeneration. Therefore, different strategies have been developed to treat SCI. One of the approaches relies on tissue engineering methods, particularly on bridging the lesion cavities. The scaffold, suitable for implantation into lesion cavity must have the appropriate chemical, physical, and mechanical properties required for cell survival and tissue formation. One of the most suitable classes of compounds for these purposes is definitely represented by hydrogels [1–3]. They are three-dimensional (3D) hydrophilic polymers held together by covalent bonds or other cohesive forces such as hydrogen or ionic bonds [3–5]. They can be either synthetic or natural in origin, or a combination of both. Synthetic polymers can be tailored in terms of composition, rate of degradation, and mechanical and chemical properties. [6]. This is much more difficult to achieve in naturally derived polymers, which, in contrast, have features supporting adhesion and cell growth.

Therefore, the presence of bioadhesive and bioactive molecules on an artificial hydrogel matrix is crucial for the successful preparation of neural biomimetic scaffolds. Synthetic materials are often coated or modified with extracellular matrix (ECM) components, e.g., laminin and fibronectin, or synthetic peptides [7–9], which can improve cell adhesion and survival by generating a permissive microenvironment within the biomaterial [10,11]. Moreover, collagen, fibronectin, and laminin are associated with wound healing and regeneration and, therefore, they can be explored for therapeutic purposes. After SCI, fibronectin is deposited within the glial scar [12]. Yet fibronectin is also known to play a role in cell differentiation, proliferation, or migration and has been used as an implant in a spinal cord lesion in some studies [13]. Fibronectin is an important glycoprotein in the developing CNS due to its involvement in cell migration [14] and it has important roles in tissue repair mainly because of its cell adhesion properties. Fibronectin was used as matrix for NSC transplants in damaged CNS and found to improve NSC survival [15]. Fibronectin can be also used in combination with other materials. For instance, poly-β-hydroxybutyrate fibers coated with alginate hydrogel and fibronectin were used for a Schwann cell transplant in the injured rat spinal cord [13]. This combination promoted axon growth across the injury.

During the last 15 years we have implanted various biomaterials inside cavities in order to provide a scaffold for the ingrowth of new tissue, especially axons and blood vessels [16–21]. In general, we have shown that hydrogels are able to provide scaffolding for new tissue to grow inside their pores. As with other studies, we have also shown that the quantity of tissue ingrowth is influenced by various adjustments of tissue scaffold, such as in combination with adhesion molecules, modifications in chemical and physical properties, or in combination with stem cells [22–25]. Such modifications may lead to motor and sensory function improvement in experimental rats after SCI [25]. Despite some improvements, the overall results are unsatisfactory, impelling the development of new scaffolds with better proregenerating qualities. In this study we implanted methacrylate hydrogel based on poly(2-hydroxyethyl methacrylate) (HEMA) modified with attached fibronectin (HEMA-Fn) and compared it with unmodified HEMA and poly[*N*-(2-hydroxypropyl) methacrylamide] (HPMA) hydrogel scaffolds in terms of functional response and tissue infiltration. We utilized a spinal cord hemisection, which provides an appropriate model for evaluating scaffolds with oriented pores as the lesion is large enough for proper orientation of the scaffold within the cavity and at the same time the functional deficit is mild enough so as to avoid excessive animal loss as opposed to other more severe experimental lesions, such as spinal cord transection or balloon-induced compression lesion. In this study we wanted to assess the long-term effect of fibronectin-enriched HEMA and compare it with plain HEMA and HPMA hydrogels. Hydrogels with oriented pores were utilized as they provide an excellent scaffold for the evaluation of newly growing axons and blood vessels within the biomaterial.

2. Results

2.1. *Hydrogel Scaffold*

Three synthetic hydrogels, namely HEMA, HEMA-Fn, and HPMA, were obtained by free-radical copolymerization producing identical inner morphology, exemplified in Figure 1A. Longitudinally shaped pores were imprinted by needle-like ammonium oxalate crystals oriented in an axial direction (Figure 1B). The pore size corresponded to the size of the starting crystals, which were 30–90 μm thick and approximately 0.3–10 mm long. According to published literature [26], this long pore size can be advantageous for the regeneration of peripheral axons, whereas their ingrowth and/or outgrowth needs much smaller pores (20–70 μm) depending on the origin of biomaterial. The pore volume calculated from an oxalate/monomer volume ratio, amounted to ~70%, which roughly corresponded to Hg porosimetry data (68.4%) [22]. The elasticity modulus of the hydrogels was ~4 and 30 kPa perpendicularly and along the pores, respectively [27].

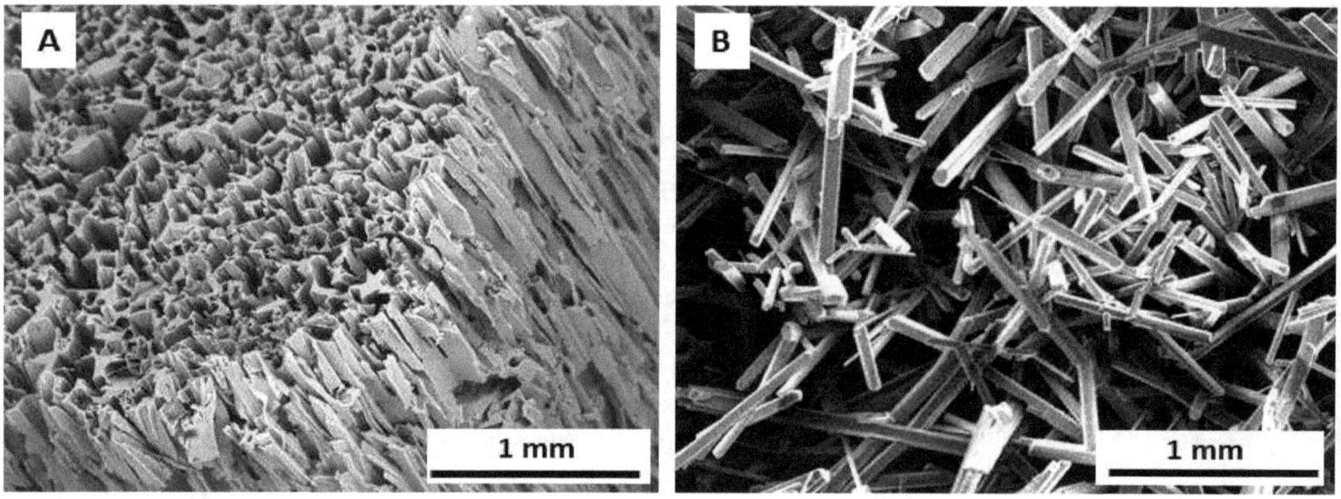

Figure 1. SEM micrographs of HEMA hydrogel (**A**) and ammonium oxalate crystals (**B**).

2.2. *Functional Tests*

All 34 animals underwent functional evaluation. The animals were tested for motor function and sensory function of the hindlimbs. The motor function was tested using the BBB score and sensory function using the plantar test. Considering the BBB testing, the right hindlimb was the injured one while the left hindlimb was considered the uninjured one. However, for the plantar test the left hindlimb was considered the injured one due to crossing of the spino-thalamic tract and the right hindlimb was considered uninjured.

2.3. *BBB*

All the animals in the study were pre-evaluated before surgery and then tested every week until week 12 after hydrogel implantation. The BBB scores for both legs were compared between the control group and the three groups of animals treated with hydrogels. During the 12 week period there were no statistically significant differences in the BBB scores for the left and right hindlimbs among any of the 4 groups (Figure 2).

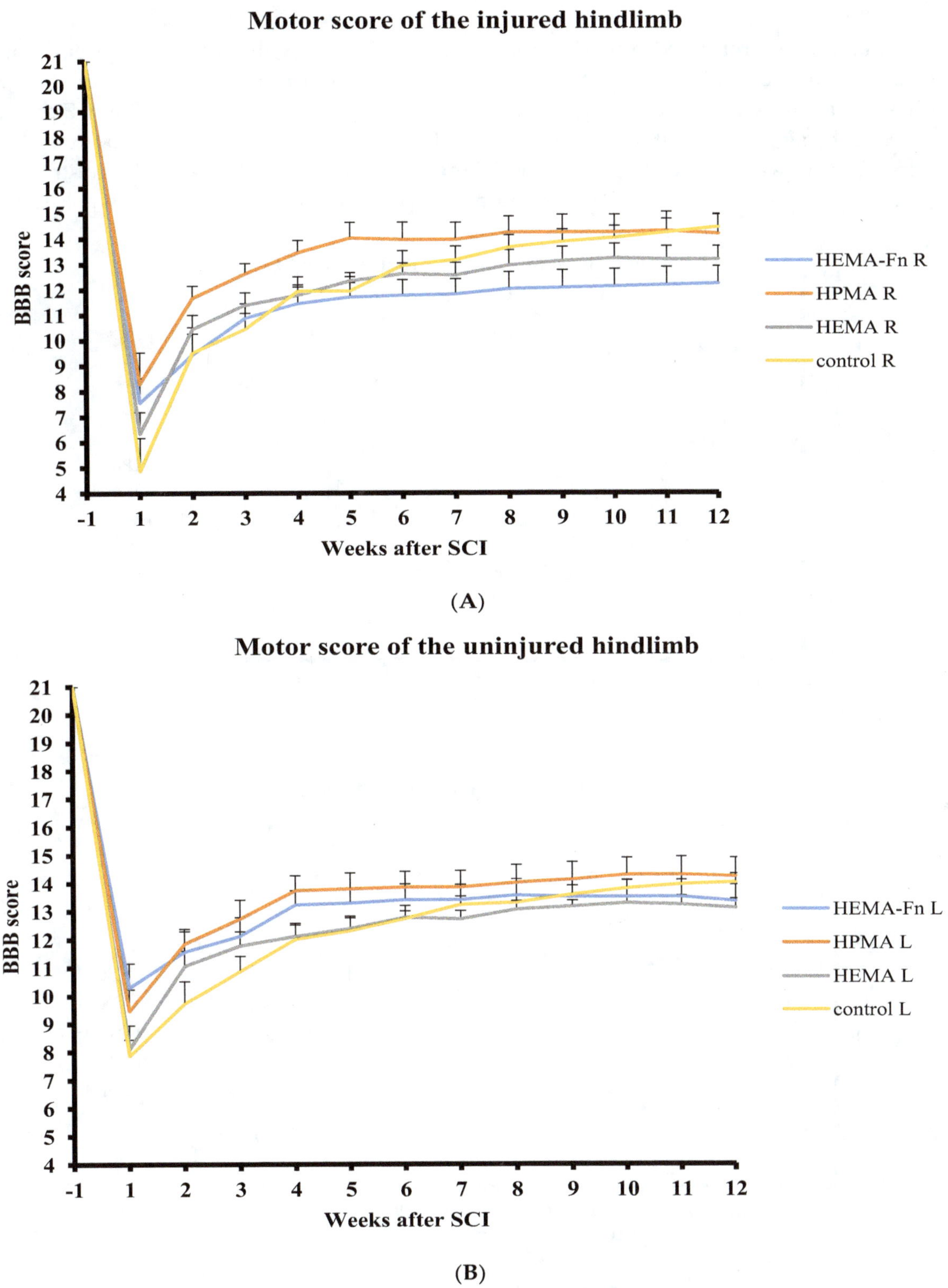

Figure 2. Comparison of motor function evaluation of the injured (**A**) and uninjured (**B**) side of hindlimbs using the BBB score. There were no statistically significant differences among the four groups (three treatment groups and one control group-hemisection only). Note the lower scores of the injured hindlimb on the side of the hemisection. The data represent mean values and error bars represent SEM.

2.4. Plantar Test

The animals were pretreated twice before surgery and then evaluated once a week until week 12 after hydrogel implantation. The plantar test for the right leg (uninjured side, Figure 3A) was not statistically significant for any of the time period. However, for the left side (injured one, Figure 3B), we found a statistically significant difference between the HEMA-Fn and the hemisection group in week 5. Furthermore, there was a statistically significant difference between the HPMA hydrogel-treated group and the hemisection group and the HPMA-treated group and the HEMA-group in week 12.

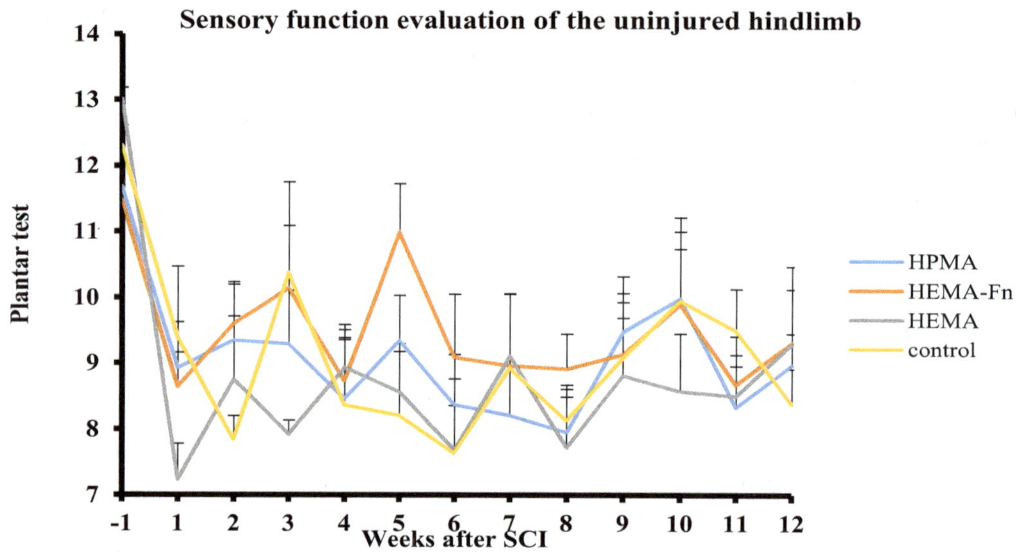

(A)

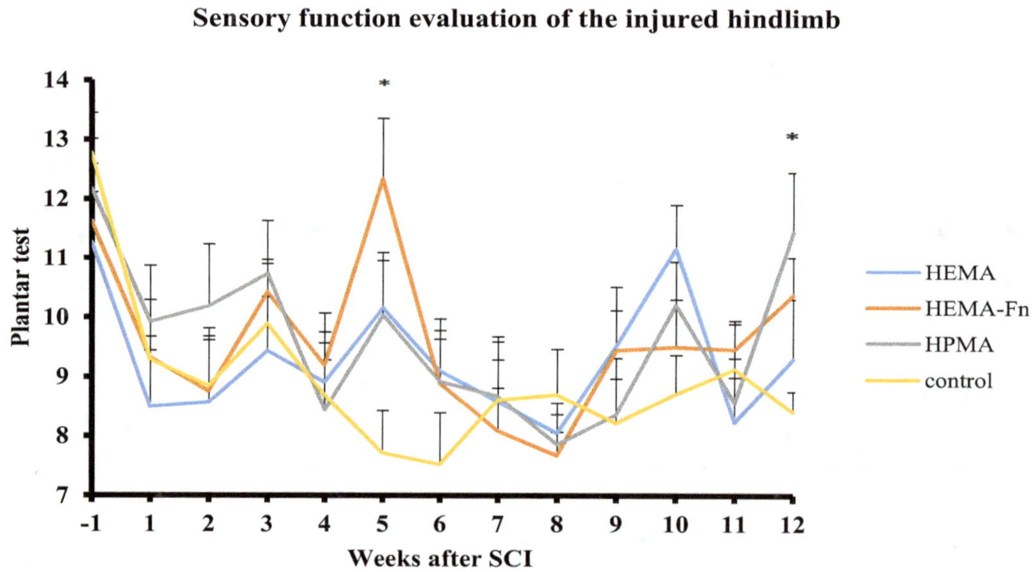

(B)

Figure 3. Sensory function evaluation of the uninjured (**A**) and injured (**B**) side of hindlimbs using the plantar test. There were statistically significant differences in the sensory response between rats treated with 2-hydroxyethylmethacrylate (HEMA)-Fn and the control group on week 5 and then between the HPMA and both the HEMA and the control group on week 12 (* $p < 0.05$). The data represent mean values and error bars represent SEM.

2.5. Microscopic Evaluation of the Hydrogel Bridge

All three hydrogel scaffolds bridged the hemisection lesion providing scaffold for tissue regrowth. In some cases small residual cysts were present on the border between the hydrogel and the spinal cord (Figure 4A). There were no signs of foreign body reactions observed in or around the hydrogels 3 months after implantation. In the control group, the lesion was represented by a large cavity with no tissue inside (Figure 4B). There was a slight narrow rim of astrogliosis with small isles of astrocytes entering the border zones of all three hydrogel scaffolds (Figure 4C). We did not observe any difference despite the fact that plain HEMA resulted in upregulation of GFAP gene (see section Gene Expression). No signs of foreign body-type giant-cell granulomatous reaction were observed 3 months after hydrogel implantation. We found no statistically significant difference in the markers of immune response among any of the 3 scaffolds (see section Gene Expression).

2.6. Connective Tissue

All 3 types of hydrogels were filled with connective tissue, however there were obvious differences. Only a little dispersed connective tissue was present in the pores of the plain HEMA hydrogels (Figure 4D). Alternatively, in both the HPMA and the HEMA-Fn hydrogels, connective tissue elements were more abundant with a rather dense infiltration of the pores (Figure 4E,F). The HPMA hydrogel promoted connective tissue infiltration inside the scaffold, in both its peripheral as well as the central part, compared to the plain HEMA scaffold (Figure 5, $p < 0.05$). The HEMA scaffold with attached fibronectin showed tendency towards higher connective tissue infiltration in both the peripheral and the central part of the hydrogel without reaching statistical significance (Figure 5, $p < 0.05$).

2.7. Axonal Regeneration

After 3 months, HPMA hydrogels were infiltrated with axonal sprouts in the peripheral areas as well as in the central parts (Figure 6). The growth of axons was guided by the oriented pores, mostly in the cranio-caudal and caudo-cranial direction. The plain HEMA scaffold did not show any neurofilaments in its pores 3 months after implantation (Figure 4G), despite its upregulation of Gap43 (see section Gene Expression). In contrast, the HEMA-Fn hydrogels showed that some axons grew into the peripheral parts of the scaffold and a minimal amount also reached the central parts of the scaffold (Figure 4H). The amount of neurofilaments in the HPMA hydrogel was significantly higher compared to both HEMA-based scaffolds (Figure 4I). There were many new axons in the peripheral part of the HPMA scaffold which extended all the way to its central area (Figure 4J).

2.8. Growth of Blood Vessels in the Hydrogels

All three hydrogels showed an extensive ingrowth of blood vessels into the periphery as well as the central part of the scaffolds—both the HEMA-based hydrogels as well as the HPMA (Figure 4K,L). Despite not reaching statistical significance, the HEMA-based hydrogel modified with fibronectin supported the highest number of blood vessels compared to the plain HEMA and the HPMA scaffolds (Figure 7). There was also no difference in the VEGFA gene during molecular analysis (see section Gene Expression). As with the axons, blood vessels also grew predominantly in an oriented fashion guided by the pores

2.9. Gene Expression

Expression of genes related to regeneration (Vegfa, Bdnf, Gap43), glial scaring (Gfap) and infiltrating macrophage phenotype (Irf5, Cd86, Mrc1) was determined 3 months after hemisection or implantation of methacrylate scaffolds. Significant upregulation of Gfap genes was detected after treatment with HEMA when compared with controls. Implantation of HEMA resulted in a trend of upregulation of M2 associated Mrc1 when compared to both HEMA-Fn and HPMA. No other statistically significant difference in any markers within the tissue of spinal cords treated with the methacrylate hydrogels or controls were observed (Figure 8).

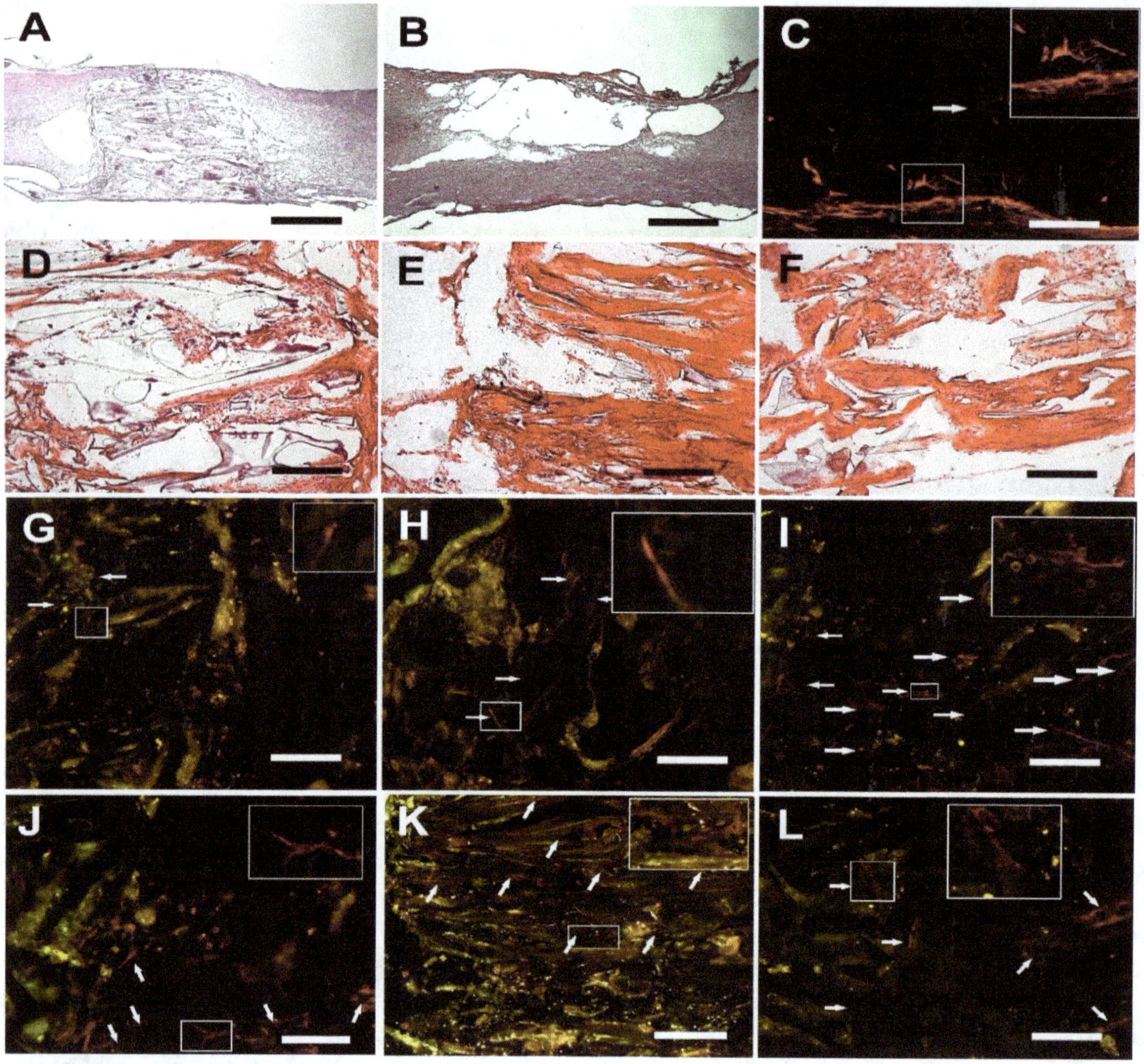

Figure 4. The mosaic presents various aspect of tissue ingrowth within the pores of the three methacrylate hydrogels. (**A**) HEMA-Fn sufficiently bridged the hemisection cavity. In some cases there were minor cavities on the border. The HEMA-Fn scaffold serves as a representative sample for all three methacrylate hydrogels (HE staining, scale bar = 1 mm). (**B**) The lesion resulted in a large pseudocystic cavity in the control group (HE staining, scale bar = 1 mm). (**C**) Subtle astrogliosis was present within the spinal cord tissue neighboring the HPMA scaffold and a few islets of astrocytes also infiltrated its peripheral part (white arrow, GFAP-Cy3 staining, scale bar = 100 μm). (**D**) Sparse connective tissue elements were found in the plain HEMA scaffold; there was a more dense infiltration within the pores of the HEMA-Fn (**E**) and the HPMA hydrogel (**F**) HE staining, scale bar = 100 μm. (**G**) No axonal sprouts were present in the HEMA scaffold, however, some axons (white arrows) reached the border zone of the spinal cord (NF160-g594 staining, scale bar = 25 μm). (**H**) A small number of sprouts (white arrows) were present within the HEMA-Fn scaffold (NF160-g594 staining, scale bar = 25 μm); significantly higher number of sprouts was present (white arrows) within the central parts (**I**) as well as the periphery (**J**) of the HPMA hydrogels (NF160-g594 staining, scale bar = 25 μm). (**K**) Blood vessels (white arrows) grew abundantly within the pores of all three hydrogels especially the HEMA-Fn scaffold, as seen in this image (RECA-g488 staining, scale bar = 50 μm). (**L**) A detailed view of the blood vessels within the HEMA-Fn scaffold (RECA-g488 staining, scale bar = 25 μm). Insert boxes depict the typical elements described in each image of the mosaic (enlarged twice to the original size).

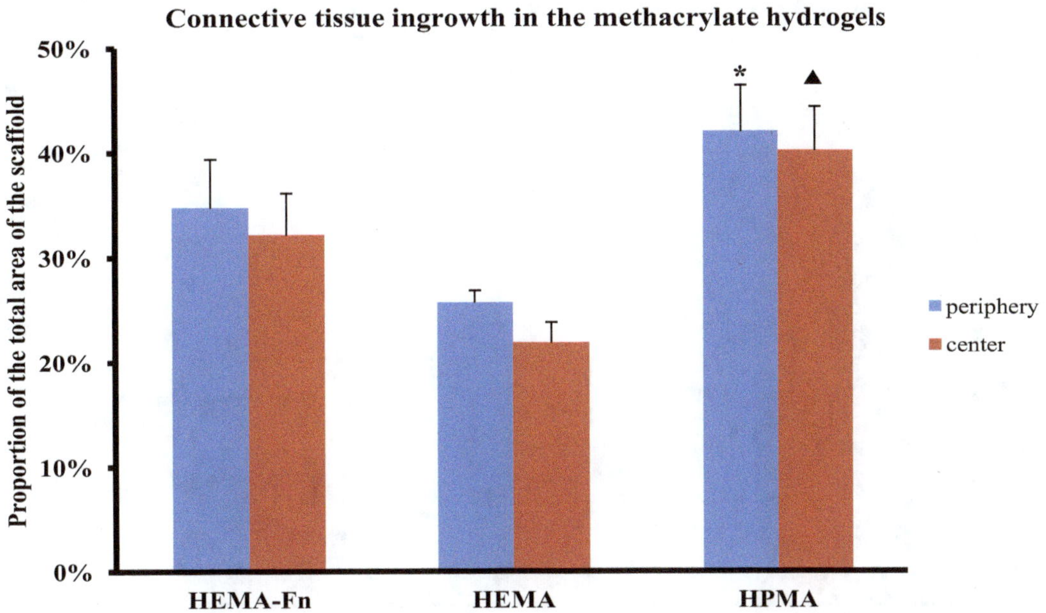

Figure 5. Comparison of connective tissue ingrowth within the three hydrogels. The graph presents the percentage of HE-positively stained tissue within the whole area of the peripheral (blue bars) and central (red bars) regions of the hydrogel. The HPMA scaffold showed higher connective tissue ingrowth within the periphery (* $p < 0.05$) as well as the central part (▲ $p < 0.05$) of the HEMA scaffold. Data shown as mean, and the error bars represent SEM. For statistical analysis, a one-way ANOVA test was used.

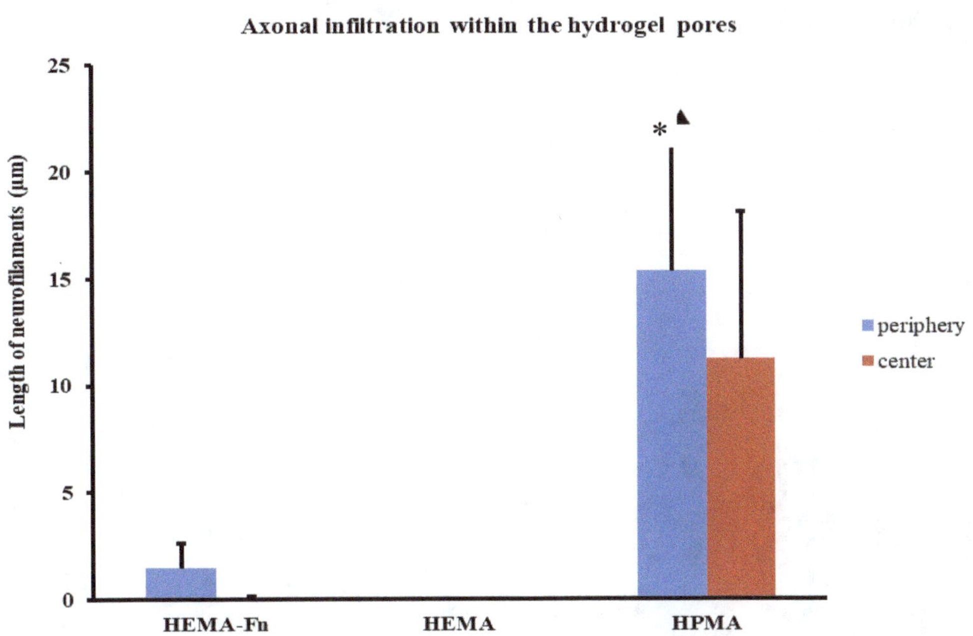

Figure 6. Comparison of axonal ingrowth within the three hydrogels. The total length of axons was assessed within the peripheral (blue bars) as well as the central (red bars) regions of the scaffold. The graph shows that the HPMA scaffold promoted statistically significant infiltration of axons within the pores of the scaffold compared to both HEMA hydrogels (* $p < 0.05$, ▲ $p < 0.05$). The graph shows that there were no axons within the HEMA scaffold, while the modification of fibronectin (HEMA-Fn) showed at least some axonal infiltration with the periphery and some even grew as far as the central parts of the scaffold. Data shown as mean and the error bars represent SEM. For statistical analysis, a one-way ANOVA test was used.

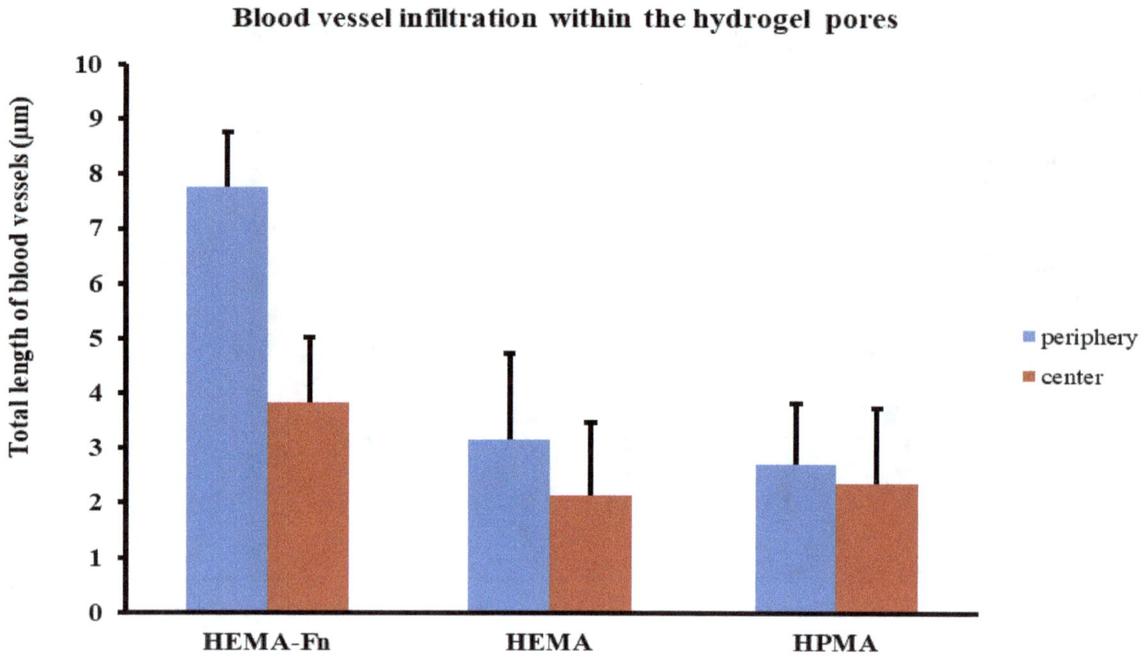

Figure 7. Comparison of blood vessels in growth within the three hydrogels. The total length of blood vessels was assessed within the peripheral (blue bars) as well as the central (red bars) regions of the scaffold. There was no statistically significant difference between the three groups but the HEMA-Fn scaffold showed a trend towards increased ingrowth of blood vessels within its pores, especially in the peripheral areas. Data shown as mean and the error bars represent SEM. For statistical analysis, a one-way ANOVA-test was used.

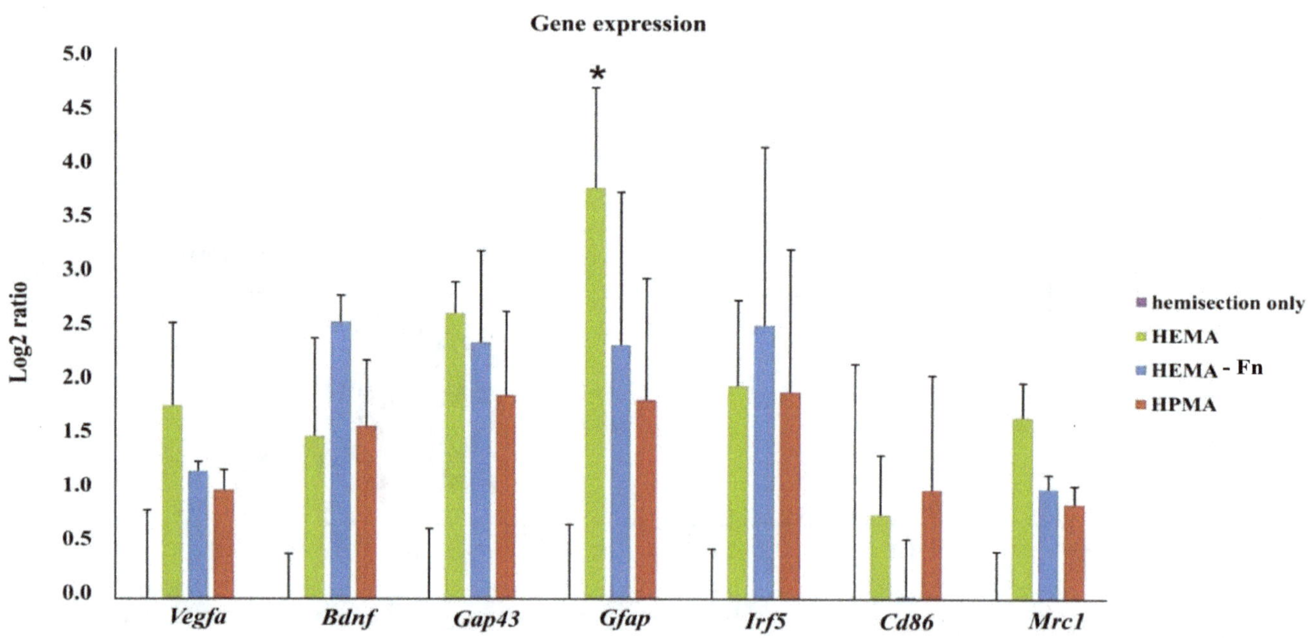

Figure 8. Gene expression in spinal cord tissue after treatment of hemisection with 3 different methacrylate scaffolds. Treatment with HEMA resulted in significant upregulation of Gfap when compared with controls (hemisection only, $n = 3$). We found no other statistically significant difference in any markers within the tissue of spinal cords treated with the methacrylate hydrogels or controls. Data shown as mean and SEM relative to hemisection (injured tissue), which was set as 0 (with * $p < 0.05$ (vs. hemisection)). For statistical analysis a one-way ANOVA test was used.

3. Discussion

SCI, especially at its chronic stage, is characterized by glial scarring and pseudocystic cavities associated with disruption of long spinal cord tracts. Experimental studies using a variety of biomaterials, including hydrogels, have been conducted during the last 20 years [16]. In this study we evaluated two methacrylate hydrogels based on HEMA and HPMA, which are considered to be excellent synthetic biomaterials resembling living tissue, in terms of water content and mechanical properties [28,29]. Their porous properties, introduced by polymerization of the respective monomers in the presence of inorganic needle-like crystals, make them suitable for neural tissue or spinal cord reconstruction as has been shown in many studies [16,20,30,31]. The advantage of synthetic hydrogels consists not only of their biological inertness, but also in the variety of possible modifications, allowing better tissue repair promoting properties [23,32,33]. Our study showed that none of the methacrylate hydrogels caused a significant immune response, as demonstrated by no upregulation of antigen-presenting cells at 3 months. There were increased signs of tissue repair in the plain HEMA scaffold 3 months after SCI as demonstrated by an upregulation of an Mrc1 gene.

In this study, one of the HEMA scaffolds was modified with attached fibronectin. Our previous study showed better bridging qualities of the HPMA scaffold when compared to HEMA. Based on our positive results with surface modification of scaffolds, we also compared fibronectin-modified HEMA, to test whether such surface modification would balance the advantage of the HPMA scaffold. Fibronectin is known to promote cellular migration, proliferation, and differentiation [34,35]. In this study we showed better connective tissue infiltration within the HPMA scaffold compared to HEMA. There was more connective tissue within HEMA modified with fibronectin when compared to plain HEMA 3 months after SCI but without reaching statistical significance. This is an extension of the finding by other authors, which demonstrated that fibronectin enhances short-term cell adhesion [36].

Several studies have also shown that fibronectin may be neuroprotective, reducing post-traumatic apoptosis while enhancing functional outcome [37,38]. King et al. showed that fibronectin promotes the growth of axons into the implant when compared to other natural molecules such as fibrin or collagen, but with the disadvantage of having large cavities at the spinal cord lesion borderline [36]. The combination of an artificial scaffold with fibronectin thus seems to be a useful type of combined therapy that may promote the regrowth of axons while creating a positive milieu for the regrowth of new axons. The combination with a HEMA scaffold ensured good integration of the implant within the knife-cut experimental cavity while fibronectin promoted the axons to cross the hydrogel-spinal cord border and infiltrate the pores in the periphery of the implant as well as in the central area. Nonetheless, none of the three methacrylate hydrogels in our study led to motor function improvement. We did not observe any differences in BBB test, except for lower BBB score on the ipsilateral side. The results from plantar test indicate that no further hyperalgesia has developed after the hydrogel implantation. HEMA-Fn and HPMA resulted in only inconsistent sensory function difference of the left hindlimb, despite the differences in the number of axons within the three scaffolds. Spinal cord hemisection is not an ideal model for testing of functional improvement. However, it is suitable for histological evaluation and quantification of cellular ingrowth into the implant.

We did not observe any axons extending across the whole scaffold and crossing the scaffold-tissue border back and re-entering the spinal cord. A higher number of axons infiltrating the scaffold but without making connections across the bridge does not therefore necessarily result in functionally meaningful improvement.

Previous studies have also shown that fibronectin enhances axonal ingrowth after SCI but the studies were restricted to a short time evaluation period. This may not, however, reflect long-term data as we have shown in our recent paper [39]. In our study, fibronectin modification of the HEMA scaffold showed some increased but statistically insignificant difference in the ingrowth of axons into the peripheral and also central parts, while there were no axonal sprouts present in the plain HEMA 3 months after SCI. When comparing the results based on the chemical backbone of the hydrogel (HEMA vs. HPMA), the HPMA scaffold supports the regrowth of axons much better compared to HEMA, even when the latter one is enriched with fibronectin. This is in line with our previous study, in which the HPMA scaffold showed improved axonal infiltration compared to HEMA [23]. Interestingly, molecular analysis showed a tendency towards increased sprouting in all three scaffolds. However, only HPMA hydrogel and partially HEMA-Fn create an environment which prevents the axon retraction from the hydrogel.

None of the tested scaffolds supported the ingrowth of astrocytes, though the GFAP protein was upregulated in the plain HEMA scaffold when compared with the hemisection. We observed only a slight astrogliosis around the 3 types of scaffolds.

New blood vessels grew into all three hydrogels; there were many of them throughout the periphery and growing further into the central parts. We found a tendency towards a denser blood vessel network in the HEMA-Fn hydrogel. This may be explained by the presence of the RGD (arginine–glycine–aspartate) peptide sequence within the fibronectin molecule, which has been shown to enhance vascular growth [23]. The presence of blood vessels within the lesion is vital as they promote axonal repair and enhance functional improvement [40,41].

Tissue engineering is based on creating a proregenerative environment for tissue repair within the lesion. The cells and their extensions (such as axons) should be properly guided in order to make functionally meaningful connections. The advantage of hydrogels with oriented pores is their ability to navigate the growth of new tissue along the long axis of their pores. However, solid hydrogels require a surgical opening of the spine and spinal cord during the process of implantation. Also, the hydrogels we evaluated were slightly stiffer compared to the scaffolds with randomly oriented pores used in our former studies, due to the need to properly retain the oriented inner structure [21,23,25]. This may be the cause of residual minor cavities on the border between the scaffold and the spinal cord. Injectable scaffolds, on the other hand, avoid the need for surgical incision and allow minimally-invasive implantation. They are also soft enough to adhere well to the spinal cord tissue. However, oriented pores within injectable scaffolds are more difficult to achieve, and therefore we cannot ensure targeted growth within such biomaterials [42]. Study of the synthesis of injectable scaffolds with oriented pores would be of interest in the future.

4. Materials and Methods

4.1. Hydrogel Scaffolds

2-Hydroxyethyl methacrylate (HEMA; Röhm, Germany) and ethylene dimethacrylate (EDMA; Ugilor S.A., France) were purified by distillation. 1-Amino-2-propanol,1,2-diaminoethan, methacryloyl chloride, 2,2′-azobisisobutyronitrile (AIBN), 2-aminoethyl methacrylate (AEMA) hydrochloride, tris (2-carboxyethyl) phosphine hydrochloride (TCEP), and *N*-γ-maleimidobutyryloxysuccinimide ester (GMBS) were purchased from Sigma-Aldrich (St. Louis, USA). Ammonium oxalate (Lach-Ner; Neratovice, Czech Republic) was crystallized from water until the formation of 30–90 μm thick and approximately 0.3–10 mm long needle-like crystals, which were used as a porogen. Fibronectin (Fn) from human plasma was obtained from Roche (Mannheim, Germany). All other chemicals were from Lach-Ner. Ultrapure Q water ultrafiltered on a Milli-Q Gradient A10 system (Millipore; Molsheim, France) was used for preparation of phosphate buffers saline (PBS) and all other experiments. *N*-(2-hydroxypropyl)methacrylamide (HPMA) and *N,N*′-ethylenebis(acrylamide) (EDMAAm) were synthetized by modification of published procedure [26]. Briefly, 1-amino-2-propanol (22.5 g), $NaNO_2$ (200 mg), and NaOH 12 g were dissolved in H_2O (300 mL), cooled at 0 °C, and dry ice (40 g) and methacryloyl chloride (31.4 g) were added. The solution was slowly heated to room temperature (RT) and stirred for 4 h until formation of ethacryloyl chloride droplets. Water was evaporated and residuum was extracted by dichloromethane, the solution was dried with $MgSO_4$, filtered through carbon black, and twice recrystallized from acetone/petroleum ether mixture. *N,N*′-ethylenebis(acrylamide) was synthetized analogously, only 1,2-diaminoethan (18 g) was used instead of 1-amino-2-propanol.

Preparation of Superporouspoly (2-Hydroxyethyl Methacrylate) (HEMA), HEMA-Fn, and Poly [(*N*-(2-Hydroxypropyl) Methacrylamide] (HPMA) Hydrogels

Three polyethylene injection syringes (5 mL) equipped with a stainless filter were filled with needle-like ammonium oxalate crystals (~70 vol %). The monomer mixtures were prepared separately, one for each syringe: (i) HEMA (2.475 g) and EDMA (0.025 g; 1 wt %); (ii) HEMA (2.450 g), EDMA (0.025 g; 1 wt %), and AEMA (0.025 g; 1 wt %); and (iii) HPMA (2.475 g) and EDMAAm (0.025 g; 1 wt %). AIBN (40 mg) was dissolved in 1,4-dioxane (5 mL) and the solution was added to each mixture, which was transferred to the syringe containing crystals. The syringe was closed and the mixture polymerized at 60°C for 16 h. At the end of the reaction, the syringe was cut lengthwise, the hydrogel cylinder was removed and immersed in 10 wt % NH_4Cl aqueous solution for 24 h, to avoid cracks and to remove 1,4-dioxane. The hydrogel was cut into 2 × 2 × 2 mm cubes, which were washed once with 0.01MHCl (100 mL) for 2 days to remove salts and finally with water. Amino groups of copolymer of HEMA and AEMA were reacted with a solution of GMBS (20 mg) in a mixture of 0.07M PBS (pH 7.4; 10.5 mL) and 1,4-dioxane (5.5 mL) at RT for 30 min to introduce maleimide (MI) groups on the surface. The product was twice washed with PBS/1,4-dioxane solution (PBS/1,4-dioxane = 10.5/5.5 *v/v*; 15 mL each), twice with water (15 mL each), and 0.1M PBS (pH 6.8; 15 mL). Fn (1 mg) containing glycine (1.126 mg) and sodium chloride (0.058 mg) were dissolved in PBS buffer (pH 7.4; 2 mL) for 2 h, a solution of TCEP (0.5 mg) in PBS (1 mL) was added and the mixture reacted at 23°C for 40 min. Poly HEMA-MI cubes were incubated in 0.1M PBS (pH 6.8; 20 mL), the solution of reduced Fn was added, and the reaction proceeded at RT for 1 h.

4.2. *Animal Handling and Surgery*

This study was performed in accordance with the European Communities Council Directive of 22 September 2010 (2010/63/EU) regarding the use of animals in research, and was approved by the Ethics Committee of the Institute of Experimental Medicine, Academy of Sciences of the Czech Republic.

4.3. *Spinal Cord Injury and Hydrogel Implantation*

Thirty-four male rats (Wistar, Anlab, Czech Republic) with a weight of 280–400 g, underwent a hemisection at the Th8 level. The animals were intraperitoneally injected with pentobarbital for anesthesia (0.06 g/1 kg i.p.); one dose of ATB (gentamicin 8 mg/1 kg i.m.), atropine (0.08 mg/1 kg s.c.), and mesocain to enhance local anesthesia (1 mg/1 kg s.c. + i.m.) was administered preoperatively. A linear skin incision was performed above the spinous processes of Th7-9; the paravertebral muscles were detached from the laminae Th7-9, and a Th8 laminectomy was performed. The dura was incised longitudinally in the midline and about a 2 mm-segment of spinal cord was dissected in its right half, creating a cavity within the spinal cord tissue. The hydrogel was implanted in such a way as to ensure that it would firmly adhere to the edges of the transection cavity without causing any undue pressure onto the surrounding spinal cord tissue. We implanted 9 rats with HEMA hydrogels with attached fragments of fibronectin, 9 rats with plain HEMA hydrogels, and 9 rats with HPMA hydrogels; 7 animals were left with hemisection only and served as controls. The muscles and skin were sutured again, and the animals were housed two in a cage with food and water ad libitum.

4.4. *Behavioral Testing*

BBB Test

The BBB open field test, originally described by Basso, Beattie, and Bresnaham [43] was used to assess basic locomotor functions (joint movement, weight support, forelimb-hindlimb coordination, paw placement, and stability of the body). All 34 rats were used for functional testing throughout the whole evaluation period. The rats were placed on the floor surrounded by boundaries making a rectangular shape once a week. Results were evaluated in the range of 0 to 21 points (0 indicated complete lack of motor capability and 21 movements indicated a healthy rat).

4.5. *Plantar*

The plantar test was performed using the plantar test instrument (Ugo Basile, Italy). A radiant thermal stimulus was applied to the plantar surface of the paws, and the latency of the paw withdrawal response was measured. Each paw was stimulated five times once a week. Hyperalgesia, as a response to the thermal stimulus, was defined as a significant decrease in the withdrawal latency.

4.6. *Tissue Processing and Histology*

The animals were sacrificed 3 months after hydrogel implantation. They were then deeply anesthetized with an intraperitoneal injection of overdose pentobarbital and perfused with physiological saline, followed by 4% paraformaldehyde in 0.1M phosphate buffer. The spinal cord was left in the bone overnight, then removed and postfixed in the same fixative for at least 1 week.

A 4 cm-long segment of the spinal cord with the lesion site in the middle was dissected, and a series of 40 mm-thick longitudinal sections were collected. Hematoxylin–eosin staining was performed, using standard protocols, and the slides were specifically evaluated using an Axio Observer D1 microscope (Carl Zeiss Microimaging GmbH, Oberkochen, Germany). For immunohistochemical studies, the following primary antibodies and dilutions were used: Cy3-conjugated anti-GFAP (1:200; Sigma-Aldrich, Saint Louis, MO, USA) to identify astrocytes, anti-NF 160 (1:200; Sigma-Aldrich, Saint Louis, MO, USA) to identify neurofilaments, and RECA-1 (1:50; Abcam, Cambridge, UK) to identify endothelial cells of blood vessels. Alexa Fluor 594 goat anti–rabbit IgG (1:200; Invitrogen) and Cy3-conjugated anti-mouse IgM (1:100; Invitrogen, Carlsbad, CA, USA) were used as secondary antibodies.

4.7. *Tissue Quantification*

The hydrogels were divided into 3 parts: the cranial end, the central part, and the caudal end. The whole surface of the scaffold per each slice was divided into 6 squares, 2 peripheral cranial and 2 peripheral caudal squares, and the central 2 squares corresponded to the hydrogel center. We calculated the number and the length of axons and blood vessels in each part of the scaffold, using the program TissueQuest Analysis Software (TissueGnostics GmbH, Vienna, Austria). Axonal fibers were manually traced within high resolution mosaic image with second channel as background. Using second channel (488 nm) as a reference channel, the combined image has shifted the background and hydrogel autofluorescence in to brown or yellow shade, whereas the specific fluorescence signal remains clear red. The mosaic was then analyzed by single squares at high magnification using a professional screen. Six spinal cords from each treatment group with 4–5 slices per spinal cord were analyzed. We then combined the data from the peripheral parts of the hydrogels (cranial and caudal ends) and evaluated them together. The central part was quantified and analyzed separately.

4.8. *qPCR*

Expression of rat target genes *Vegfa*, *Bdnf*, *Gap43*, *Gfap*, *Irf5*, *Cd86*, and *Mrc1* at 3 months after hemisection with or without implanted hydrogel (n = 3–5), was measured using quantitative real-time reverse transcription polymerase chain reaction (qRT-PCR). RNA was isolated from frozen spinal cord tissue sections, using the High Pure RNA Kit (Roche, Penzberg, Germany). RNA was quantified with spectrophotometer (NanoPhotometerTM P-Class, Munchen, Germany), and isolated RNA was reverse transcribed into cDNA using Transcriptor Universal cDNA Master (Roche, Penzberg, Germany) and a thermal cycler (T100™ Thermal Cycler, Bio-Rad, Hercules, CA, USA). Reactions were performed using cDNA solution, FastStart Universal Probe Master (Roche, Penzberg, Germany), and TaqMan® Gene Expression Assays (Life Technologies, Carlsbad, CA, USA): glyceraldehyde-3-phosphate dehydrogenase/Gapdh/Rn01775763_g1, vascular endothelial growth factor/Vegf/Rn01511602_m1, brain-derived neurotrophic factor/Bdnf/Rn02531967_s1, growth associated protein 43/Gap43/Rn01474579_m1, glial fibrillary acidic protein/Gfap/Rn00566603_m1, interferon regulatory factor 5/Irf5/Rn01500522_m1, macrophage mannose receptor 1/Mrc1/Rn01487342_m1, and CD86/Rn00571654_m1. The final reaction volume was 10 μL containing 25 ng of extracted RNA. Real-time PCR cycler (StepOnePlus™, Life Technologies, Carlsbad, CA, USA) was used for amplification. The following cycling conditions were used, 2 min at 50 °C, 10 min at 95 °C, followed by 40 cycles of 15 s at 95 °C and 1 min at 60 °C. Relative quantification of gene expression was determined using the ΔΔCt method. Data was analyzed with StepOnePlus® software (v2.3) Life Technologies, Carlsbad, CA, USA). For normalization of gene expression levels Gapdh gene was used. A log2 scale was used to display the symmetric magnitude for up- and downregulated genes. From obtained values of control animals (hemi-section only), the arithmetical mean was calculated and this value was set as zero. The statistical analysis (*t*-test) was performed from ΔCt values of controls as well as treated animals.

4.9. Statistical Analysis

The mean values are reported as mean ± SEM. For behavioral tests histological analysis and gene markers intergroup differences were analyzed using one-way ANOVA (probability values <0.05).

5. Conclusions

The HPMA hydrogel shows better potential for SCI repair compared to HEMA hydrogel. The attachment of fibronectin improves limited connective tissue and axonal ingrowth, however without any long-term functional improvement. More sophisticated modifications of future scaffolds would be needed if we want to achieve functionally relevant long-term results.

Author Contributions: A.H., D.H., Š.K. and P.J. designed the study, H.M., V.P. and D.H. participated in preparing the three methacrylate hydrogel scaffolds, A.H. performed the surgical procedures (hydrogel implantation), K.K. (Kristýna Kekulová) and B.S. performed functional testing, J.R. and K.J. did tissue analysis, J.C. and A.H. participated in data analysis and statistical evaluation, A.H., Š.K. and P.J. wrote the paper and performed final revision and evaluation of the manuscript. K.K. (Kristýna Kárová) and L.M.U. did qPCR analysis.

Acknowledgments: We would like to thank Frances Zatřepálková for proofreading the manuscript.

References

1. Atala, R.; Langer, R.; Thomson, J.; Nerem, R. *Principles of Regenerative Medicine*; Academic Press: Burlington, MA, USA, 2008.
2. Hu, B.H.; Su, J.; Messersmith, P.B. Hydrogels cross-linked by native chemical ligation. *Biomacromolecules* **2009**, *10*, 2194–2200. [CrossRef] [PubMed]
3. Slaughter, B.V.; Khurshid, S.S.; Fisher, O.Z.; Khademhosseini, A.; Peppas, N.A. Hydrogels in regenerative medicine. *Adv. Mater.* **2009**, *21*, 3307–3329. [CrossRef] [PubMed]
4. Drury, J.L.; Mooney, D.J. Hydrogels for tissue engineering: Scaffold design variables and applications. *Biomaterials* **2003**, *24*, 4337–4351. [CrossRef]
5. Hoffman, A.S. Hydrogels for biomedical applications. *Adv. Drug Deliv. Rev.* **2002**, *54*, 3–12. [CrossRef]
6. Shoichet, M. Polymer scaffolds for Biomaterials Applications. *Macromolecules* **2010**, *43*, 581–591. [CrossRef]
7. Ahuja, C.S.; Fehlings, M. Concise Review: Bridging the Gap: Novel Neuroregenerative and Neuroprotective Strategies in Spinal Cord Injury. *Stem Cells Transl. Med.* **2016**, *5*, 914–924. [CrossRef] [PubMed]
8. Estrada, V.; Brazda, N.; Schmitz, C.; Heller, S.; Blazyca, H.; Martini, R.; Muller, H.W. Long-lasting significant functional improvement in chronic severe spinal cord injury following scar resection and polyethylene glycol implantation. *Neurobiol. Dis.* **2014**, *67*, 165–179. [CrossRef] [PubMed]
9. Evans, A.R.; Euteneuer, S.; Chavez, E.; Mullen, L.M.; Hui, E.E.; Bhatia, S.N.; Ryan, A.F. Laminin and fibronectin modulate inner ear spiral ganglion neurite outgrowth in an in vitro alternate choice assay. *Dev. Neurobiol.* **2007**, *67*, 1721–1730. [CrossRef] [PubMed]

10. Chen, B.K.; Knight, A.M.; de Ruiter, G.C.; Spinner, R.J.; Yaszemski, M.J.; Currier, B.L.; Windebank, A.J. Axon regeneration through scaffold into distal spinal cord after transection. *J. Neurotrauma* **2009**, *26*, 1759–1771. [CrossRef] [PubMed]
11. Miller, C.; Shanks, H.; Witt, A.; Rutkowski, G.; Mallapragada, S. Oriented Schwann cell growth on micropatterned biodegradable polymer substrates. *Biomaterials* **2001**, *22*, 1263–1269. [CrossRef]
12. Zhu, Y.; Soderblom, C.; Trojanowsky, M.; Lee, D.H.; Lee, J.K. Fibronectin Matrix Assembly after Spinal Cord Injury. *J. Neurotrauma* **2015**, *32*, 1158–1167. [CrossRef] [PubMed]
13. Novikova, L.N.; Pettersson, J.; Brohlin, M.; Wiberg, M.; Novikov, L.N. Biodegradable poly-beta-hydroxybutyrate scaffold seeded with Schwann cells to promote spinal cord repair. *Biomaterials* **2008**, *29*, 1198–1206. [CrossRef] [PubMed]
14. Venstrom, K.A.; Reichardt, L.F. Extracellular matrix. 2: Role of extracellular matrix molecules and their receptors in the nervous system. *Off. Publ. Fed. Am. Soc. Exp. Biol.* **1993**, *7*, 996–1003. [CrossRef]
15. Tysseling-Mattiace, V.M.; Sahni, V.; Niece, K.L.; Birch, D.; Czeisler, C.; Fehlings, M.G.; Stupp, S.I.; Kessler, J.A. Self-assembling nanofibers inhibit glial scar formation and promote axon elongation after spinal cord injury. *J. Neurosci.* **2008**, *28*, 3814–3823. [CrossRef] [PubMed]
16. Hejcl, A.; Lesny, P.; Pradny, M.; Michalek, J.; Jendelova, P.; Stulik, J.; Sykova, E. Biocompatible hydrogels in spinal cord injury repair. *Physiol. Res.* **2008**, *57* (Suppl. 3), S121–S132. [PubMed]
17. Pradny, M.; Michalek, J.; Lesny, P.; Hejcl, A.; Vacik, J.; Slouf, M.; Sykova, E. Macroporous hydrogels based on 2-hydroxyethyl methacrylate. Part 5: Hydrolytically degradable materials. *J. Mater. Sci. Mater. Med.* **2006**, *17*, 1357–1364. [CrossRef] [PubMed]
18. Kubinova, S.; Horak, D.; Hejcl, A.; Plichta, Z.; Kotek, J.; Sykova, E. Highly superporous cholesterol-modified poly(2-hydroxyethyl methacrylate) scaffolds for spinal cord injury repair. *J. Biomed. Mater. Res. A* **2011**, *99*, 618–629. [CrossRef] [PubMed]
19. Zaviskova, K.; Tukmachev, D.; Dubisova, J.; Vackova, I.; Hejcl, A.; Bystronova, J.; Pravda, M.; Scigalkova, I.; Sulakova, R.; Velebny, V.; et al. Injectable hydroxyphenyl derivative of hyaluronic acid hydrogel modified with rgd as scaffold for spinal cord injury repair. *J. Biomed. Mater. Res. A* **2018**, *106*, 1129–1140. [CrossRef] [PubMed]
20. Sykova, E.; Jendelova, P.; Urdzikova, L.; Lesny, P.; Hejcl, A. Bone marrow stem cells and polymer hydrogels—Two strategies for spinal cord injury repair. *Cell Mol. Neurobiol.* **2006**, *26*, 1113–1129. [CrossRef] [PubMed]
21. Hejcl, A.; Urdzikova, L.; Sedy, J.; Lesny, P.; Pradny, M.; Michalek, J.; Burian, M.; Hajek, M.; Zamecnik, J.; Jendelova, P.; et al. Acute and delayed implantation of positively charged 2-hydroxyethyl methacrylate scaffolds in spinal cord injury in the rat. *J. Neurosurg. Spine* **2008**, *8*, 67–73. [CrossRef] [PubMed]
22. Kubinova, S.; Horak, D.; Hejcl, A.; Plichta, Z.; Kotek, J.; Proks, V.; Forostyak, S.; Sykova, E. SIKVAV-modified highly superporous PHEMA scaffolds with oriented pores for spinal cord injury repair. *J. Tissue Eng. Regen. Med.* **2015**, *9*, 1298–1309. [CrossRef] [PubMed]
23. Hejcl, A.; Ruzicka, J.; Kapcalova, M.; Turnovcova, K.; Krumbholcova, E.; Pradny, M.; Michalek, J.; Cihlar, J.; Jendelova, P.; Sykova, E. Adjusting the chemical and physical properties of hydrogels leads to improved stem cell survival and tissue ingrowth in spinal cord injury reconstruction: A comparative study of four methacrylate hydrogels. *Stem Cells Dev.* **2013**, *22*, 2794–2805. [CrossRef] [PubMed]
24. Hejcl, A.; Lesny, P.; Pradny, M.; Sedy, J.; Zamecnik, J.; Jendelova, P.; Michalek, J.; Sykova, E. Macroporous hydrogels based on 2-hydroxyethyl methacrylate. Part 6: 3D hydrogels with positive and negative surface charges and polyelectrolyte complexes in spinal cord injury repair. *J. Mater. Sci. Mater. Med.* **2009**, *20*, 1571–1577. [CrossRef] [PubMed]
25. Hejcl, A.; Sedy, J.; Kapcalova, M.; Toro, D.A.; Amemori, T.; Lesny, P.; Likavcanova-Masinova, K.; Krumbholcova, E.; Pradny, M.; Michalek, J.; et al. HPMA-RGD hydrogels seeded with mesenchymal stem cells improve functional outcome in chronic spinal cord injury. *Stem Cells Dev.* **2010**, *19*, 1535–1546. [CrossRef] [PubMed]
26. Filippov, S.; Hruby, M.; Konak, C.; Mackova, H.; Spirkova, M.; Stepanek, P. Novel pH-responsive nanoparticles. *Langmuir* **2008**, *24*, 9295–9301. [CrossRef] [PubMed]
27. Bruzauskaite, I.; Bironaite, D.; Bagdonas, E.; Bernotiene, E. Scaffolds and cells for tissue regeneration: Different scaffold pore sizes-different cell effects. *Cytotechnology* **2016**, *68*, 355–369. [CrossRef] [PubMed]

28. Flynn, L.; Dalton, P.D.; Shoichet, M.S. Fiber templating of poly(2-hydroxyethyl methacrylate) for neural tissue engineering. *Biomaterials* **2003**, *24*, 4265–4272. [CrossRef]
29. Woerly, S.; Pinet, E.; de Robertis, L.; Van Diep, D.; Bousmina, M. Spinal cord repair with PHPMA hydrogel containing RGD peptides (NeuroGel). *Biomaterials* **2001**, *22*, 1095–1111. [CrossRef]
30. Hejcl, A.; Jendelova, P.; Sykova, E. Experimental reconstruction of the injured spinal cord. *Adv. Technol. Stand. Neurosurg.* **2011**, *37*, 65–95.
31. Loh, N.K.; Woerly, S.; Bunt, S.M.; Wilton, S.D.; Harvey, A.R. The regrowth of axons within tissue defects in the CNS is promoted by implanted hydrogel matrices that contain BDNF and CNTF producing fibroblasts. *Exp. Neurol.* **2001**, *170*, 72–84. [CrossRef] [PubMed]
32. Plant, G.W.; Woerly, S.; Harvey, A.R. Hydrogels containing peptide or aminosugar sequences implanted into the rat brain: Influence on cellular migration and axonal growth. *Exp. Neurol.* **1997**, *143*, 287–299. [CrossRef] [PubMed]
33. Kang, C.E.; Baumann, M.D.; Tator, C.H.; Shoichet, M.S. Localized and sustained delivery of fibroblast growth factor-2 from a nanoparticle-hydrogel composite for treatment of spinal cord injury. *Cells Tissues Organs* **2013**, *197*, 55–63. [CrossRef] [PubMed]
34. Danen, E.H.; Yamada, K.M. Fibronectin, integrins, and growth control. *J. Cell Physiol.* **2001**, *189*, 1–13. [CrossRef] [PubMed]
35. To, W.S.; Midwood, K.S. Plasma and cellular fibronectin: Distinct and independent functions during tissue repair. *Fibrog. Tissue Repair* **2011**, *4*, 21. [CrossRef] [PubMed]
36. King, V.R.; Alovskaya, A.; Wei, D.Y.; Brown, R.A.; Priestley, J.V. The use of injectable forms of fibrin and fibronectin to support axonal ingrowth after spinal cord injury. *Biomaterials* **2010**, *31*, 4447–4456. [CrossRef] [PubMed]
37. Sakai, T.; Johnson, K.J.; Murozono, M.; Sakai, K.; Magnuson, M.A.; Wieloch, T.; Cronberg, T.; Isshiki, A.; Erickson, H.P.; Fassler, R. Plasma fibronectin supports neuronal survival and reduces brain injury following transient focal cerebral ischemia but is not essential for skin-wound healing and hemostasis. *Nat. Med.* **2001**, *7*, 324–330. [CrossRef] [PubMed]
38. King, V.R.; Hewazy, D.; Alovskaya, A.; Phillips, J.B.; Brown, R.A.; Priestley, J.V. The neuroprotective effects of fibronectin mats and fibronectin peptides following spinal cord injury in the rat. *Neuroscience* **2010**, *168*, 523–530. [CrossRef] [PubMed]
39. Hejcl, A.; Ruzicka, J.; Proks, V.; Mackova, H.; Kubinova, S.; Tukmachev, D.; Cihlar, J.; Horak, D.; Jendelova, P. Dynamics of tissue ingrowth in SIKVAV-modified highly superporous PHEMA scaffolds with oriented pores after bridging a spinal cord transection. *J. Mater. Sci. Mater. Med.* **2018**, *29*, 89. [CrossRef] [PubMed]
40. Iida, T.; Nakagawa, M.; Asano, T.; Fukushima, C.; Tachi, K. Free vascularized lateral femoral cutaneous nerve graft with anterolateral thigh flap for reconstruction of facial nerve defects. *J. Reconstr. Microsurg.* **2006**, *22*, 343–348. [CrossRef] [PubMed]
41. Glaser, J.; Gonzalez, R.; Sadr, E.; Keirstead, H.S. Neutralization of the chemokine CXCL10 reduces apoptosis and increases axon sprouting after spinal cord injury. *J. Neurosci. Res.* **2006**, *84*, 724–734. [CrossRef] [PubMed]
42. Macaya, D.; Spector, M. Injectable hydrogel materials for spinal cord regeneration: A review. *Biomed. Mater.* **2012**, *7*, 012001. [CrossRef] [PubMed]
43. Basso, D.M.; Beattie, M.S.; Bresnahan, J.C. A sensitive and reliable locomotor rating scale for open field testing in rats. *J. Neurotrauma* **1995**, *12*, 1–21. [CrossRef] [PubMed]

5

Stem Cells Therapy for Spinal Cord Injury

Marina Gazdic [1], Vladislav Volarevic [2], C. Randall Harrell [3], Crissy Fellabaum [3], Nemanja Jovicic [4], Nebojsa Arsenijevic [2] and Miodrag Stojkovic [1,5,*]

1 Faculty of Medical Sciences, Department of Genetics, University of Kragujevac, 34000 Kragujevac, Serbia; marinagazdic87@gmail.com

2 Faculty of Medical Sciences, Department of Microbiology and immunology, Center for Molecular Medicine and Stem Cell Research, University of Kragujevac, 34000 Kragujevac, Serbia; drvolarevic@yahoo.com (V.V.); arne@medf.kg.ac.rs (N.A.)

3 Regenerative Processing Plant, LLC, 34176 US Highway 19 N Palm Harbor, Palm Harbor, FL 34684, USA; dr.harrell@regenerativeplant.org (C.R.H.); crissy@regenerativeplant.org (C.F.)

4 Faculty of Medical Sciences, Department of Histology and embryology, University of Kragujevac, 34000 Kragujevac, Serbia; nemanjajovicic.kg@gmail.com

5 Spebo Medical, 16 Norvezanska, 16000 Leskovac, Serbia

* Correspondence: mstojkovic@spebo.com

Abstract: Spinal cord injury (SCI), a serious public health issue, most likely occurs in previously healthy young adults. Current therapeutic strategies for SCI includes surgical decompression and pharmacotherapy, however, there is still no gold standard for the treatment of this devastating condition. Inefficiency and adverse effects of standard therapy indicate that novel therapeutic strategies are required. Because of their neuroregenerative and neuroprotective properties, stem cells are a promising tool for the treatment of SCI. Herein, we summarize and discuss the promising therapeutic potential of human embryonic stem cells (hESC), induced pluripotent stem cells (iPSC) and ependymal stem/progenitor cells (epSPC) for SCI.

Keywords: spinal cord injury; stem cells; embryonic stem cells; induced pluripotent stem cells; ependymal stem/progenitor cells

1. Introduction

Spinal cord injury (SCI), a serious public health issue, most likely occurs in previously healthy young adults. Country-level incidence studies show that incidenceof SCI ranges from 40 to 80 per million people per year [1]. The aim of modern society is to prevent traumatic SCI usually caused by road traffic accidents, falls from heights, and violence (gunshot or stab wound), as well as nontraumatic SCI resulting from cancer, spinal disk degeneration, or arthritis. Gray and white matter damage after SCI leads to partial or complete motor, sensory, or autonomic deficit in parts of the body distal to the lesion site. In accordance, the most devastating of all SCIs are injuries of the cervical spine, accompanied by high-grade dysfunction of the central nervous system (CNS). In order to determine the severity of SCI, the American Spinal Injury Association (ASIA) defined international standards for neurological classification and formulated impairment scale for neurological assessment of individuals with SCI [2]. The most severe SCI is complete, irreversible and characterized by increased mortality risk compared to the general population due to cardiovascular, respiratory and genitourinary complications, deep venous thrombosis, chronic neuropathic pain, pressure ulcers, and infections [3].

Although a detailed understanding of molecular mechanisms involved in the pathophysiology of SCI provides great promise for improving therapeutic strategies for spinal cord repair, there is still no gold standard for the treatment of this devastating condition. Because of their differentiation abilities and secretion of a variety of cytokines and growth factors, stem cells have been extensively studied as a novel neuroregenerative and neuroprotective agents for the treatment of SCI. A large number of murine models of acute, subacute and chronic SCI, that resemble lesions that develop in the adult human spinal cord following exposure to trauma, have demonstrated not only therapeutic role of in vitro-expanded stem cell-derived progenitor, but also the cellular and molecular mechanism of spinal cord repair and neurological improvements through activation of endogenous stem cells.

In this review, we summarize the advantages and disadvantages of current surgical and pharmacological approaches and discuss promising therapeutic potential of human embryonic stem cells (hESC), induced pluripotent stem cells (iPSC) and ependymal stem/progenitor cells (epSPC) for SCI. We hope that the data highlighted in this report may be of relevance to stem cell researchers and clinicians as a backdrop to future development of stem cell-based therapy of SCI.

2. Pathophysiology

Neurological outcome after SCI is associated with mechanical destruction of spinal tissue and secondary injury mediated by multiple pathophysiological processes (reviewed in [4]). Displacement of the anatomical structures of the spinal cord, following the initial mechanical events underlies the onset of SCI and refers to the primary injury phase. Physical forces such as compression, contusion, laceration, and acute stretch, damage nerve cells and their axons, leading to the disruption of descending neuronal pathways [5]. During the secondary phase of SCI, the series of destructive pathological processes occur, leading to massive cellular dysfunction and death, aberrant molecular signaling and generation of harmful metabolic products. Immediately after sudden mechanical trauma, focal microhemorrhage, vasospasm and reduction in blood flow, are seen within the injured cord. Disturbance in ion chomeostasis, glutamaterelease, and lipid peroxidation in the lesion site contribute to further progression of neurological dysfunction in patients with SCI by activating consequential cascade of destructive pathophysiological mechanisms [6–8]. Electrolytic disbalance in SCI is characterized by elevated extracellular concentration of potassium (K^+) and increased intracellular concentration of sodium (Na^+) and calcium (Ca^{2+}) [9]. As a result of the high amount of potassium in the extracellular area, the transmission of a nerve impulse is blocked. Intracellular acidosis promotes excessive water influx into the neurons, resulting in cytotoxic edema and neuronal death (reviewed in [10,11]. Damaged cells massively release various toxic metabolites as well as excitatory amino acid glutamate, which trigger autodestructive free-radical generation and excitotoxicity [9,12]. Reactive oxygen species cause oxidative damage of DNA, and lipid peroxidation in the cellular membranes. These pathological changes observed in the lesion site lead to further progression of neurons and glia cells necrosis and apoptosis [13]. It is well known that immune response significantly contributes to pathogenesis of SCI. Interestingly, the inflammatory process has both aggressive and protective effects on damaged spinal cord. Mechanical trauma breaks the integrity and increases permeability of the blood-spinal cord barrier, thus contributing to inflammatory cell invasion, and edema generation at the lesion site. Neutrophils, macrophages, T cells and microglia infiltrate the spinal parenchyma, and produce wide range of proinflammatory cytokines tumor necrosis factor alpha (TNF-α), interleukin-1 beta (IL-1β), interleukin-1 alpha (IL-1α), and interleukin-6 (IL-6) [14–17]. Expression of ion channels included in the family of connexins (Cx) is augmented at early stages after traumatic SCI and contributes to secondary damage of spinal cord and neuropathic pain [18]. Neuroinflammation causes the development of a necrotic cavity surrounded by a glial scar that prevents SCI progression [19]. At the same time, activated macrophages and microglia are involved in phagocytosis of necrotic and destroyed tissue. This rapid removal of cellular debris is significant for establishing an environment beneficial for neuroregeneration [20,21].

3. Current Therapeutic Strategies for Spinal Cord Injury

3.1. Surgical Decompression

Surgical Timing in Acute Spinal Cord Injury Study (STASCIS) showed that urgent surgical decompression within 24 h after injury significantly increased post-operative motor and sensory functions according to American Spinal Injury Association (ASIA) score [22,23]. Although early decompression reduces the risk of respiratory failure and sepsis [24], neurological surgery for the treatment of SCI is still associated with complications such as incidental durotomy or meningitis [25]. These limitations indicate that STASCIS and urgent neurological surgery in SCI as a widely adopted treatment requires further improvement.

3.2. Therapeutic Hypothermia

Beneficial effects of modest (32–34 °C) systemic hypothermia induced by intravascular cooling catheter have been clearly demonstrated in SCI [26,27]. Problems related to the safety of invasive systemic treatment and relation between temperature at the spinal cord lesion and core body temperature have been successfully resolved by localized cooling of the injury site during surgical decompression [28]. Systemic hypothermia as well as local cooling attenuate main pathophysiological processes during SCI including neuronal metabolism, neuroinflammation, oxidative stress, excitotoxicity, and apoptosis [29,30]. At the same time, decreased temperature protects the spinal cord from further injury by preserving the blood-spinal cord barrier (BSCB) and reducing edema, and induces neurorepair by enhancing angiogenesis and neurogenesis [29]. However, the effects of timing and duration of hypothermia as well as the best rewarming method on endogenous mechanisms and mobilization of stem cells are still the main challenges in the use of therapeutic hypothermia for the treatment of SCI [31].

3.3. Pharmacotherapy

Because of their anti-inflammatory effects and capacity to reduce oxidative stress and excitotoxicity, corticosteroids are used in many preclinical and clinical studies as therapeutic agents for the treatment of SCI [32]. Although it was expected that methylprednisolone would have the ability to suppress immune-mediated damage after SCI by decreasing the inflammatory cytokine production, several clinical studies failed to demonstrate functional repair after methylprednisolone administration [33–37]. Use of methylprednisolone in patients with SCI has become controversial, because of high rate of complications such as sepsis, pulmonary embolism, and gastrointestinal hemorrhage [33–37]. In order to improve pharmacological treatment of secondary injury phase, neuroprotective and regenerative effects of various agents were evaluated in clinical trials during the last decade. Several prospective, multicenter human studies demonstrated neurologic improvement in patients with spinal cord trauma who received riluzole [38], GM1 ganglioside [39], BA-210 [40], minocycline [41] or granulocyte-colony stimulating factor (G-CSF) [42], suggesting the potential of these agents for application in routine clinical practice.

4. Stem Cells—New Hope for Spinal Cord Injury

4.1. Human Embryonic Stem Cells

Human embryonic stem cells (hESC) are derived from the inner cell mass of the preimplantation blastocysts, by removing the trophectoderm cells by immunosurgery [43]. hESC are positive for pluripotent stem cell surface antigens such as stage specific embryonic antigens 3 and 4 (SSEA-3 and SSEA-4), TRA-1-60, TRA-1-81, and express well-known pluripotency-associated genes octamer-binding transcription factor 3/4 (*OCT3/4*), sex determining region Y box-containing gene 2 (*SOX2*), and *NANOG* [44,45]. Elevated alkaline phosphatase and telomerase activity are associated with their unlimited proliferative potential [44,45]. These markers are used to verify the successful isolation of a new hESC line and confirm the maintenance of an undifferentiated pluripotent state for established hESC.

In addition to remarkable proliferative capacity, hESC exhibit pluripotency both in vitro and in vivo. Because of their ability for differentiation into cells of ectodermal origin such as neuronal and glial cells, hESC are used in many preclinical studies (reviewed in [46]) as a new therapeutic option for SCI (Figure 1A). Several previously published papers have shown that transplantation of hESC-derived oligodendrocyte progenitor cells (OPC) to SCI models resulted in cell survival and clinically relevant recovery of neurological functions with no evidence of harmful effects [47–49].

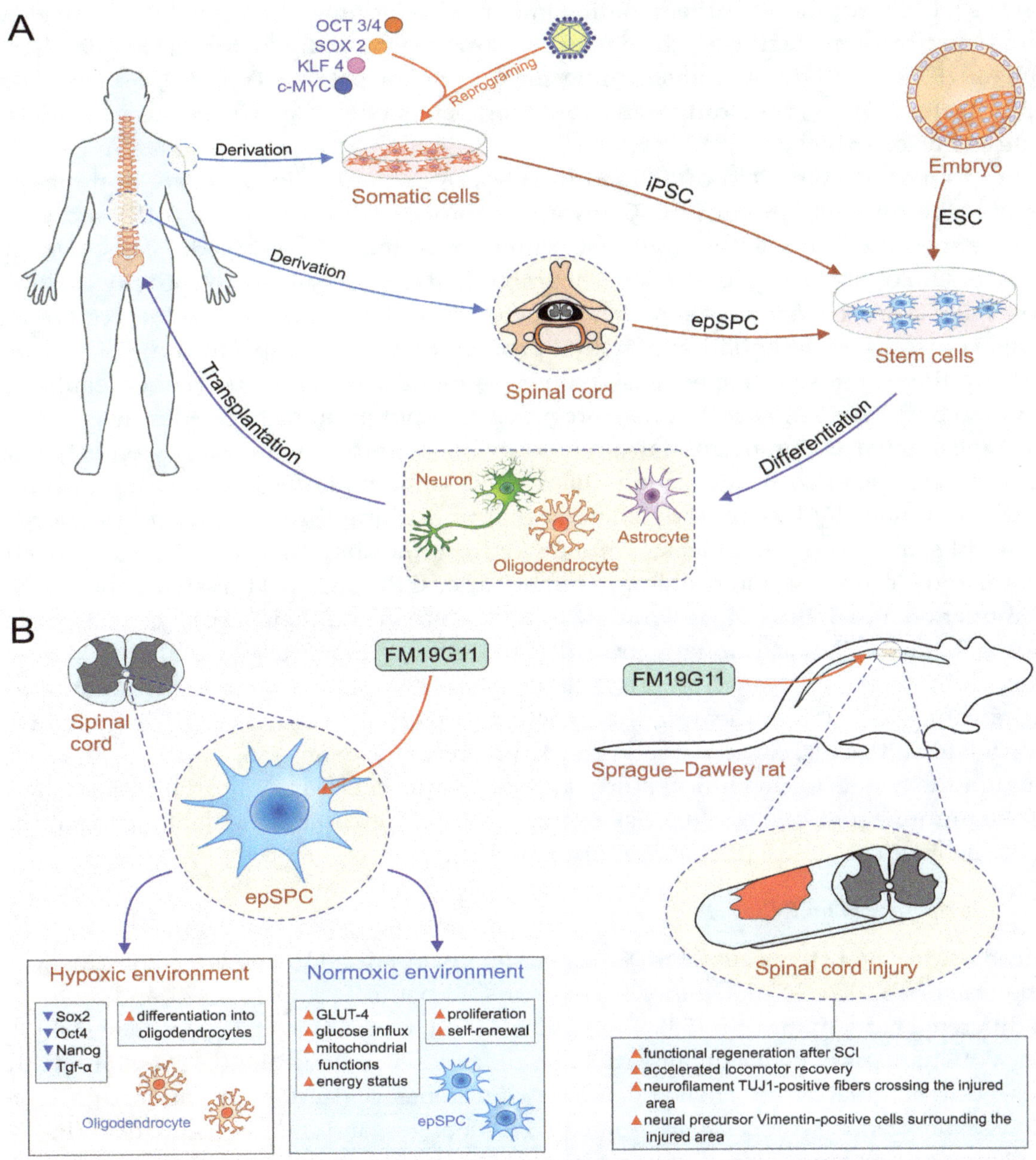

Figure 1. (**A**)Human embryonic stem cells (hESC), induced pluripotent stem cells (iPSC) and ependymal stem/progenitor cells (epSPC) as a promising tool in the therapy of SCI; (**B**) the role of FM19G11, an inhibitor of hypoxia inducible factor (HIFα), to mobilize epSPC. OCT3/4, octamer-binding transcription factor 3/4; SOX2, sex determining region Y box-containing gene 2; KLF4, Krüppel-like factor 4; TGF-α, transforming growth factor-alpha; GLUT-4, glucose transporter type 4.

Keirstead and coworkers demonstrated that hESC-derived OPC transplanted seven days after SCI in rats differentiate into mature oligodendrocytes, induce myelin sheath regeneration and significantly improve locomotor function [48]. In contrast, OPC administration ten months after injury, did not manage to improve neurological outcome in injured animals compared with controls, suggesting that first week after SCI is the optimal time point for OPC transplantation [48]. Neural stem cells (NSC) clonally derived from murine embryonic stem cells (dNSCs), without embryoid bodies formation, survive and differentiate into neurons, oligodendrocytes, and astrocytes after injection into the spinal cord lesion one week after SCI in mice. Salewski et al. provided the evidence that transplanted dNSCs have broad spectrum of beneficial neuroregenerative effects associated with enhanced remyelination of damage axons [50]. In addition to differentiation into myelin-forming oligodendrocytes, hESC-derived OPC express neurotrophic factors such as neurite growth-promoting factor 2 (NEGF2), hepatocyte growth factor (HGF), activin A, transforming growth factor-beta 2 (TGF-β2), and brain-derived neurotrophic factor (BDNF), providing significant therapeutic effects in SCI such as neuronal survival and neurite extension [51,52].

In order to increase the yield of defined hESC-derived neural lineages, we optimized in vitro conditions for the differentiation of hESC towards motoneuron progenitors (MP) and OPC using chemically defined mediums without animal components and without feeder cells. This protocol induces conversion of hESC into rosettes and neural tube-like structures with capacity to differentiate into region specific and functional neurons, astrocytes, and oligodendrocytes [53]. For the first time, we achieved controlled differentiation of neural progenitors towards specific type of neuronal cells by stimulating the rosettes with specific signaling factors in vitro [53]. Promising results obtained under in vitro conditions suggest that neuroregenerative potential of hESC-derived OPC and MP should be investigated using an animal model of SCI. Therefore, we used a well-established rat model of complete spinal cord transection, that resemble the pathology of the most severe clinical cases of SCI in humans [54]. Our study showed that transplanted cells OPC and MP survived for at least 4 months, and migrated at least 3 mm away from the site of injury [55]. Main mechanisms of behavioral and electrophysiological improvement after OPC and MP transplantation in SCI were their differentiation into mature oligodendrocytes and neurons and their capacity to produce various neurotrophic factors [55]. Additionally, transplanted OPC and MP triggered Janus kinase/signal transducers and activators of transcription (JAK/STAT) and Notch signaling in the lesion site leading to enhanced astrogliosis [56] indicating that reactive astrocytes in synergy with transplanted cells promote survival and growth of serotonergic and dopaminergic axons [56].

Although the results of preclinical study are promising, there are important issues such as the possibility of immune rejection and the risk of tumor formation after transplantation that should be addressed to achieve successful hESC-based therapy [57].

4.2. Induced Pluripotent Stem Cells

Induced pluripotent stem cells (iPSC) were originally obtained by the viral transduction of four transcription factors: *SOX2*, *OCT3/4*, tumor suppressor Krüppel-like factor 4 [*KLF4*], and proto-oncogene *c-MYC* in differentiated somatic cells [58]. The standard viral integrative reprogramming techniques are associated with many risks including insertional mutagenesis, uncontrolled expression of integrated transgenes—downregulation or silencing of the transgenes or tumor formation due to residual reactivation of transgenes, senescence-associated DNA changes, and immunogenicity of iPSC-derived cells [59]. Huge efforts have been devoted toward the development of novel protocols in order to improve quality and efficiency of reprogramming technology and to bring iPSC-derived cells closer to clinic. During the last decade, several studies suggested alternative non-integrative delivery methods for more safety iPSC generation such as use of adenovirus and Sendai virus as well as non-viral-mediated molecular strategies (*Cre-loxP*-mediated recombination, *PiggyBac*-transposition episomal DNA vectors, and direct miRNA transfection) [60–64]. All these technologies provide an opportunity to derive pluripotent cells similar to hESC in terms of morphology, karyotype, and phenotype without destruction of human embryos. The use of patient-specific iPSC for treatment of SCI is particularly attractive, given that they avoid the ethical considerations and immunological rejection of hESC and represent a source of autologous cells that can be differentiated to neural progenitor cells (NPC), neurons, oligodendrocytes, and astrocytes at the same time underlining the integration of transplanted cells into the site of injury as an important issue of successful cell-based therapy (Figure 1A). Several research groups reported that iPSC are capable of generating mature dopaminergic neurons [65,66], motor neurons (MN) [67–69], and GABAergic interneurons [70], however, it is known that transplantation of mature neurons is characterized by poor cellular engraftment versus transplantation of neural progenitors. Consequently, transplantation of neural progenitors has been a focus, and seems to be a promising approach for the treatment of SCI. Several groups reported that autologous iPSC derived neural precursor cells (iPSC-NPC) could be efficiently derived [71,72] and used for transplantation into rodents with SCI [73,74]. Transplanted NPC predominantly gave rise to myelin-producing oligodendrocytes, leading to remyelination and improvement of nerve conduction [73]. Moreover, iPSC-NPC migrated long distances, integrated into the spinal cord and differentiated into mature neurons and glia, resulting in synaptic reconstruction and locomotor recovery [75–77]. In addition, neurotrophic factors produced by iPSC-NPC, modulate immunopathological events following SCI [78]. Hayashi and colleagues found that iPSC-derived astrocytes injected into the injured rodent spinal cord increased the sensitivity to mechanical stimulus but did not affect locomotor functions [79].

Although patient-specific iPSC are a revolutionary tool which could pave the way to personalized medicine, many issues remain to be improved including reprogramming techniques as well as protocols for targeted differentiation.

4.3. Ependymal Stem/Progenitor Cells

It has been demonstrated that OPC, astrocytes, and ependymal cells are the most important dividing cells in the adult spinal cord [80–82]. Astrocytes and OPC have the capacity to self-renew, however they cannot give rise to different types of specialized cells, indicating that they are not NSC [83]. Ependymal stem/progenitor cells (epSPC) are adult multipotent stem cells characterized by the ability to differentiate into the both glial cells and neurons [18,56] and can be found around the spinal central canal [4] (Figure 1A, Table 1).

Table 1. The capacity of engraftment and differentiation, contribution to functional recovery and risk of tumorigenesis of transplanted hESC, iPSC and epSPC in animal model of spinal cord injury Stem cell source.

Stem Cell Source	Differentiation	Engraftment	Contribution to Functional Recovery	Tumorigenesis
hESC	differentiation into neurons and glia [53,64]	hESC-derived OPCs and MPs engraft for at least 4 months in the lesion site [55]	significant improvement of behavioral and electrophysiological, function of injured animals at early time points after SCI [55,56]	risk of teratoma formation [46,57]
iPSC	differentiation into neural progenitor cells, neurons, oligodendrocytes, and astrocytes [72–77]	integration for at least 12 weeks after transplantation into injured spinal cord tissue [74]	iPSC-derived cells promote functional recovery in an early SCI model [72–77]	more tumorigenic than hESC due to genetic and epigenetic aberrations [46]
epSPC	differentiation into glial cells (oligodendrocytes and astrocytes) and neurons [18,34]	detected 2 months after transplantation [56]	accelerates recovery of motor activity 1 week after injury [56]	low rates of tumorigenesis [4]

hESC, human embryonic stem cells; OPC, oligodendrocyte progenitor cells; MP, motoneuron progenitors; iPSC, induced pluripotent stem cells; epSPC, ependymal stem/progenitor cells; SCI, spinal cord injury.

OPC, present in the white and gray matter in the adult CNS, are the main proliferating cell types in the intact spinal cord [80]. Under homeostatic conditions, neural/glial antigen 2 (NG2)—expressing OPC proliferate and differentiate into mature oligodendrocytes maintaining tissue integrity over the lifespan. Following SCI, OPC migrate to the spinal cord lesion sites, and extensively contribute to remyelination [80,81]. The recent studies [84,85] have shown that glial growth factor 2 (GGF2) and ferritin administration promote oligodendrogenesis and improve functional recovery after SCI. Thus, enhancing the endogenous OPC response to injury could be a potential therapeutic approach to manage tissue repair and regeneration without the transplantation of exogenous cells.

It is well known that astrocyte turnover is low in healthy spinal cords, however, these cells respond to SCI by intensive dividing and forming the border of glial scar with fibromeningeal and $NG2^{+}$glia cells [80,86]. Astrocytes in the scar's periphery inhibit axonal growth in the environment of SCI through secretion of inhibitory molecules such as heparan sulphate proteoglycan, dermatan sulphate proteoglycan, keratan sulphate proteoglycan and chondroitin sulphate proteoglycan (CSPG) [87]. In addition to the extracellular matrix components, semaphorin 3, ephrin-B2 and its receptor EPHB2 and the Slit proteins produced by reactive astrocytes, have largely negative effects on nerve regeneration [87]. Following these observations, several in vivo studies provided the evidence that application of chondroitinase ABC (ChABC) as an individual therapy or in combination with other treatments degraded CSPG in scar tissue, enhanced growth and regeneration of axons, and re-established neural pathways below the lesion (reviewed in [88]). Enzyme-based treatments may provide new opportunities to overcome detrimental effects of glial scar and may offer new hope for success in therapy of SCI.

However, as we mentioned, reactive astrocytes surrounding the spinal cord lesion prevent an excessive inflammatory cell infiltration leading to decrease in immune-mediated damage of spinal cord. Interestingly, during the last two decades, there is growing evidence suggesting novel cellular and molecular mechanisms underlying neuroprotective effect of astrogliosis after SCI. The fact that glial scar is composed of at least two phenotypically and developmentally different populations of astrocytes, may explain a dual role of scar tissue on spinal cord regeneration. Although the most extensive proliferation of epSPC occurs during embryogenesis and the early postnatal period, there are data suggesting slow proliferation rate of epSPC surrounding spinal cord in adulthood [89–91]. More importantly, endogenous epSPC are activated 72 h after SCI to migrate from spinal central canal towards the lesion site, divide extensively, and generate astrocytes, as well as a small number of oligodendrocytes [80,82,92,93]. Only small portion of epSPC differentiate toward oligodendrocytes responsible for myelin production, typically located in white matter areas of spinal cord [94]. Most of the epSPC-derived progeny express astrocytic markers [82], however, these reactive astrocytes are glial fibrillary acidic protein (GFAP) negative, invade glial scar center and promote axonal growth and regeneration [80,82,95]. In contrast to astrocytes constituting the glial scar border, epSPC-derived reactive astrocytes actively maintain extracellular homeostasis. In particular, astrocytic uptake of glutamate prevents glutamate-mediated neuronal loss, suggesting that pharmacological stimulation of astrocytes may be a promising therapeutic target for SCI as well as other pathologies involving excitotoxicity. In addition, astrocytes provide significant metabolic support to neurons, regulate extracellular potassium level, and prevent generation of free radicals [96]. The neuroprotective capacity of astrocytes is mediated by wide variety of soluble factors including brain-derived neurotrophic factor, ciliary neurotrophic factor, nerve growth factor (NGF), and basic fibroblast growth factor (FGF-2) and the extracellular matrix molecules laminin and fibronectin [97]. Thus, specific modulation of two reactive astrocyte subpopulations in the injured spinal cord, protective in the core and harmful at the periphery of glial scar, could represent a new regeneration strategy for SCI.

Although the precise mechanism for improved functional recovery after intrathecal administration of epidermal growth factor (EGF) and fibroblast growth factor 2 (FGF-2) is not known [98], these findings suggested that stimulation of resident NSC might be used as a possible new therapeutic approach for SCI treatment. Endogenous cell-based therapeutic approach avoids the risks of exogenous cell transplantation such as risk of tumor formation after engraftment, and possible immunogenicity that requires immunosuppression. Thus, we explored a new chemical entity, FM19G11 as a new pharmacological agent for spinal cord regeneration (Figure 1B). FM19G11, by HIF2α-mediated mechanisms, inhibits the transcriptional and protein expression of pluripotency markers *Sox2*, *Oct4*, *Nanog*, and *Tgf-α* in epSPC, leading to increased differentiation of epSPC into oligodendrocytes in a hypoxic environment [99]. However, under normoxic conditions, FM19G11 stimulates glucose intake and mitochondrial functions in epSPC, causing an increased energy status and high proliferation of epSPC (Figure 1B, left panel). Furthermore, we confirmed neuroregenerative properties of FM19G11 using an animal model of SCI [100]. In line with previous findings, paralysis of hind limbs was significantly reversed in FM19G11-treated rats with SCI compared to vehicle treated animals [100] (Figure 1B, right panel). Furthermore, we showed that epSPC isolated from rats with an SCI (epSPCi) display enhanced capability for self-renewal and differentiation toward oligodendrocyte progenitors compared to epSPC from healthy animals [56]. This isconsistent with the fact that the inflammatory environment to which quiescent epSPCare exposed after SCI modulates gene expression profile and induces recruitment of endogenous epSPCto the lesion site [82,92]. In order to delineate the molecular mechanisms responsible for higher regeneration ability of epSPCi after injury, we analyzed the role of Cx50, an ion channel involved in differentiation of stem cells into glial cells within the injured area. In non-pathological conditions, epSPC show high expression levels of Cx50, however, activated epSPCi express low levels of Cx50, indicating adverse effects of Cx50 in spinal cord regeneration [18,101]. An additional molecular mechanism of increased regenerative capacities of epSPCi versus epSPC could be changes in purinergic receptors (P2Y) expression in stem cells. We showed that downregulation of P2Y1 receptor and an upregulation of P2Y4 receptor increases differentiation potential and proliferation ability of epSPCi, respectively [102]. Hence, transplantation of epSPCi or epSPCi-derived oligodendrocyte precursors [OPCi] immediately after spinal cord contusion was a more efficient therapeutic strategy for the locomotor recovery one week after treatment than epSPC or OPC transplantation [56]. Therefore, our studies revealed that transplanted epSPCi differentiated rarely and that beneficial effect of transplanted epSPCi in SCI was primarily based on their release of trophic and immunomodulatory factors that alter function of immune cells [56]. Combination of epSPCi transplantation and local application of FM19G11 reduced glial scar and enhanced generation of oligodendrocyte precursor, however, did not significantly improve the neurological outcome compared to the individual treatments [103]. Therefore, to treat SCI as complex disorder, new hope might be found in a combination of cell transplantation, pharmacotherapy, mobilization of endogenous stem cells and bioscaffolds [103,104].

5. Conclusions

Stem cell therapy in SCI provides a clue to solve the challenges which currently used medical procedures cannot treat. Because of their neuroregenerative, neuroprotective and immunomodulatory properties, stem cells are an innovative approach for the therapy of SCI. The presence of NSC in the adult CNS raises the possibility of the modulation of an endogenous regenerative process. Although further investigations are necessary to confirm neurological benefits by adjusting doses and drug administrations, treatments for mobilization of endogenous stem cell population have been considered as a promising therapeutic approach to enhance repair mechanisms in SCI. Additionally, results of preclinical studies indicate that application of stem cell-derived progenitors significantly reduces neurological disability in most severe SCIs. However, the main safety issue regarding pluripotent stem cell-based transplantation is still a lack of efficient protocols to obtain pure cell populations without the presence of unwanted cell types, and undifferentiated hESC/iPSC. It is important to highlight that stem cell transplantation alone is not sufficient to bridge a spinal cord lesion, therefore, a repair strategy based on combination of well-established therapeutic modalities, including surgery and medications, and stem cell-derived neural cells is an extremely attractive option for the treatment of this devastating injuries. Therefore, it is critical to develop new modalities such as directly applied pharmacology and biomaterials that support stem cell survival and provide better tissue integration. Future studies must be focused on resolving issues such as ideal sources of stem cells and safety of stem cell-based therapy with the aim to utterly exploit the promising therapeutic potential of both exogenous and endogenous stem cells in SCI.

Acknowledgments: This study was supported by Serbian Ministry of Science (ON175069 and ON175103).

Author Contributions: Marina Gazdic, Vladislav Volarevic, C. Randall Harrell, Crissy Fellabaum, Nemanja Jovicic, Nebojsa Arsenijevic, Miodrag Stojkovic designed and wrote the manuscript.

References

1. International Perspectives on Spinal Cord Injury. Available online: http://apps.who.int/iris/bitstream/10665/94190/1/9789241564663_eng.pdf (accessed on 15 January 2018).
2. Available online: http://asia-spinalinjury.org (accessed on 15 January 2018).
3. Hagen, E.M. Acute complications of spinal cord injuries. *World J. Orthop.* **2015**, *6*, 17–23. [CrossRef] [PubMed]
4. Ronaghi, M.; Erceg, S.; Moreno-Manzano, V.; Stojkovic, M. Challenges of stem cell therapy for spinal cord injury: Human embryonic stem cells, endogenous neural stem cells, or induced pluripotent stem cells? *Stem Cells* **2010**, *28*, 93–99. [CrossRef] [PubMed]
5. Ackery, A.; Tator, C.; Krassioukov, A. A global perspective on spinal cord injury epidemiology. *J. Neurotrauma* **2004**, *21*, 1355–1370. [CrossRef] [PubMed]
6. Beattie, M.S.; Li, Q.; Bresnahan, J.C. Cell death and plasticity after experimental spinal cord injury. *Prog. Brain Res.* **2000**, *128*, 9–21. [PubMed]
7. Blight, A.R. Spinal cord injury models: Neurophysiology. *J. Neurotrauma* **1992**, *9*, 147–150. [CrossRef] [PubMed]
8. Grossman, S.D.; Rosenberg, L.J.; Wrathall, J.R. Relationship of altered glutamate receptor subunit mRNA expression to acute cell loss after spinal cord contusion. *Exp. Neurol.* **2001**, *168*, 283–289. [CrossRef] [PubMed]
9. Fehlings, M.G.; Nakashima, H.; Nagoshi, N.; Chow, D.S.; Grossman, R.G.; Kopjar, B. Rationale, design and critical end points for the Riluzole in Acute Spinal Cord Injury Study (RISCIS): A randomized, double-blinded, placebo-controlled parallel multi-center trial. *Spinal Cord* **2016**, *54*, 8–15. [CrossRef] [PubMed]
10. Garcia, E.; Aguilar-Cevallos, J.; Silva-Garcia, R.; Ibarra, A. Cytokine and Growth Factor Activation In Vivo and In Vitro after Spinal Cord Injury. *Mediat. Inflamm.* **2016**, *2016*. [CrossRef] [PubMed]
11. Hayta, E.; Elden, H. Acute spinal cord injury: A review of pathophysiology and potential of non-steroidal anti-inflammatory drugs for pharmacological intervention. *J. Chem. Neuroanat.* **2017**, *87*, 25–31. [CrossRef] [PubMed]
12. Li, S.; Stys, P.K. Mechanisms of ionotropic glutamate receptor-mediated excitotoxicity in isolated spinal cord white matter. *J. Neurosci.* **2000**, *20*, 1190–1198. [PubMed]
13. Visavadiya, N.P.; Patel, S.P.; VanRooyen, J.L.; Sullivan, P.G.; Rabchevsky, A.G. Cellular and subcellular oxidative stress parameters following severe spinal cord injury. *Redox Biol.* **2016**, *8*, 59–67. [CrossRef] [PubMed]
14. Pineau, I.; Lacroix, S. Proinflammatory cytokine synthesis in the injured mouse spinal cord: Multiphasic expression pattern and identification of the cell types involved. *J. Comp. Neurol.* **2007**, *500*, 267–285. [CrossRef] [PubMed]
15. Kettenmann, H.; Hanisch, U.K.; Noda, M.; Verkhratsky, A. Physiology of microglia. *Physiol. Rev.* **2001**, *91*, 461–553. [CrossRef] [PubMed]
16. Oyinbo, C.A. Secondary injury mechanisms in traumatic spinal cord injury: A nugget of this multiply cascade. *Acta Neurobiol. Exp. (Wars)* **2011**, *71*, 281–299. [PubMed]
17. Kong, X.; Gao, J. Macrophage polarization: A key event in the secondary phase of acute spinal cord injury. *J. Cell Mol. Med.* **2017**, *21*, 941–954. [CrossRef] [PubMed]
18. Rodriguez-Jimenez, F.J.; Alastrue, A.; Stojkovic, M.; Erceg, S.; Moreno-Manzano, V. Connexin 50 modulates Sox2 expression in spinal-cord-derived ependymal stem/progenitor cells. *Cell Tissue Res.* **2016**, *365*, 295–307. [CrossRef] [PubMed]

19. Gris, P.; Tighe, A.; Levin, D.; Sharma, R.; Brown, A. Transcriptional regulation of scar gene expression in primary astrocytes. *Glia* **2007**, *55*, 1145–1155. [CrossRef] [PubMed]
20. Allison, D.J.; Ditor, D.S. Immune dysfunction and chronic inflammation following spinal cord injury. *Spinal Cord* **2015**, *53*, 14–18. [CrossRef] [PubMed]
21. David, S.; Wee Yong, V. Harmful and beneficial effects of inflammation after spinal cord injury: Potential therapeutic implications. *Handb. Clin. Neurol.* **2012**, *109*, 485–502. [PubMed]
22. Yılmaz, T.; Kaptanoğlu, E. Current and future medical therapeutic strategies for the functional repair of spinal cord injury. *World J. Orthop.* **2015**, *6*, 42–55. [CrossRef] [PubMed]
23. Wilson, J.R.; Forgione, N.; Fehlings, M.G. Emerging therapies for acute traumatic spinal cord injury. *CMAJ* **2013**, *185*, 485–492. [CrossRef] [PubMed]
24. Cengiz, S.L.; Kalkan, E.; Bayir, A.; Ilik, K.; Basefer, A. Timing of thoracolomber spine stabilization in trauma patients; impact on neurological outcome and clinical course. A real prospective (rct) randomized controlled study. *Arch. Orthop. Trauma Surg.* **2008**, *128*, 959–966. [CrossRef] [PubMed]
25. Saxler, G.; Krämer, J.; Barden, B.; Kurt, A.; Pförtner, J.; Bernsmann, K. The long-term clinical sequelae of incidental durotomy in lumbar disc surgery. *Spine* **2005**, *30*, 2298–2302. [CrossRef] [PubMed]
26. Dididze, M.; Green, B.A.; Dietrich, W.D.; Vanni, S.; Wang, M.Y.; Levi, A.D. Systemic hypothermia in acute cervical spinal cord injury: A case-controlled study. *Spinal Cord* **2013**, *51*, 395–400. [CrossRef] [PubMed]
27. Levi, A.D.; Casella, G.; Green, B.A.; Dietrich, W.D.; Vanni, S.; Jagid, J.; Wang, M.Y. Clinical outcomes using modest intravascular hypothermia after acute cervical spinal cord injury. *Neurosurgery* **2010**, *66*, 670–677. [CrossRef] [PubMed]
28. Hansebout, R.R.; Hansebout, C.R. Local cooling for traumatic spinal cord injury: Outcomes in 20 patients and review of the literature. *J. Neurosurg. Spine* **2014**, *20*, 550–561. [CrossRef] [PubMed]
29. Wang, J.; Pearse, D.D. Therapeutic Hypothermia in Spinal Cord Injury: The Status of Its Use and Open Questions. *Int. J. Mol. Sci.* **2015**, *16*, 16848–16879. [CrossRef] [PubMed]
30. Polderman, K.H. Mechanisms of action, physiological effects, and complications of hypothermia. *Crit. Care Med.* **2009**, *37* (Suppl. 7), S186–S202. [CrossRef] [PubMed]
31. Rogers, W.K.; Todd, M. Acute spinal cord injury. *Best Pract. Res. Clin. Anaesthesiol.* **2016**, *30*, 27–39. [CrossRef] [PubMed]
32. Coutinho, A.E.; Chapman, K.E. The anti-inflammatory and immunosuppressive effects of glucocorticoids, recent developments and mechanistic insights. *Mol. Cell. Endocrinol.* **2011**, *335*, 2–13. [CrossRef] [PubMed]
33. Bracken, M.B.; Shepard, M.J.; Collins, W.F.; Holford, T.R.; Young, W.; Baskin, D.S.; Eisenberg, H.M.; Flamm, E.; Leo-Summers, L.; Maroon, J.; et al. A randomized, controlled trial of methylprednisolone or naloxone in the treatment of acute spinal-cord injury: Results of the second National Acute Spinal Cord Injury Study. *N. Engl. J. Med.* **1990**, *322*, 1405–1411. [CrossRef] [PubMed]
34. Bracken, M.B.; Shepard, M.J.; Holford, T.R.; Leo-Summers, L.; Aldrich, E.F.; Fazl, M.; Fehlings, M.; Herr, D.L.; Hitchon, P.W.; Marshall, L.F.; et al. Administration of methyl prednisolone for 24 or 48 hours or tirilazad mesylate for 48 hours in the treatment of acute spinal cord injury: Results of the third National Acute Spinal Cord Injury randomized controlled trial. *JAMA* **1997**, *277*, 1597–1604. [CrossRef] [PubMed]
35. Ito, Y.; Sugimoto, Y.; Tomioka, M.; Kai, N.; Tanaka, M. Does high dose methylprednisolone sodium succinate really improve neurological status in patient with acute cervical cord injury? A prospective study about neurological recovery and early complications. *Spine* **2009**, *34*, 2121–2124. [CrossRef] [PubMed]
36. Pointillart, V.; Petitjean, M.E.; Wiart, L.; Vital, J.M.; Lassié, P.; Thicoipé, M.; Dabadie, P. Pharmacological therapy of spinal cord injury during the acute phase. *Spinal Cord* **2000**, *38*, 71–76. [CrossRef] [PubMed]
37. Matsumoto, T.; Tamaki, T.; Kawakami, M.; Yoshida, M.; Ando, M.; Yamada, H. Earlycomplications of high-dose methylprednisolone sodium succinate treatment in the follow-up of acute cervical spinal cord injury. *Spine* **2001**, *26*, 426–430. [CrossRef] [PubMed]
38. Grossman, R.G.; Fehlings, M.G.; Frankowski, R.F.; Burau, K.D.; Chow, D.S.; Tator, C.; Teng, A.; Toups, E.G.; Harrop, J.S.; Aarabi, B.; et al. A prospective, multicenter, phase I matched-comparison group trial of safety, pharmacokinetics, and preliminary efficacy of riluzole in patients with traumatic spinal cord injury. *J. Neurotrauma* **2014**, *31*, 239–255. [CrossRef] [PubMed]
39. Geisler, F.H.; Coleman, W.P.; Grieco, G.; Poonian, D. Sygen Study Group: The Sygen multicenter acute spinal cord injury study. *Spine* **2001**, *26* (Suppl. 24), S87–S98. [CrossRef] [PubMed]

40. Fehlings, M.G.; Theodore, N.; Harrop, J.; Maurais, G.; Kuntz, C.; Shaffrey, C.I.; Kwon, B.K.; Chapman, J.; Yee, A.; Tighe, A.; et al. A phase I/IIa clinical trial of a recombinant Rho protein antagonist in acute spinal cord injury. *J. Neurotrauma* **2011**, *28*, 787–796. [CrossRef] [PubMed]
41. Casha, S.; Zygun, D.; McGowan, M.D.; Bains, I.; Yong, V.W.; Hurlbert, R.J. Results of a phase II placebo-controlled randomized trial of minocycline in acute spinal cord injury. *Brain* **2012**, *135 Pt 4*, 1224–1236. [CrossRef] [PubMed]
42. Inada, T.; Takahashi, H.; Yamazaki, M.; Okawa, A.; Sakuma, T.; Kato, K.; Hashimoto, M.; Hayashi, K.; Furuya, T.; Fujiyoshi, T.; et al. Multicenter prospective nonrandomized controlled clinical trial to prove neurotherapeutic effects of granulocyte colony-stimulating factor for acute spinal cord injury: Analyses of follow-up cases after at least 1 year. *Spine* **2014**, *39*, 213–219. [CrossRef] [PubMed]
43. Smith, A.G. Embryo-derived stem cells: Of mice and men. *Annu. Rev. Cell Dev. Biol.* **2001**, *17*, 435–462. [CrossRef] [PubMed]
44. Thomson, J.A.; Itskovitz-Eldor, J.; Shapiro, S.S.; Waknitz, M.A.; Swiergiel, J.J.; Marshall, V.S.; Jones, J.M. Embryonic stem cell lines derived from human blastocysts. *Science* **1998**, *28*, 1145114–1145117. [CrossRef]
45. Reubinoff, B.E.; Pera, M.F.; Fong, C.Y.; Trounson, A.; Bongso, A. Embryonic stem cell lines from human blastocysts: Somatic differentiation in vitro. *Nat. Biotechnol.* **2000**, *18*, 399–404. [CrossRef] [PubMed]
46. Lukovic, D.; Moreno Manzano, V.; Stojkovic, M.; Bhattacharya, S.S.; Erceg, S. Concise review: Human pluripotent stem cells in the treatment of spinal cord injury. *Stem Cells* **2012**, *30*, 1787–1792. [CrossRef] [PubMed]
47. Nistor, G.I.; Totoiu, M.O.; Haque, N.; Carpenter, M.K.; Keirstead, H.S. Human embryonic stem cells differentiate into oligodendrocytes in high purity and myelinate after spinal cord transplantation. *Glia* **2005**, *49*, 385–396. [CrossRef] [PubMed]
48. Keirstead, H.S.; Nistor, G.; Bernal, G.; Totoiu, M.; Cloutier, F.; Sharp, K.; Steward, O. Human embryonic stem cell derived oligodendrocyte progenitor cell transplants remyelinate and restore locomotion after spinal cord injury. *J. Neurosci.* **2005**, *25*, 4694–4705. [CrossRef] [PubMed]
49. Cloutier, F.; Siegenthaler, M.M.; Nistor, G.; Keirstead, H.S. Transplantation of human embryonic stem cell-derived oligodendrocyte progenitors into rat t spinal cord injuries does not cause harm. *Regen. Med.* **2006**, *1*, 469–479. [CrossRef] [PubMed]
50. Salewski, R.P.; Mitchell, R.A.; Shen, C.; Fehlings, M.G. Transplantation of neural stem cells clonally derived from embryonic stem cells promotes recovery after murine spinal cord injury. *Stem Cells Dev.* **2015**, *24*, 36–50. [CrossRef] [PubMed]
51. Faulkner, J.; Keirstead, H.S. Human embryonic stem cell-derived oligodendrocyte progenitors for the treatment of spinal cord injury. *Transpl. Immunol.* **2005**, *15*, 131–142. [CrossRef] [PubMed]
52. Zhang, Y.W.; Denham, J.; Thies, R.S. Oligodendrocyte progenitor cells derived from human embryonic stem cells express neurotrophic factors. *Stem Cells* **2006**, *15*, 943–952. [CrossRef] [PubMed]
53. Erceg, S.; Laínez, S.; Ronaghi, M.; Stojkovic, P.; Pérez-Aragó, M.A.; Moreno-Manzano, V.; Moreno-Palanques, R.; Planells-Cases, R.; Stojkovic, M. Differentiation of human embryonic stem cells to regional specific neural precursors in chemically defined medium conditions. *PLoS ONE* **2008**, *3*, e2122. [CrossRef] [PubMed]
54. Lukovic, D.; Moreno-Manzano, V.; Lopez-Mocholi, E.; Rodriguez-Jiménez, F.J.; Jendelova, P.; Sykova, E.; Oria, M.; Stojkovic, M.; Erceg, S. Complete rat spinal cord transection as a faithful model of spinal cord injury for translational cell transplantation. *Sci. Rep.* **2015**, *5*, 9640. [CrossRef] [PubMed]
55. Erceg, S.; Ronaghi, M.; Oria, M.; Roselló, M.G.; Aragó, M.A.; Lopez, M.G.; Radojevic, I.; Moreno-Manzano, V.; Rodríguez-Jiménez, F.J.; Bhattacharya, S.S.; et al. Transplanted oligodendrocytes and motoneuron progenitors generated from human embryonic stem cells promote locomotor recovery after spinal cord transection. *Stem Cells* **2010**, *28*, 1541–1549. [CrossRef] [PubMed]
56. Moreno-Manzano, V.; Rodríguez-Jiménez, F.J.; García-Roselló, M.; Laínez, S.; Erceg, S.; Calvo, M.T.; Ronaghi, M.; Lloret, M.; Planells-Cases, R.; Sánchez-Puelles, J.M.; et al. Activated spinal cord ependymal stem cells rescue neurological function. *Stem Cells* **2009**, *27*, 733–743. [CrossRef] [PubMed]
57. Tetzlaff, W.; Okon, E.B.; Karimi-Abdolrezaee, S.; Hill, C.E.; Sparling, J.S.; Plemel, J.R.; Plunet, W.T.; Tsai, E.C.; Baptiste, D.; Smithson, L.J.; et al. A systematic review of cellular transplantation therapies for spinal cord injury. *J. Neurotrauma* **2011**, *28*, 1611–1682. [CrossRef] [PubMed]
58. Takahashi, K.; Yamanaka, S. Induction of pluripotent stem cells from mouse embryonic and adult fibroblast cultures by defined factors. *Cell* **2006**, *126*, 663–676. [CrossRef] [PubMed]

59. Volarevic, V.; Markovic, B.S.; Gazdic, M.; Volarevic, A.; Jovicic, N.; Arsenijevic, N.; Armstrong, L.; Djonov, V.; Lako, M.; Stojkovic, M. Ethical and Safety Issues of Stem Cell-Based Therapy. *Int. J. Med. Sci.* **2018**, *15*, 36–45. [CrossRef] [PubMed]
60. Stadtfeld, M.; Nagaya, M.; Utikal, J.; Weir, G.; Hochedlinger, K. Induced pluripotent stem cells generated without viral integration. *Science* **2008**, *322*, 945–949. [CrossRef] [PubMed]
61. Okita, K.; Nakagawa, M.; Hyenjong, H.; Ichisaka, T.; Yamanaka, S. Generation of mouse induced pluripotent stem cells without viral vectors. *Science* **2008**, *322*, 949–953. [CrossRef] [PubMed]
62. Soldner, F.; Hockemeyer, D.; Beard, C.; Gao, Q.; Bell, G.W.; Cook, E.G.; Hargus, G.; Blak, A.; Cooper, O.; Mitalipova, M.; et al. Parkinson's disease patient-derived induced pluripotent stem cells free of viral reprogramming factors. *Cell* **2009**, *136*, 964–977. [CrossRef] [PubMed]
63. Plath, K.; Lowry, W.E. Progress in understanding reprogramming to the induced pluripotent state. *Nat. Rev. Genet.* **2011**, *12*, 253–265. [CrossRef] [PubMed]
64. Woltjen, K.; Michael, I.P.; Mohseni, P.; Desai, R.; Mileikovsky, M.; Hämäläinen, R.; Cowling, R.; Wang, W.; Liu, P.; Gertsenstein, M.; et al. piggyBac transposition reprograms fibroblasts to induced pluripotent stem cells. *Nature* **2009**, *458*, 766–770. [CrossRef] [PubMed]
65. Zhang, Y.; Pak, C.; Han, Y.; Ahlenius, H.; Zhang, Z.; Chanda, S.; Marro, S.; Patzke, C.; Acuna, C.; Covy, J.; et al. Rapid single-step induction of functional neurons from human pluripotent stem cells. *Neuron* **2013**, *78*, 785–798. [CrossRef] [PubMed]
66. Hallett, P.J.; Deleidi, M.; Astradsson, A.; Smith, G.A.; Cooper, O.; Osborn, T.M.; Sundberg, M.; Moore, M.A.; Perez-Torres, E.; Brownell, A.L.; et al. Successful function of autologous iPSC-derived dopamine neurons following transplantation in an on-human primate model of Parkinson's Disease. *Cell Stem Cell* **2015**, *16*, 269–274. [CrossRef] [PubMed]
67. Sareen, D.; O'Rourke, J.G.; Meera, P.; Muhammad, A.K.; Grant, S.; Simpkinson, M.; Bell, S.; Carmona, S.; Ornelas, L.; Sahabian, A.; et al. Targeting RNA foci in iPSC-derived motor neurons from ALS patients with a C9ORF72 repeat expansion. *Sci. Transl. Med.* **2013**, *5*, 208ra149. [CrossRef] [PubMed]
68. Karumbayaram, S.; Novitch, B.G.; Patterson, M.; Umbach, J.A.; Richter, L.; Lindgren, A.; Conway, A.E.; Clark, A.T.; Goldman, S.A.; Plath, K.; et al. Directed differentiation of human-induced pluripotent stem cells generates active motor neurons. *Stem Cells* **2009**, *27*, 806–811. [CrossRef] [PubMed]
69. Jha, B.S.; Rao, M.; Malik, N. Motor neuron differentiation from pluripotent stem cells and other intermediate proliferative precursors that can be discriminated by lineage specific reporters. *Stem Cell Rev.* **2015**, *11*, 194–204. [CrossRef] [PubMed]
70. Nicholas, C.R.; Chen, J.; Tang, Y.; Southwell, D.G.; Chalmers, N.; Vogt, D.; Arnold, C.M.; Chen, Y.J.; Stanley, E.G.; Elefanty, A.G.; et al. Functional maturation of hPSC-derived forebrain interneurons requires an extended timeline and mimics human neural development. *Cell Stem Cell* **2013**, *12*, 573–586. [CrossRef] [PubMed]
71. Chambers, S.M.; Mica, Y.; Lee, G.; Studer, L.; Tomishima, M.J. Dual-SMAD Inhibition/WNT Activation-Based Methods to Induce Neural Crest and Derivatives from Human Pluripotent Stem Cells. *Methods Mol. Biol.* **2016**, *1307*, 329–343. [PubMed]
72. Muratore, C.R.; Srikanth, P.; Callahan, D.G.; Young-Pearse, T.L. Comparison and optimization of hiPSC forebrain cortical differentiation protocols. *PLoS ONE* **2014**, *9*, e105807. [CrossRef] [PubMed]
73. Salewski, R.P.; Mitchell, R.A.; Li, L.; Shen, C.; Milekovskaia, M.; Nagy, A.; Fehlings, M.G. Transplantation of Induced Pluripotent Stem Cell-Derived Neural Stem Cells Mediate Functional Recovery Following Thoracic Spinal Cord Injury Through Remyelination of Axons. *Stem Cells Transl. Med.* **2015**, *4*, 743–754. [CrossRef] [PubMed]
74. Nagoshi, N.; Okano, H. Applications of induced pluripotent stem cell technologies in spinal cord injury. *J. Neurochem.* **2017**, *141*, 848–860. [CrossRef] [PubMed]
75. Fujimoto, Y.; Abematsu, M.; Falk, A.; Tsujimura, K.; Sanosaka, T.; Juliandi, B.; Semi, K.; Namihira, M.; Komiya, S.; Smith, A.; et al. Treatment of a mouse model of spinal cord injury by transplantation of human induced pluripotent stem cell-derived long-term self-renewing neuroepithelial-like stem cells. *Stem Cells* **2012**, *30*, 1163–1173. [CrossRef] [PubMed]

76. Kobayashi, Y.; Okada, Y.; Itakura, G.; Iwai, H.; Nishimura, S.; Yasuda, A.; Nori, S.; Hikishima, K.; Konomi, T.; Fujiyoshi, K.; et al. Pre-evaluated safe human iPSC-derived neural stem cells promote functional recovery after spinal cord injury in common marmoset without tumorigenicity. *PLoS ONE* **2012**, *7*, e52787. [CrossRef] [PubMed]
77. Nutt, S.E.; Chang, E.A.; Suhr, S.T.; Schlosser, L.O.; Mondello, S.E.; Moritz, C.T.; Cibelli, J.B.; Horner, P.J. Caudalized human iPSC-derived neural progenitor cells produce neurons and glia but fail to restore function in an early chronic spinal cord injury model. *Exp. Neurol.* **2013**, *248*, 491–503. [CrossRef] [PubMed]
78. Amemori, T.; Ruzicka, J.; Romanyuk, N.; Jhanwar-Uniyal, M.; Sykova, E.; Jendelova, P. Comparison of intraspinal and intrathecal implantation of induced pluripotent stem cell-derived neural precursors for the treatment of spinal cord injury in rats. *Stem Cell Res. Ther.* **2015**, *6*, 257. [CrossRef] [PubMed]
79. Hayashi, K.; Hashimoto, M.; Koda, M.; Naito, A.T.; Murata, A.; Okawa, A.; Takahashi, K.; Yamazaki, M. Increase of sensitivity to mechanical stimulus after transplantation of murine induced pluripotent stem cell-derived astrocytes in a rat spinal cord injury model. *J. Neurosurg. Spine* **2011**, *15*, 582–593. [CrossRef] [PubMed]
80. Barnabé-Heider, F.; Göritz, C.; Sabelström, H.; Takebayashi, H.; Pfrieger, F.W.; Meletis, K.; Frisén, J. Origin of new glial cells in intact and injured adult spinal cord. *Cell Stem Cell* **2010**, *7*, 470–482. [CrossRef] [PubMed]
81. Horner, P.; Power, A.; Kempermann, G.; Kuhn, H.; Palmer, T.; Winkler, J.; Thal, L.; Gage, F. Proliferation and differentiation of progenitor cells throughout the intact adult rat spinal cord. *J. Neurosci.* **2000**, *20*, 2218–2228. [PubMed]
82. Meletis, K.; Barnabé-Heider, F.; Carlén, M.; Evergren, E.; Tomilin, N.; Shupliakov, O.; Frisén, J.; Abeliovich, A. Spinal cord injury reveals multilineage differentiation of ependymal cells. *PLoS Biol.* **2008**, *6*, e182. [CrossRef] [PubMed]
83. Burda, J.E.; Sofroniew, M.V. Reactive gliosis and the multicellular response to CNS damage and disease. *Neuron* **2014**, *81*, 229–248. [CrossRef] [PubMed]
84. Whittaker, M.T.; Zai, L.J.; Lee, H.J.; Pajoohesh-Ganji, A.; Wu, J.; Sharp, A.; Wyse, R.; Wrathall, J.R. GGF2 (Nrg1-beta3) treatment enhances NG2+ cell response and improves functional recovery after spinal cord injury. *Glia* **2012**, *60*, 281–294. [CrossRef] [PubMed]
85. Schonberg, D.L.; Goldstein, E.Z.; Sahinkaya, F.R.; Wei, P.; Popovich, P.G.; McTigue, D.M. Ferritin stimulates oligodendrocyte genesis in the adult spinal cord and can be transferred from macrophages to NG2 cells in vivo. *J. Neurosci.* **2012**, *32*, 5374–5384. [CrossRef] [PubMed]
86. Lee-Liu, D.; Edwards-Faret, G.; Tapia, V.S.; Larraín, J. Spinal cord regeneration: Lessons for mammals from non-mammalian vertebrates. *Genesis* **2013**, *51*, 529–544. [CrossRef] [PubMed]
87. Silver, J.; Miller, J.H. Regeneration beyond the glial scar. *Nat. Rev. Neurosci.* **2004**, *5*, 146–156. [CrossRef] [PubMed]
88. Bradbury, E.J.; Carter, L.M. Manipulating the glial scar: Chondroitinase ABC as a therapy for spinal cord injury. *Brain Res. Bull.* **2011**, *84*, 306–316. [CrossRef] [PubMed]
89. Bruni, J.E. Ependymal development, proliferation, and functions: A review. *Microsc. Res. Tech.* **1998**, *41*, 2–13. [CrossRef]
90. Dromard, C.; Guillon, H.; Rigau, V.; Ripoll, C.; Sabourin, J.C.; Perrin, F.E.; Scamps, F.; Bozza, S.; Sabatier, P.; Lonjon, N.; et al. Adult human spinal cord harbors neural precursor cells that generate neurons and glial cells in vitro. *J. Neurosci. Res.* **2008**, *86*, 1916–1926. [CrossRef] [PubMed]
91. Blasko, J.; Martoncikova, M.; Lievajova, K.; Saganova, K.; Korimova, A.; Racekova, E. Regional differences of proliferation activity in the spinal cord ependyma of adult rats. *Open Life Sci.* **2012**, *7*, 397–403. [CrossRef]
92. Johansson, C.B.; Momma, S.; Clarke, D.L.; Risling, M.; Lendahl, U.; Frisén, J. Identification of a neural stem cell in the adult mammalian central nervous system. *Cell* **1999**, *96*, 25–34. [CrossRef]
93. Mothe, A.J.; Tator, C.H. Proliferation, migration, and differentiation of endogenous ependymal region stem/progenitor cells following minimal spinal cord injury in the adult rat. *Neuroscience* **2005**, *131*, 177–187. [CrossRef] [PubMed]
94. Duan, H.; Song, W.; Zhao, W.; Gao, Y.; Yang, Z.; Li, X. Endogenous neurogenesis in adult mammals after spinal cord injury. *Sci. China Life Sci.* **2016**, *59*, 1313–1318. [CrossRef] [PubMed]
95. Frisén, J.; Johansson, C.B.; Török, C.; Risling, M.; Lendahl, U. Rapid, widespread, and longlasting induction of nestin contributes to the generation of glial scar tissue after CNS injury. *J. Cell Biol.* **1995**, *131*, 453–464. [CrossRef] [PubMed]

96. Bélanger, M.; Magistretti, P.J. The role of astroglia in neuroprotection. *Dialogues Clin. Neurosci.* **2009**, *11*, 281–295. [PubMed]
97. Wiese, S.; Karus, M.; Faissner, A. Astrocytes as a source for extracellular matrix molecules and cytokines. *Front. Pharmacol.* **2012**, *3*, 120. [CrossRef] [PubMed]
98. Hamann, M.C.J.; Tator, C.H.; Shoichet, M.S. Injectable intrathecal delivery system for localized administration of EGF and FGF-2 to the injured rat spinal cord. *Exp. Neurol.* **2005**, *194*, 106–119. [CrossRef] [PubMed]
99. Moreno-Manzano, V.; Rodríguez-Jiménez, F.J.; Aceña-Bonilla, J.L.; Fustero-Lardíes, S.; Erceg, S.; Dopazo, J.; Montaner, D.; Stojkovic, M.; Sánchez-Puelles, J.M. FM19G11, a new hypoxia-inducible factor (HIF) modulator, affects stem cell differentiation status. *J. Biol. Chem.* **2010**, *285*, 1333–1342. [CrossRef] [PubMed]
100. Rodríguez-Jimnez, F.J.; Alastrue-Agudo, A.; Erceg, S.; Stojkovic, M.; Moreno-Manzano, V. FM19G11 favors spinal cord injury regeneration and stem cell self-renewal by mitochondrial uncoupling and glucose metabolism induction. *Stem Cells* **2012**, *30*, 2221–2233. [CrossRef] [PubMed]
101. Rodriguez-Jimenez, F.J.; Alastrue-Agudo, A.; Stojkovic, M.; Erceg, S.; Moreno-Manzano, V. Connexin 50 Expression in Ependymal Stem Progenitor Cells after Spinal Cord Injury Activation. *Int. J. Mol. Sci.* **2015**, *16*, 26608–26618. [CrossRef] [PubMed]
102. Gómez-Villafuertes, R.; Rodríguez-Jiménez, F.J.; Alastrue-Agudo, A.; Stojkovic, M.; Miras-Portugal, M.T.; Moreno-Manzano, V. Purinergic Receptors in Spinal Cord-Derived Ependymal Stem/Progenitor Cells and Their Potential Role in Cell-Based Therapy for Spinal Cord Injury. *Cell Transpl.* **2015**, *24*, 1493–1509. [CrossRef] [PubMed]
103. Alastrue-Agudo, A.; Rodriguez-Jimenez, F.J.; Mocholi, E.L.; De Giorgio, F.; Erceg, S.; Moreno-Manzano, V. FM19G11 and Ependymal Progenitor/Stem Cell Combinatory Treatment Enhances Neuronal Preservation and Oligodendrogenesis after Severe Spinal Cord Injury. *Int. J. Mol. Sci.* **2018**, *19*, 200. [CrossRef] [PubMed]
104. Valdes-Sánchez, T.; Rodriguez-Jimenez, F.J.; García-Cruz, D.M.; Escobar-Ivirico, J.L.; Alastrue-Agudo, A.; Erceg, S.; Monleón, M.; Moreno-Manzano, V. Methacrylate-endcapped caprolactone and FM19G11 provide a proper niche for spinal cord-derived neural cells. *J. Tissue Eng. Regen. Med.* **2015**, *9*, 734–739. [CrossRef] [PubMed]

6

Level-Specific Differences in Systemic Expression of Pro- and Anti-Inflammatory Cytokines and Chemokines after Spinal Cord Injury

James Hong [1,2], Alex Chang [1,2], Mohammad-Masoud Zavvarian [1,2], Jian Wang [1], Yang Liu [1] and Michael G. Fehlings [1,3,*]

1 Division of Genetics and Development, Toronto Western Research Institute, University Health Network, Toronto, ON M5T 2S8, Canada; james.hong@live.com (J.H.); le.chang@mail.utoronto.ca (A.C.); Mohammad.zavvarian@mail.utoronto.ca (M.-M.Z.); jianw@uhnres.utoronto.ca (J.W.); Yang.Liu@uhnresearch.ca (Y.L.)

2 Institute of Medical Science, University of Toronto, Toronto, ON M5S 1A8, Canada

3 Spinal Program, University Health Network, Toronto Western Hospital, Toronto, ON M5T 2S8, Canada

* Correspondence: Michael.Fehlings@uhn.ca

Abstract: While over half of all spinal cord injuries (SCIs) occur in the cervical region, the majority of preclinical studies have focused on models of thoracic injury. However, these two levels are anatomically distinct—with the cervical region possessing a greater vascular supply, grey-white matter ratio and sympathetic outflow relative to the thoracic region. As such, there exists a significant knowledge gap in the secondary pathology at these levels following SCI. In this study, we characterized the systemic plasma markers of inflammation over time (1, 3, 7, 14, 56 days post-SCI) after moderate-severe, clip-compression cervical and thoracic SCI in a rat model. Using high-throughput ELISA panels, we observed a clear level-specific difference in plasma levels of VEGF, leptin, IP10, IL18, GCSF, and fractalkine. Overall, cervical SCI had reduced expression of both pro- and anti-inflammatory proteins relative to thoracic SCI, likely due to sympathetic dysregulation associated with higher level SCIs. However, contrary to the literature, we did not observe level-dependent splenic atrophy with our incomplete SCI model. This is the first study to compare the systemic plasma-level changes following cervical and thoracic SCI using level-matched and time-matched controls. The results of this study provide the first evidence in support of level-targeted intervention and also challenge the phenomenon of high SCI-induced splenic atrophy in incomplete SCI models.

Keywords: spinal cord injury; inflammation; plasma

---

1. Introduction

Traumatic spinal cord injury (SCI)—despite breakthroughs in pre-operative, surgical and post-operative care—continues to be a life-threatening injury, both acutely and chronically [1]. After primary mechanical injury, a dual-edged cascade of inflammatory and vascular events—collectively referred to as the secondary injury phase—ensues [2,3]. While it is difficult to determine the causative mechanism of secondary injury, several mechanisms including vascular disruption [4], glutamate excitoxicity [5,6], lipid peroxidation [7–9], blood-spinal-cord-barrier disruption [10–12] and ionic imbalance [13,14] have been the focus of therapeutic targeting. The ultimate consequence of these events is apoptosis, neuronal and axonal death, and de/dys-myelination manifesting as grey and white matter loss at the injury epicenter [1].

Preclinical SCI studies thus far, driven by post-operative care requirements and ease-of-use, have most commonly employed thoracic SCI (tSCI) models despite the increased prevalence and incidence of cervical SCI (cSCI) [15]. A central rationale for specifically investigating cSCI models is the appreciation that critical anatomical differences exist between the cervical and thoracic spinal cord resulting in different pathophysiological responses to injury and treatment [16]. For instance, the cervical spine is composed of smaller vertebrae with increased mobility, has increased central and peripheral vascular supply and flow, a higher gray-white matter ratio, and contains the neural circuitry crucial for respiration, forelimb motion, and sympathetic outflow to the heart. Pathophysiologically, the cervical gray matter vasculature has less pericyte coverage than the thoracic cord, resulting in a blood spinal cord barrier (BSCB) predisposed to increased permeability [10]. Further, in high-thoracic transection models of SCI, removal of spinal sympathetic preganglionic neurons from supraspinal control results in autonomic dysreflexia [17]. This in turn has been shown to instigate immunosuppressive effects—known as SCI-induced immune depression syndrome (SCI-IDS)—that stem directly from early splenocyte death and splenic atrophy due to acute and repeated chronic exposure to glucocorticoids and intrasplenic norepinephrine [18].

As cSCI has a direct neurological impact on cardiovascular function and peripheral immunity [19–21], we aimed to characterize the temporal profile (3–56 days) of vascular and inflammatory markers after cSCI and tSCI and elucidate any level-specific changes in their expression. Further, as robust spleen-mass changes were observed in the aforementioned transection studies on SCI-IDS, we also evaluated time and sham-normalized spleen-body weight ratios in our model.

2. Results

Of the 35 proteins surveyed in this study, 19 passed our initial filtering criteria, while 16 proteins that contained interpolated, extrapolated or out-of-range values were removed. All comparisons below are presented in order from thoracic to cervical.

2.1. *Level-Specific Differences in Plasma Protein Levels after Cervical and Thoracic Laminectomy*

To investigate whether there were baseline differences in the expression of any of these proteins after cervical and thoracic laminectomy, heat-mapping and statistical analyses of protein concentrations were carried out with naïve plasma shown as a reference (excluded from cluster analyses). Heat-mapping (Figure 1A) demonstrated several clusters of expression. While several proteins had trending differences (RANTES, $p = 0.06$ at 14 days; LIX, $p = 0.052$ at 14 days; and IL10, $p = 0.068$), two proteins within cluster 5 showed significant differences in the expression of IP10 (56 days, 131.5 ± 11.2 vs. 450.3 ± 15.8 pg/mL, $p = 0.003$) and IL18 (3 days, 745.1 ± 84.8 vs. 400.2 ± 47.5 pg/mL, $p = 0.036$). The time-series expression of these three proteins is shown in Figure 1B.

2.2. *Level-Specific Differences in Plasma Protein Levels after Cervical and Thoracic SCI*

Of the 19 proteins analyzed (Figure 2), six showed significant differences at one or more time-points between time-matched, level-matched, laminectomy-normalized cSCI and tSCI groups (expressed as fold-change to laminectomy). The six proteins that showed level-specific differences were VEGF (day 7, -0.1 ± 0.2 vs. 1.325 ± 0.1, $p = 0.03$), leptin (day 1, 1.2 ± 0.4 vs. -0.05 ± 0.3, $p = 0.04$; day 56, -0.1 ± 0.4 vs. -2.0 ± 0.4, $p = 0.0009$), IP10 (day 1, 0.3 ± 0.3 vs. -0.7 ± 0.04, $p = 0.02$; day 7, -0.891 ± 0.3 vs. 0.4 ± 0.2, $p = 0.0005$; day 56, 0.9 ± 0.2 vs. -1.0 ± 0.3, $p < 0.0001$), IL18 (day 56, -1.5 ± 0.3 vs. -0.05 ± 0.4, $p = 0.02$), GCSF (day 7, 1.010 ± 0.187 vs. 3.943 ± 1.663, $p = 0.006$), and fractalkine (day 1, 0.3 ± 0.1 vs. -0.6 ± 0.2, $p = 0.004$). Both of the proteins (IP10 and IL18) that showed level-specific baseline differences were significant after SCI. However, while differences in the 56-day baseline of IP10 contributed to a significant result, the 3-day baseline difference in IL18 did not.

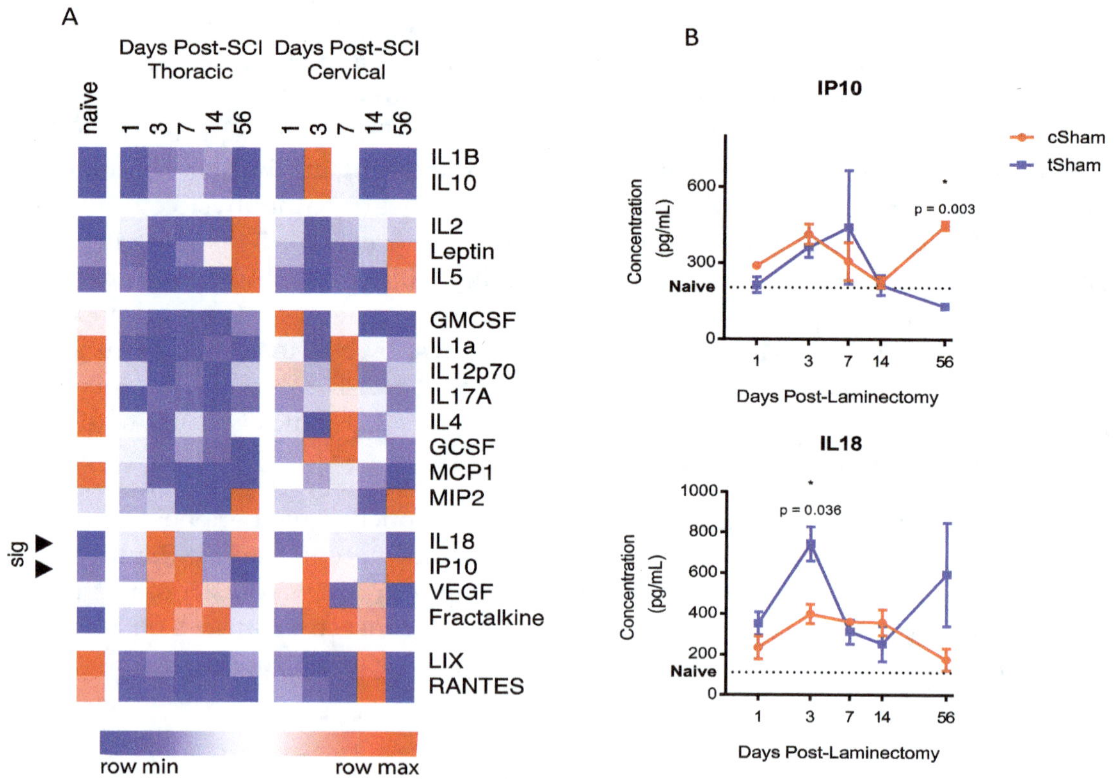

Figure 1. (**A**) Heat map and hierarchical cluster analyses reveal six clusters of temporal expression amongst cSham and tSham groups. Of the proteins analyzed, two proteins (marked with arrows) within cluster 4 reached statistical significance (IL18 and IP10). Naive data are shown as a baseline reference. Data are shown with relative color coding, with blue associated with the row minimum and red with the row maximum; all data are based on raw concentration in pg/mL; (**B**) Temporal expression of the two significant level-distinct proteins. Error bars represent SEM.

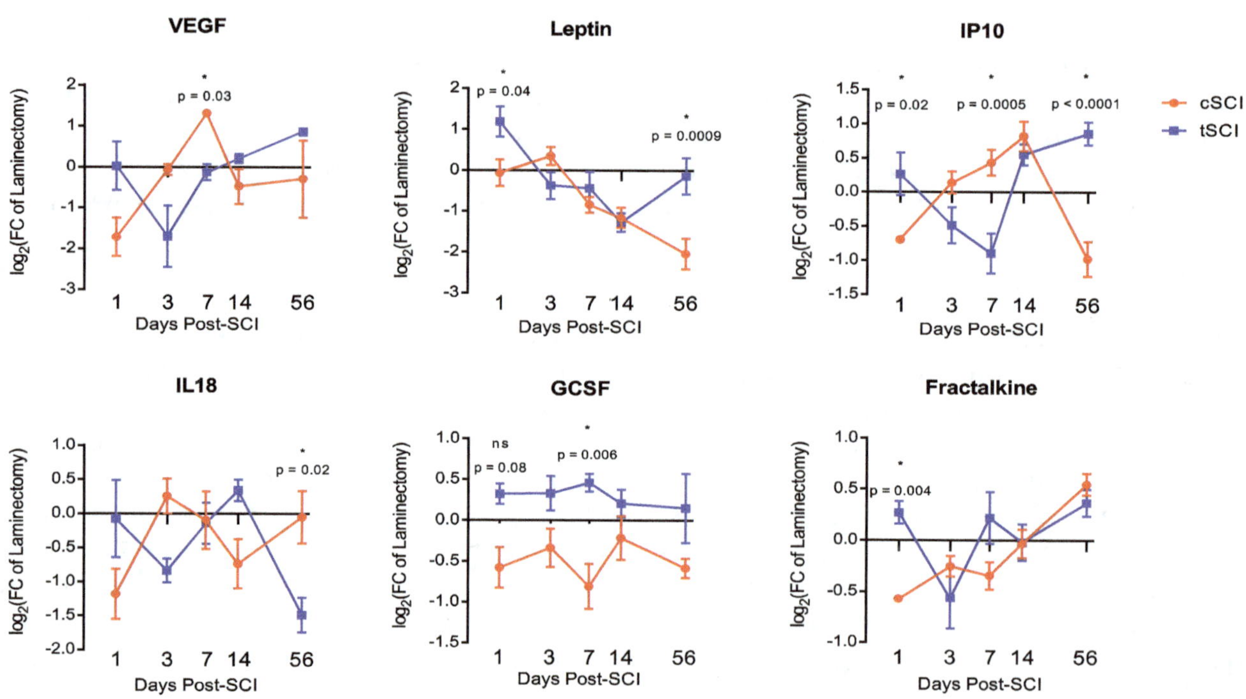

Figure 2. Temporal expression profile of the six significant differentially-expressed proteins: VEGF, leptin, IP10, IL18, GCSF and fractalkine. Error bars represent SEM.

2.3. Temporal Expression Patterns of Plasma Proteins after SCI

To dissect the various temporal expression patterns after cSCI and tSCI, heatmap and *k*-means cluster analysis were performed (Figure 3). In tSCI, three main clusters were found with cluster 1 showing acute/chronic upregulation with subacute downregulation; cluster 2 showing an acute/subacute upregulation with chronic downregulation; and cluster 3 consisting of a single member showing constitutive upregulation. Similarly, in cSCI, three major clusters were defined with cluster 1 showing constitutive downregulation with some acute upregulation; cluster 2 showing proteins with acute/subacute downregulation with chronic upregulation; and cluster 3 showing proteins that had acute/subacute upregulation followed by chronic downregulation.

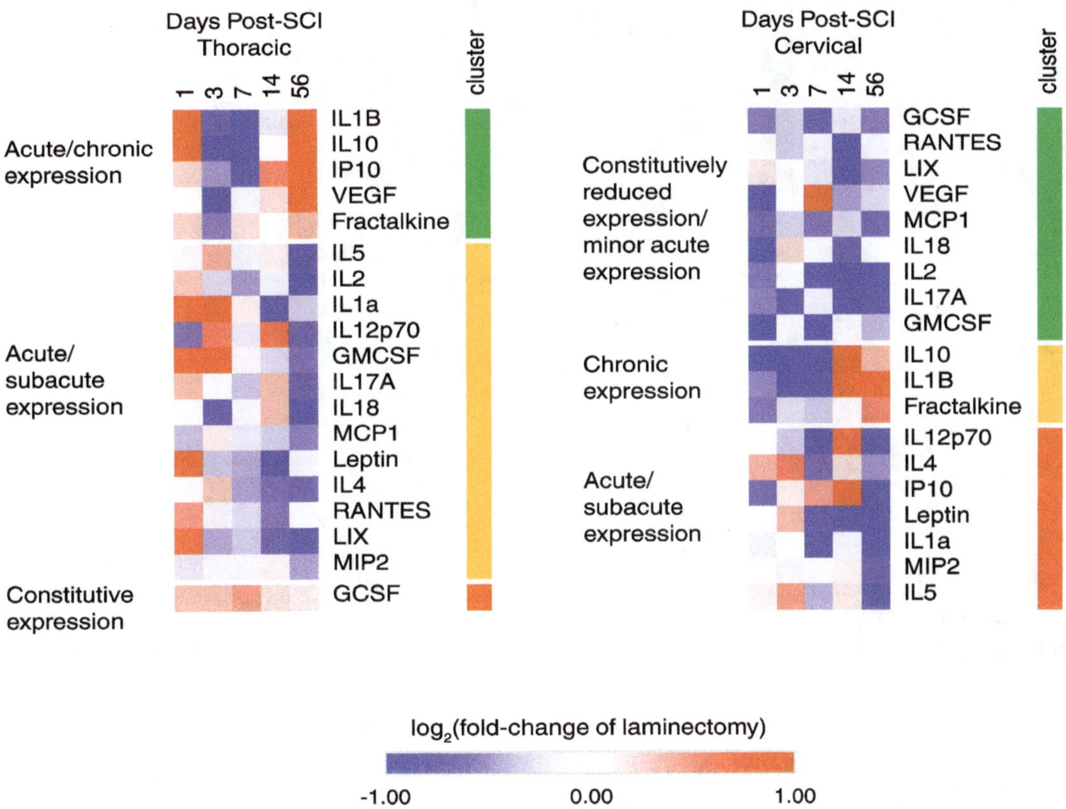

Figure 3. Heatmap and *k*-means clustering reveals three major clusters of temporal expression in cSCI and tSCI. Expression is displayed as log2 (fold-change of laminectomy) with blue indicating downregulation and red indicating upregulation.

2.4. Functional Classification of Serum Protein after SCI

Using several reviews and meta-analyses articles [22–29], pro-inflammatory and anti-inflammatory functions were assigned to each of the 19 proteins to survey the overall inflammatory status after cSCI and tSCI (Figure 4). It is evident that overall, tSCI has increased expression of both pro- and anti-inflammatory proteins over time compared to cSCI. While most of these proteins are strikingly upregulated in the acute phase of thoracic relative to cervical SCI, a few of these differences equilibrated chronically (e.g., IL1b, fractalkine, IL10).

2.5. Spleen Weight

To identify whether splenic atrophy was observed in our model of incomplete SCI, mass-normalized spleen weights were measured and expressed as a fold-change of time-matched laminectomized shams (Figure 5). While a decrease in weight between injured and time-matched laminectomized shams was seen in both cSCI and tSCI, this did not reach statistical significance.

However, a significant increase in spleen weight was observed between 3 and 14 days in cSCI (0.862 ± 0.078 vs. 1.188 ± 0.113, $p = 0.03$), but only trended for tSCI ($p = 0.06$).

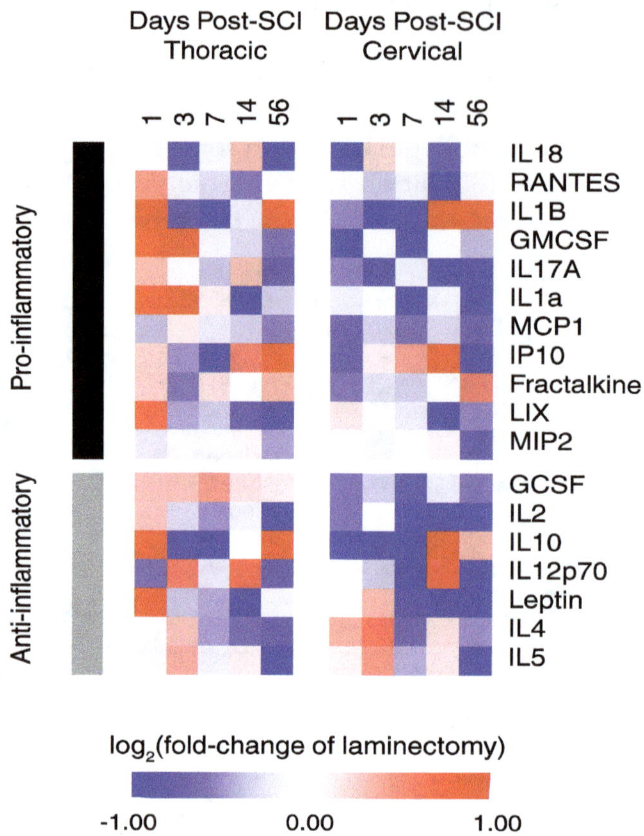

Figure 4. Heat map of functionally-segregated proteins after cSCI and tSCI. Expression is displayed as log2 (fold-change of laminectomy) with blue indicating downregulation and red indicating upregulation.

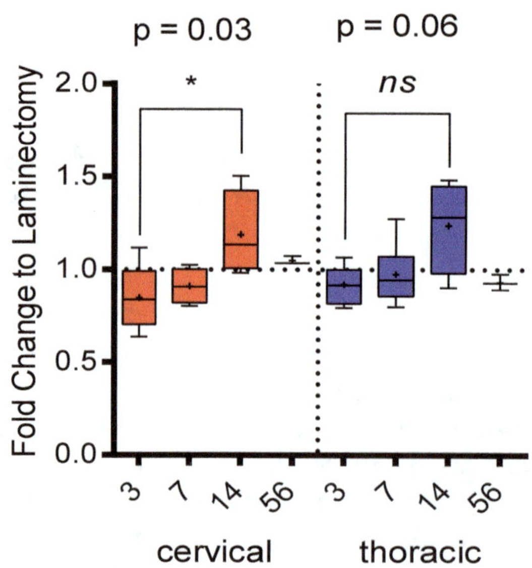

Figure 5. Mass: spleen ratios expressed as fold-change of time-matched laminectomized shams. Error bars represent SEM, and means are indicated by +. A significant change in spleen weight was observed in cSCI between day 3 and day 14.

3. Discussion

In summary, this is the first study to characterize the temporal plasma expression profile of multiple cytokines, chemokines and growth factors after SCI. It is also the first study to use clinically-relevant models of cSCI and tSCI to determine level-specific differences in the expression of these inflammation-related molecules. This study establishes three main points: (1) time and level-matched laminectomy controls are essential for accurate data interpretation after SCI; (2) there exist both acute and chronic differences in plasma protein expression between cSCI and tSCI; and (3) splenic atrophy is not a robust phenomenon after incomplete cSCI, and as there continues to be evidence of peripheral immune depression after cSCI, it is also not a conclusive diagnostic tool for assessing the state of SCI-IDS.

Inflammation after SCI is considered one of the major drivers of secondary injury and tissue loss, and is often considered a dual-edged sword [30,31]. Our current results examined a small percentage of the cytokine/chemokines/growth factors involved, however, due to the spectrum of cells that secrete these factors, we cannot accurately pinpoint the cellular mediators of the temporal and level-specific changes that we have observed. With regards to the cause of level-differences between laminectomized shams, it is likely they are due to the degree of invasiveness and its associated fibrosis above the site of laminectomy and its differential impact on the cord over time between the two levels.

Studies on five of the six level-distinct proteins have already been conducted in the rodent tSCI model, with IL18 being the only exception with no SCI-associated studies. VEGF is well-known as a potent angiogenic factor that promotes the growth and development of endothelial cells. Our lab was one of the first to study the role of VEGF as a therapeutic agent after acute tSCI [32,33]. In these studies, transcriptionally-enhancing VEGF expression resulted in increased axon preservation, reduced necrosis, and an increase in blood vessels that ultimately translated to increased functional recovery as measured by Catwalk gait analyses. Another study using a contusion tSCI model [34], found that acute intraspinal infusion of VEGF into the lesion epicentre induced autophagy and reduced inflammation in the spinal cord, ultimately resulting in functional recovery as measured by the BBB motor scale. In this study, they showed that VEGF administration reduced the expression of IL1b, IL10 and TNFa in in vitro cultures of LPS-treated neuro-glia co-cultures. In our study, VEGF was upregulated at day 7 relative to tSCI and this change did indeed coincide with striking systemic reductions in IL1b and IL10. Further, an upregulation of these proteins was observed at 14- and 56-days post-cSCI when VEGF expression returned to baseline. Perhaps one of the major underlying factors of this level-dependent change after cSCI is the impact of cervical injury on the systemic vasculature as autonomic dysreflexia contributes directly to frequent vascular stress. Overall, there is significant evidence to suggest that VEGF therapy would be effective in both acute cSCI and tSCI, with the potential to also reduce chronic inflammation in both models.

As a hormone produced mainly by adipose cells, leptin is crucial for energetic balance in the central nervous system. Previous studies into leptin have shown that it is often upregulated both locally and systemically after tSCI [35–37]. While these acute studies were severely limited by the lack of time-matched controls, we observed a striking upregulation of plasma leptin in tSCI, but not cSCI at 1- and 56-days post-SCI. As leptin is regulated by the sympathetic nervous system, a study has shown that patients with high level SCIs have dysfunctional leptin expression [38]—thus supporting our data. A study [39] that acutely administered purified leptin in a rodent model of tSCI showed increased expression of neuroprotective genes, reduced inflammation and improved BBB, Catwalk and von Frey metrics suggesting that acute and chronic leptin deficiency may be a potent therapeutic target in SCI.

An upregulation in systemic and local IP10 has been demonstrated in both human and rodent SCI [40–42], and while no time-matched controls were used, this upregulation persisted as long as 14 days post-SCI in the murine tSCI model. IP10, is a chemokine secreted by a wide array of immune cells, endothelial cells and fibroblasts in response to IFNg [43]. In our study, IP10 expression was inversely expressed between the two levels, with cSCI experiencing a peak of expression during the subacute phase (days 3–14), and tSCI in the acute and chronic phases (day 1 and 56). Studies that neutralized the expression of IP10 showed markedly reduced inflammation, apoptosis, tissue loss and showed modestly improved BBB and BMS outcomes [42,44,45].

While GCSF has had no reported systemic or local expression in the SCI literature, here we find that the expression of GCSF is opposite in cSCI and tSCI. That is, while GCSF is upregulated in tSCI, it is downregulated in cSCI with time-to-time changes also in contrary motion with the exception of day 56. As purified GCSF administration alone and in combination with adipose- and bone-marrow-derived stem and neural stem cells has been shown to be highly beneficial in rodent and human tSCI—including increased tissue preservation, reduced apoptosis and scarring, and improved BBB, BMS and A [46–56]—such a paradigm may prove to be even more effective in the all stages of cSCI where a deficiency in GCSF is seen.

Receptor knockouts of the fractalkine receptor CX3CR1 have resulted in reduced $iNOS^+/Ly6C^{low}/MHCII^+/CD11c^-$ macrophages and activated microglia that have reduced expression of IL6 and iNOS. In these studies, the authors observed modest improvements in the BMS score [57–59]. In our study, the systemic fractalkine ligand is significantly upregulated in tSCI at 1-day post-SCI relative to cSCI, with both tSCI and cSCI experiencing late peaks 56-days post-SCI. Fractalkine is present in both a cell-bound and soluble form, and while both forms are potent chemo-attractants for migrating monocytes, the soluble form is also known to attract T cells. As such, while fractalkine receptor antagonism may be an ideal therapeutic target for acute tSCI, it may also be a valuable target for chronic tSCI and cSCI.

Two potential mechanisms by which cSCI induces an overall decrease in circulating protein are (1) SCI-IDS [20,21] and (2) increased cellular localization (and as such cytokine/chemokines) to the site of injury [26,28,41]. SCI-IDS is a phenomenon characterized by rapid splenic atrophy due to repeated bouts of autonomic dysreflexia in higher-level injuries. Interestingly, level-dependent splenic atrophy was not observed between our two incomplete models of cSCI and tSCI (Figure 5). The latter cytokine/chemokine "sink" concept is well-supported by the literature, as recent characterizations of cytokine/chemokine profiles in the spinal cord of SCI rodents and individuals show a striking acute and chronically-persistent expression of many pro- and anti-inflammatory cytokines. This, in conjunction with the increased BSCB permeability after cSCI, may well result in the formation of an inflammatory *milieu* that can be a potent trigger for secondary injury—especially chronic inflammation. All in all, we have shown striking evidence of level-specific differences in the systemic plasma expression of various cytokines and chemokines. In light of these results, preclinical researchers should adapt time-matched laminectomized controls and consider the impact of anatomical level on the therapeutic target of interest.

4. Materials and Methods

All animal experiments were approved by the Animal Care Committee of the University Health Network (Project ID Code: #2212, Date of Approval: 17 May 2017) in compliance with the Canadian Council on Animal Care.

4.1. Clip-Compression SCI and Spleen Weight

Female adult Wistar rats (12-weeks old, 250–300 g, $n = 5$/group for injured, $n = 3$/group for laminectomy and naïve) were used (Charles River Laboratories, Wilmington, MA, USA, http://www.criver.com). Prior to surgery, 0.05 mg/kg of buprenorphine and 5 mL of saline were administered subcutaneously. 1–2% of isoflurane in a 1:1 mixture of O_2 and N_2O was used for anesthesia, and a laminectomy was performed at C6-7 and T6-7, respectively. Following this, a moderate-severe injury was induced for 1-min at the cervical or thoracic level as described previously [15,60]. Until the endpoint (1, 3, 7, 14, 56 days post-SCI), the animals were given subcutaneous buprenorphine (0.05 mg/kg, bid), oral amoxicillin trihydrate/clavulanate potassium (Apotex Pharmaceuticals, Toronto, ON, Canada) and subcutaneous saline injections (0.9%, 5 mL sid). Animals were housed individually in cages at 27 °C, and their bladders were manually expressed thrice daily until recovery.

Prior to sacrifice and perfusion, animal mass and spleens were collected from anesthetized rats and their weight recorded and normalized to their body mass.

4.2. Neurobehavioural Assessments

Starting at 7 days post-SCI, weekly forelimb and hindlimb function were assessed with the grip strength meter (SDI Grip Strength System DFM-10, San Diego Instruments, San Diego, CA, USA, http://www.sandiegoinstruments.com) and the BBB Locomotor Rating Scale [61] for cSCI and tSCI, respectively (Figure 6).

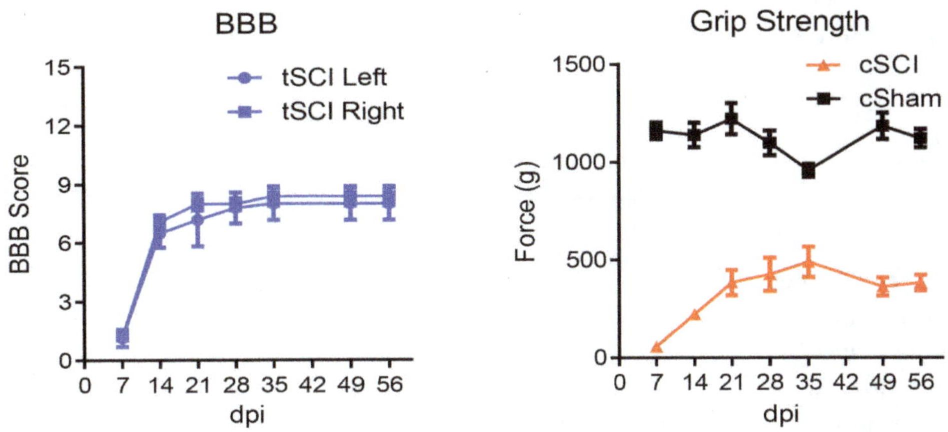

Figure 6. Hindlimb (BBB) and forelimb (Grip strength) assessments following tSCI and cSCI, respectively. No statistical outliers were detected using Grubb's test ($\alpha > 0.05$) indicating good homogeneity of data. Error bars represent SEM.

4.3. Blood Collection and High-Throughput ELISA

Blood was collected via a cardiac puncture prior to perfusion using a BD-Vacutainer® Safety-Lok™ (Franklin Lakes, New Jersey, US) blood collection set containing EDTA. The blood samples were kept on ice and immediately centrifuged at 3000 rpm (Eppendorf 5810R) for 10 min at 4 °C. The plasma (supernatant) was then carefully aspirated and transferred to a Protein Lo-Bind tube (Eppendorf, Hamburg, Germany). 100 µL of the sample was then sent to Eve Technologies (Calgary, AB, Canada, https://www.evetechnologies.com) for high-throughput ELISA profiling using their rat Discovery Assays™ for cytokine/chemokines (RD27) and vascular injury markers (P1, P2). All proteins that contained interpolated/extrapolated/out-of-range values were removed from the study. The concentration of these proteins was calculated using a standard curve and expressed in pg/mL.

4.4. Clustering and Statistical Analysis

Data are presented as mean±SEM and comparisons are presented in order from cervical to thoracic. Heatmap, *k*-means and hierarchical row clustering (1−Cosine Similarity) was performed using the Morpheus software package from the Broad Institute (Cambridge, MA, USA, https://software.broadinstitute.org/morpheus/). Assessment of normality was performed for each group using the Shapiro-Wilk test of the *Rfit* package. All protein level comparisons between cSCI and tSCI were performed in GraphPad using either the one-way ANOVA function with post-hoc Sidak's for multiple corrections (parametric, p-adjusted threshold = 0.05) or Krustal-Wallis test with post-hoc Dunn's for multiple corrections (non-parametric, p-adjusted threshold = 0.05). Spleen-body mass ratio comparisons were done in GraphPad using a one-way ANOVA with post-hoc Sidak for multiple corrections (p-adjusted threshold = 0.05).

Author Contributions: J.H.: conception and design, collection and/or assembly of data, data analysis and interpretation, manuscript writing, final approval of manuscript; A.C.: collection and/or assembly of data, data analysis, final approval of manuscript; M.-M.Z.: collection and/or assembly of data, final approval of manuscript; J.W.: collection and/or assembly of data, final approval of manuscript; Y.L.: collection and/or assembly of data, final approval of manuscript; M.G.F.: conception and design, data analysis and interpretation, financial support, manuscript editing, final approval of manuscript.

Acknowledgments: We thank Paul Bradshaw and Tim Worden for project management and manuscript review.

Abbreviations

BBB	Basso, Beattie and Bresnahan
BMS	Basso Mouse Scale
BSCB	Blood-spinal-cord-barrier
PBS	Phosphate buffer solution
SCI	Spinal cord injury
GMCSF	Granulocyte-macrophage colony-stimulating factor
IL1a	Interleukin 1 alpha
IL1b	Interleukin 1 beta
IL2	Interleukin-2
IL17A	Interleukin-17A
IL18	Interleukin-18
MCP1	Monocyte chemoattractant protein-1
IP10	Interferon gamma-induced protein 10
LIX	Lipopolysaccharide-induced CXC chemokine
MIP2	macrophage inflammatory protein 2
RANTES	regulated on activation, normal T cell expressed and secreted
GCSF	Granulocyte-colony stimulating factor
IL4	Interleukin-4
IL10	Interleukin-10
IL12	Interleukin-12
IL5	Interleukin-5
IFNg	Interferon gamma
VEGF	Vascular endothelial growth factor

References

1. Ahuja, C.S.; Wilson, J.R.; Nori, S.; Kotter, M.R.N.; Druschel, C.; Curt, A.; Fehlings, M.G. Traumatic spinal cord injury. *Nat. Rev. Dis. Primers* **2017**, *3*, 17018. [CrossRef] [PubMed]
2. Tator, C.H.; Fehlings, M.G. Review of the secondary injury theory of acute spinal cord trauma with emphasis on vascular mechanisms. *J. Neurosurg.* **1991**, *75*, 15–26. [CrossRef] [PubMed]
3. Tator, C.H.; Koyanagi, I. Vascular mechanisms in the pathophysiology of human spinal cord injury. *J. Neurosurg.* **1997**, *86*, 483–492. [CrossRef] [PubMed]
4. Figley, S.A.; Khosravi, R.; Legasto, J.M.; Tseng, Y.-F.; Fehlings, M.G. Characterization of vascular disruption and blood-spinal cord barrier permeability following traumatic spinal cord injury. *J. Neurotrauma* **2014**, *31*, 541–552. [CrossRef] [PubMed]
5. Rothstein, J.D.; Dykes-Hoberg, M.; Pardo, C.A.; Kanai, Y.; Bristol, L.A.; Kuncl, R.W.; Welty, D.F.; Jin, L.; Hediger, M.A.; Wang, Y.; et al. Knockout of Glutamate Transporters Reveals a Major Role for Astroglial Transport in Excitotoxicity and Clearance of Glutamate. *Neuron* **1996**, *16*, 675–686. [CrossRef]
6. Agrawal, S.K.; Fehlings, M.G. Role of NMDA and Non-NMDA Ionotropic Glutamate Receptors in Traumatic Spinal Cord Axonal Injury. *J. Neurosci.* **1997**, *17*, 1055–1063. [CrossRef] [PubMed]

7. Braughler, J.M.; Duncan, L.A.; Chase, R.L. Interaction of lipid peroxidation and calcium in the pathogenesis of neuronal injury. *Cent. Nerv. Syst. Trauma* **1985**, *2*, 269–283. [CrossRef] [PubMed]
8. Diaz-Ruiz, A.; Rios, C.; Duarte, I.; Correa, D.; Guizar-Sahagun, G.; Grijalva, I.; Ibarra, A. Cyclosporin-A inhibits lipid peroxidation after spinal cord injury in rats. *Neurosci. Lett.* **1999**, *266*, 61–64. [CrossRef]
9. Kaptanoglu, E.; Solaroglu, I.; Okutan, O.; Surucu, H.S.; Akbiyik, F.; Beskonakli, E. Erythropoietin exerts neuroprotection after acute spinal cord injury in rats: Effect on lipid peroxidation and early ultrastructural findings. *Neurosurg. Rev.* **2004**, *27*, 113–120. [CrossRef] [PubMed]
10. Winkler, E.A.; Sengillo, J.D.; Bell, R.D.; Wang, J.; Zlokovic, B.V. Blood-spinal cord barrier pericyte reductions contribute to increased capillary permeability. *J. Cereb. Blood Flow Metab.* **2012**, *32*, 1841–1852. [CrossRef] [PubMed]
11. Whetstone, W.D.; Hsu, J.-Y.C.; Eisenberg, M.; Werb, Z.; Noble-Haeusslein, L.J. Blood-spinal cord barrier after spinal cord injury: Relation to revascularization and wound healing. *J. Neurosci. Res.* **2003**, *74*, 227–239. [CrossRef] [PubMed]
12. Noble, L.J.; Wrathall, J.R. Blood-spinal cord barrier disruption proximal to a spinal cord transection in the rat: Time course and pathways associated with protein leakage. *Exp. Neurol.* **1988**, *99*, 567–578. [CrossRef]
13. Fehlings, M.G.; Agrawal, S. Role of sodium in the pathophysiology of secondary spinal cord injury. *Spine* **1995**, *20*, 2187–2191. [CrossRef] [PubMed]
14. Schwartz, G.; Fehlings, M.G. Evaluation of the neuroprotective effects of sodium channel blockers after spinal cord injury: Improved behavioral and neuroanatomical recovery with riluzole. *J. Neurosurg. Spine* **2001**, *94*, 245–256. [CrossRef]
15. Wilcox, J.T.; Satkunendrarajah, K.; Nasirzadeh, Y.; Laliberte, A.M.; Lip, A.; Cadotte, D.W.; Foltz, W.D.; Fehlings, M.G. Generating level-dependent models of cervical and thoracic spinal cord injury: Exploring the interplay of neuroanatomy, physiology, and function. *Neurobiol. Dis.* **2017**, *105*, 194–212. [CrossRef] [PubMed]
16. Ulndreaj, A.; Badner, A.; Fehlings, M.G. Promising neuroprotective strategies for traumatic spinal cord injury with a focus on the differential effects among anatomical levels of injury. *F1000Res* **2017**, *6*, 1907. [CrossRef] [PubMed]
17. Zhang, Y.; Guan, Z.; Reader, B.; Shawler, T.; Mandrekar-Colucci, S.; Huang, K.; Weil, Z.; Bratasz, A.; Wells, J.; Powell, N.D.; et al. Autonomic Dysreflexia Causes Chronic Immune Suppression after Spinal Cord Injury. *J. Neurosci.* **2013**, *33*, 12970–12981. [CrossRef] [PubMed]
18. Lucin, K.M.; Sanders, V.M.; Popovich, P.G. Stress hormones collaborate to induce lymphocyte apoptosis after high level spinal cord injury. *J. Neurochem.* **2009**, *110*, 1409–1421. [CrossRef] [PubMed]
19. Partida, E.; Mironets, E.; Hou, S.; Tom, V.J. Cardiovascular dysfunction following spinal cord injury. *Neural Regen. Res.* **2016**, *11*, 189–194. [PubMed]
20. Brommer, B.; Engel, O.; Kopp, M.A.; Watzlawick, R.; Müller, S.; Prüss, H.; Chen, Y.; DeVivo, M.J.; Finkenstaedt, F.W.; Dirnagl, U.; et al. Spinal cord injury-induced immune deficiency syndrome enhances infection susceptibility dependent on lesion level. *Brain* **2016**, *139*, 692–707. [CrossRef] [PubMed]
21. Schwab, J.M.; Zhang, Y.; Kopp, M.A.; Brommer, B.; Popovich, P.G. The paradox of chronic neuroinflammation, systemic immune suppression, autoimmunity after traumatic chronic spinal cord injury. *Exp. Neurol.* **2014**, *258*, 121–129. [CrossRef] [PubMed]
22. Waykole, Y.P.; Doiphode, S.S.; Rakhewar, P.S.; Mhaske, M. Anticytokine therapy for periodontal diseases: Where are we now? *J. Indian Soc. Periodontol.* **2009**, *13*, 64–68. [CrossRef] [PubMed]
23. Audet, M.-C.; Anisman, H. Interplay between pro-inflammatory cytokines and growth factors in depressive illnesses. *Front. Cell. Neurosci.* **2013**, *7*, 68. [CrossRef] [PubMed]
24. Kofler, S.; Nickel, T.; Weis, M. Role of cytokines in cardiovascular diseases: A focus on endothelial responses to inflammation. *Clin. Sci.* **2005**, *108*, 205–213. [CrossRef] [PubMed]
25. Mukhamedshina, Y.O.; Akhmetzyanova, E.R.; Martynova, E.V.; Khaiboullina, S.F.; Galieva, L.R.; Rizvanov, A.A. Systemic and Local Cytokine Profile following Spinal Cord Injury in Rats: A Multiplex Analysis. *Front. Neurol.* **2017**, *8*, 581. [CrossRef] [PubMed]
26. Bartholdi, D.; Schwab, M.E. Expression of pro-inflammatory cytokine and chemokine mRNA upon experimental spinal cord injury in mouse: An in situ hybridization study. *Eur. J. Neurosci.* **1997**, *9*, 1422–1438. [CrossRef] [PubMed]

27. Klusman, I.; Schwab, M.E. Effects of pro-inflammatory cytokines in experimental spinal cord injury. *Brain Res.* **1997**, *762*, 173–184. [CrossRef]
28. Schnell, L.; Fearn, S.; Schwab, M.E.; Perry, V.H.; Anthony, D.C. Cytokine-induced acute inflammation in the brain and spinal cord. *J. Neuropathol. Exp. Neurol.* **1999**, *58*, 245–254. [CrossRef] [PubMed]
29. Francos Quijorna, I.; Santos-Nogueira, E.; Gronert, K.; Sullivan, A.B.; Kopp, M.A.; Brommer, B.; David, S.; Schwab, J.M.; Lopez Vales, R. Maresin 1 promotes inflammatory resolution, neuroprotection and functional neurological recovery after spinal cord injury. *J. Neurosci.* **2017**, *29*, 11731–11743. [CrossRef] [PubMed]
30. Anderson, A.J.; Robert, S.; Huang, W.; Young, W.; Cotman, C.W. Activation of complement pathways after contusion-induced spinal cord injury. *J. Neurotrauma* **2004**, *21*, 1831–1846. [CrossRef] [PubMed]
31. Kasinathan, N.; Vanathi, M.B.; Subrahmanyam, V.M.; Rao, J.V. A review on response of immune system in spinal cord injury and therapeutic agents useful in treatment. *Curr. Pharm. Biotechnol.* **2015**, *16*, 26–34. [CrossRef] [PubMed]
32. Figley, S.A.; Liu, Y.; Karadimas, S.K.; Satkunendrarajah, K.; Fettes, P.; Spratt, S.K.; Lee, G.; Ando, D.; Surosky, R.; Giedlin, M.; et al. Delayed administration of a bio-engineered zinc-finger VEGF-A gene therapy is neuroprotective and attenuates allodynia following traumatic spinal cord injury. *PLoS ONE* **2014**, *9*, e96137. [CrossRef] [PubMed]
33. Liu, Y.; Figley, S.; Spratt, S.K.; Lee, G.; Ando, D.; Surosky, R.; Fehlings, M.G. An engineered transcription factor which activates VEGF-A enhances recovery after spinal cord injury. *Neurobiol. Dis.* **2010**, *37*, 384–393. [CrossRef] [PubMed]
34. Wang, H.; Wang, Y.; Li, D.; Liu, Z.; Zhao, Z.; Han, D.; Yuan, Y.; Bi, J.; Mei, X. VEGF inhibits the inflammation in spinal cord injury through activation of autophagy. *Biochem. Biophys. Res. Commun.* **2015**, *464*, 453–458. [CrossRef] [PubMed]
35. Wang, L.; Tang, X.; Zhang, H.; Yuan, J.; Ding, H.; Wei, Y. Elevated leptin expression in rat model of traumatic spinal cord injury and femoral fracture. *J. Spinal Cord Med.* **2011**, *34*, 501–509. [CrossRef] [PubMed]
36. Gezici, A.R.; Ergun, R.; Karakas, A.; Gunduz, B. Serum leptin levels following acute experimental spinal cord injury. *J. Spinal Cord Med.* **2009**, *32*, 416–421. [CrossRef] [PubMed]
37. Garshick, E.; Walia, P.; Goldstein, R.L.; Teylan, M.; Lazzari, A.A.; Tun, C.G.; Hart, J.E. Plasma Leptin and Reduced FEV1 and FVC in Chronic Spinal Cord Injury. *PM R* **2017**, *10*, 276–285. [CrossRef] [PubMed]
38. Jeon, J.Y.; Steadward, R.D.; Wheeler, G.D.; Bell, G.; McCargar, L.; Harber, V. Intact sympathetic nervous system is required for leptin effects on resting metabolic rate in people with spinal cord injury. *J. Clin. Endocrinol. Metab.* **2003**, *88*, 402–407. [CrossRef] [PubMed]
39. Fernández-Martos, C.M.; González, P.; Rodriguez, F.J. Acute leptin treatment enhances functional recovery after spinal cord injury. *PLoS ONE* **2012**, *7*, e35594. [CrossRef] [PubMed]
40. Kwon, B.K.; Streijger, F.; Fallah, N.; Noonan, V.K.; Bélanger, L.M.; Ritchie, L.; Paquette, S.J.; Ailon, T.; Boyd, M.C.; Street, J.; et al. Cerebrospinal Fluid Biomarkers To Stratify Injury Severity and Predict Outcome in Human Traumatic Spinal Cord Injury. *J. Neurotrauma* **2017**, *34*, 567–580. [CrossRef] [PubMed]
41. Lee, Y.L.; Shih, K.; Bao, P.; Ghirnikar, R.S.; Eng, L.F. Cytokine chemokine expression in contused rat spinal cord. *Neurochem. Int.* **2000**, *36*, 417–425. [CrossRef]
42. Glaser, J.; Gonzalez, R.; Sadr, E.; Keirstead, H.S. Neutralization of the chemokine CXCL10 reduces apoptosis and increases axon sprouting after spinal cord injury. *J. Neurosci. Res.* **2006**, *84*, 724–734. [CrossRef] [PubMed]
43. Di Lernia, V. Targeting the IFN-γ/CXCL10 pathway in lichen planus. *Med. Hypotheses* **2016**, *92*, 60–61. [CrossRef] [PubMed]
44. Glaser, J.; Gonzalez, R.; Perreau, V.M.; Cotman, C.W.; Keirstead, H.S. Neutralization of the chemokine CXCL10 enhances tissue sparing and angiogenesis following spinal cord injury. *J. Neurosci. Res.* **2004**, *77*, 701–708. [CrossRef] [PubMed]
45. Gonzalez, R.; Hickey, M.J.; Espinosa, J.M.; Nistor, G.; Lane, T.E.; Keirstead, H.S. Therapeutic neutralization of CXCL10 decreases secondary degeneration and functional deficit after spinal cord injury in mice. *Regen. Med.* **2007**, *2*, 771–783. [CrossRef] [PubMed]
46. Min, J.; Kim, J.H.; Choi, K.H.; Yoon, H.H.; Jeon, S.R. Is There Additive Therapeutic Effect When GCSF Combined with Adipose-Derived Stem Cell in a Rat Model of Acute Spinal Cord Injury? *J. Korean Neurosurg. Soc.* **2017**, *60*, 404–416. [CrossRef] [PubMed]

47. Nishio, Y.; Koda, M.; Kamada, T.; Someya, Y.; Kadota, R.; Mannoji, C.; Miyashita, T.; Okada, S.; Okawa, A.; Moriya, H.; et al. Granulocyte colony-stimulating factor attenuates neuronal death and promotes functional recovery after spinal cord injury in mice. *J. Neuropathol. Exp. Neurol.* **2007**, *66*, 724–731. [CrossRef] [PubMed]
48. Kato, K.; Koda, M.; Takahashi, H.; Sakuma, T.; Inada, T.; Kamiya, K.; Ota, M.; Maki, S.; Okawa, A.; Takahashi, K.; et al. Granulocyte colony-stimulating factor attenuates spinal cord injury-induced mechanical allodynia in adult rats. *J. Neurol. Sci.* **2015**, *355*, 79–83. [CrossRef] [PubMed]
49. Dittgen, T.; Pitzer, C.; Plaas, C.; Kirsch, F.; Vogt, G.; Laage, R.; Schneider, A. Granulocyte-colony stimulating factor (G-CSF) improves motor recovery in the rat impactor model for spinal cord injury. *PLoS ONE* **2012**, *7*, e29880. [CrossRef] [PubMed]
50. Kadota, R.; Koda, M.; Kawabe, J.; Hashimoto, M.; Nishio, Y.; Mannoji, C.; Miyashita, T.; Furuya, T.; Okawa, A.; Takahashi, K.; et al. Granulocyte colony-stimulating factor (G-CSF) protects oligodendrocyte and promotes hindlimb functional recovery after spinal cord injury in rats. *PLoS ONE* **2012**, *7*, e50391. [CrossRef] [PubMed]
51. Guo, Y.; Liu, S.; Wang, P.; Zhang, H.; Wang, F.; Bing, L.; Gao, J.; Yang, J.; Hao, A. Granulocyte colony-stimulating factor improves neuron survival in experimental spinal cord injury by regulating nucleophosmin-1 expression. *J. Neurosci. Res.* **2014**, *92*, 751–760. [CrossRef] [PubMed]
52. Koda, M.; Nishio, Y.; Kamada, T.; Someya, Y.; Okawa, A.; Mori, C.; Yoshinaga, K.; Okada, S.; Moriya, H.; Yamazaki, M. Granulocyte colony-stimulating factor (G-CSF) mobilizes bone marrow-derived cells into injured spinal cord and promotes functional recovery after compression-induced spinal cord injury in mice. *Brain Res.* **2007**, *1149*, 223–231. [CrossRef] [PubMed]
53. Lee, J.-S.; Yang, C.-C.; Kuo, Y.-M.; Sze, C.-I.; Hsu, J.-Y.C.; Huang, Y.-H.; Tzeng, S.-F.; Tsai, C.-L.; Chen, H.-H.; Jou, I.-M. Delayed granulocyte colony-stimulating factor treatment promotes functional recovery in rats with severe contusive spinal cord injury. *Spine* **2012**, *37*, 10–17. [CrossRef] [PubMed]
54. Takahashi, H.; Yamazaki, M.; Okawa, A.; Sakuma, T.; Kato, K.; Hashimoto, M.; Hayashi, K.; Furuya, T.; Fujiyoshi, T.; Kawabe, J.; et al. Neuroprotective therapy using granulocyte colony-stimulating factor for acute spinal cord injury: A phase I/IIa clinical trial. *Eur. Spine J.* **2012**, *21*, 2580–2587. [CrossRef] [PubMed]
55. Kamiya, K.; Koda, M.; Furuya, T.; Kato, K.; Takahashi, H.; Sakuma, T.; Inada, T.; Ota, M.; Maki, S.; Okawa, A.; et al. Neuroprotective therapy with granulocyte colony-stimulating factor in acute spinal cord injury: A comparison with high-dose methylprednisolone as a historical control. *Eur. Spine J.* **2015**, *24*, 963–967. [CrossRef] [PubMed]
56. Yoon, S.H.; Shim, Y.S.; Park, Y.H.; Chung, J.K.; Nam, J.H.; Kim, M.O.; Park, H.C.; Park, S.R.; Min, B.-H.; Kim, E.Y.; et al. Complete Spinal Cord Injury Treatment Using Autologous Bone Marrow Cell Transplantation and Bone Marrow Stimulation with Granulocyte Macrophage-Colony Stimulating Factor: Phase I/II Clinical Trial. *Stem Cells* **2007**, *25*, 2066–2073. [CrossRef] [PubMed]
57. Poniatowski, Ł.A.; Wojdasiewicz, P.; Krawczyk, M.; Szukiewicz, D.; Gasik, R.; Kubaszewski, Ł.; Kurkowska-Jastrzębska, I. Analysis of the Role of CX3CL1 (Fractalkine) and Its Receptor CX3CR1 in Traumatic Brain and Spinal Cord Injury: Insight into Recent Advances in Actions of Neurochemokine Agents. *Mol. Neurobiol.* **2017**, *54*, 2167–2188. [CrossRef] [PubMed]
58. Donnelly, D.J.; Longbrake, E.E.; Shawler, T.M.; Kigerl, K.A.; Lai, W.; Tovar, C.A.; Ransohoff, R.M.; Popovich, P.G. Deficient CX3CR1 signaling promotes recovery after mouse spinal cord injury by limiting the recruitment and activation of Ly6Clo/iNOS+ macrophages. *J. Neurosci.* **2011**, *31*, 9910–9922. [CrossRef] [PubMed]
59. Freria, C.M.; Hall, J.C.E.; Wei, P.; Guan, Z.; McTigue, D.M.; Popovich, P.G. Deletion of the Fractalkine Receptor, CX3CR1, Improves Endogenous Repair, Axon Sprouting, and Synaptogenesis after Spinal Cord Injury in Mice. *J. Neurosci.* **2017**, *37*, 3568–3587. [CrossRef] [PubMed]
60. Wilcox, J.T.; Fehlings, M.G. Acute Clip Compression Model of SCI. In *Experimental Neurosurgery in Animal Models*; Neuromethods; Springer: New York, NY, USA, 2016; Volume 116, pp. 111–117.
61. Basso, D.M.; Beattie, M.S.; Bresnahan, J.C. A Sensitive and Reliable Locomotor Rating Scale for Open Field Testing in Rats. *J. Neurotrauma* **1995**, *12*, 1–21. [CrossRef] [PubMed]

7

FM19G11 and Ependymal Progenitor/Stem Cell Combinatory Treatment Enhances Neuronal Preservation and Oligodendrogenesis after Severe Spinal Cord Injury

Ana Alastrue-Agudo [1], Francisco Javier Rodriguez-Jimenez [1], Eric López Mocholi [1], Francesca De Giorgio [1], Slaven Erceg [2] and Victoria Moreno-Manzano [1,*]

1 Neuronal and Tissue Regeneration Laboratory, Príncipe Felipe Research Center, 46012 Valencia, Spain; aalastrue@cipf.es (A.A.-A.); frodriguez@cipf.es (F.J.R.-J.); elopezm@cipf.es (E.L.M.); f.degiorgio85@gmail.com (F.D.G.)

2 Stem Cell Therapies in Neurodegenerative Diseases Laboratory, Centro de Investigación Príncipe Felipe, 46012 Valencia, Spain; serceg@cipf.es

* Correspondence: vmorenom@cipf.es

Abstract: Spinal cord injury (SCI) suffers from a lack of effective therapeutic strategies. We have previously shown that individual therapeutic strategies, transplantation of ependymal stem/progenitor cells of the spinal cord after injury (epSPCi) or FM19G11 pharmacological treatment, induce moderate functional recovery after SCI. Here, the combination of treatments has been assayed for functional and histological analysis. Immediately after severe SCI, one million epSPCi were intramedullary injected, and the FM19G11 compound or dimethyl sulfoxide (DMSO) (as the vehicle control) was administrated via intrathecal catheterization. The combination of treatments, epSPCi and FM19G11, improves locomotor tasks compared to the control group, but did not significantly improve the Basso, Beattie, Bresnahan (BBB) scores for locomotor analysis in comparison with the individual treatments. However, the histological analysis of the spinal cord tissues, two months after SCI and treatments, demonstrated that when we treat the animals with both epSPCi and FM19G11, an improved environment for neuronal preservation was generated by reduction of the glial scar extension. The combinatorial treatment also contributes to enhancing the oligodendrocyte precursor cells by inducing the expression of Olig1 in vivo. These results suggest that a combination of therapies may be an exciting new therapeutic treatment for more efficient neuronal activity recovery after severe SCI.

Keywords: FM19G11; spinal cord injury; ependymal progenitor stem cells; oligodendrogenesis; locomotion; neuronal regeneration; axon growth

---

1. Introduction

Traumatic spinal cord injury (SCI) is a devastating disorder with loss of neurological function immediately below the affected segment with no currently effective treatment for the subsequent paralysis. The failure to recover from SCI in adult mammals is attributed to both extrinsic and intrinsic factors [1]. The extrinsic factors include a lack of appropriate trophic support like brain-derived neurotrophic factor (BDNF), basic-fibroblastic growth factor (bFGF), vascular endothelial growth factor (VEGF) [2], stromal derived factor 1 (SDF1) [3] or insulin-like growth factor 1 (IGF-1) [4], since among others, they have shown neuroprotective effects when added ectopically.

In the primary injury phase, the direct impact causes cell death at the injury site with axonal damage leading to the interruption of the ascending and descending spinal pathways. The blockade of nerve conduction generates paralysis and temporary loss of neural functions by spinal shock. The primary injury leads to massive cell death of neurons, glial cells and endothelial cells lining the blood vessels. The surviving neurons at the lesion site respond with a barrage of action potentials that create significant local shifts in ion levels and cause also the release of excitatory neurotransmitters (i.e., glutamate), resulting in the death of more nearby neurons [5]. The inflammatory response after SCI is initiated by peripherally-derived immune cells (macrophages-monocytes, neutrophils and T-cells) and glial activation (astrocytes and microglia) [6–8]. Macrophages and microglia contribute to the inflammatory response through the release of cytokines like tumor necrosis factor α (TNF-α), interleukin 1 or 6 (IL1 or IL6) [9] in an initial phase; however, later, additional anti-inflammatory cytokines like IL10 are known to contribute to tissue remodeling [10,11]. The secondary phase is also marked by the massive death of oligodendrocytes. The combination of demyelination and altered ion channel function may lead to changes in surviving neurons that can produce central chronic pain. The lesion site forms a fluid-filled cavity delimited by the reactive scar acting as a containment barrier forming an impenetrable wall with extracellular matrix proteins and chondroitin sulfate limiting the axonal regrowth [12], thereby inhibiting the regenerative potential of those axons to reconnect with the distal segments [13]. SCI is a complex and multifactorial cascade of events that progressively reduces the chances of the limited endogenous regenerative capacity to rescue the lost connections. Therefore, therapeutic interventions need to rapidly interfere with this degenerative cascade via powerful neuroprotective activities, promoting in addition functional neuronal plasticity. A combination of neuroprotective and neuroregenerative treatments constitutes the current key strategies for the creation of an efficient SCI treatment. Several strategies have already shown the efficiency of the combination of cell therapy and pharmacological approaches [14]. Transplantation of neural stem/progenitor cells (NSPCs) has shown promising results in the repair and regeneration of lost neural tissues and the associated restoration of neurological deficits [14–16]. NSPCs include multipotent stem cells present in the periventricular subependymal layer and the subgranular zone of the dentate gyrus in the brain, as well as in the ependymal regions lining the central canal of the spinal cord (epSPCs) [13]. NSPCs represent an ideal candidate for stem cell-based SCI therapy based on noted functional improvements after transplantation and the absence of malignant transformation, offering a safe and relevant cell type for clinical applications. After SCI, epSPCs proliferate and migrate to the injured area and produce new oligodendrocyte progenitors [14]. We previously showed that acute transplantation of undifferentiated epSPCs from SCI donors (epSPCi) or in vitro differentiated OPCs into a rat model of severe spinal cord contusion produced significant locomotion recovery from one week after injury [15]. Moreover, we recently demonstrated the advantages of the synergistic activity of the polyacetal curcumin (PA-curcumin), a new polymeric conjugate of curcumin, with epSPCi in rats with chronic SCI. A single administration of the combinatory treatment into the intrathecal space significantly rescued the locomotor activity of the paralyzed rats, as opposed to ineffective individual treatments [17]. The PA-curcumin produced neuroprotective and anti-inflammatory capabilities, as previously reported [18–22], but also showed regenerative activity by increasing axonal elongation-related mechanisms. The epSPCi, with multipotent characteristics, lining the central canal of the spinal cord [15], after SCI, proliferate and migrate to the injured zone, giving rise to new oligodendrocyte progenitors [23]. Acute transplantation of epSPCi efficiently reversed the paralysis associated with acute SCI in rats [24,25]. The transplanted cells migrated long distances from the rostral and caudal regions to reach the neurofilament-labeled axons in and around the lesion zone, while epSPC transplanted animals always showed fewer cavities and a smaller scar area [25]. In the chronic scenario, although epSPCi improved the locomotion, only partial success was found in comparison with the acute treatment [26]. However, the combination of treatments, for instance by combining PA-curcumin and epSPCi, significantly induced both β-tubulin-III (neurofilament marker for neuronal projections) and GAP43 (axon growth marker) expression at the epicenter of the injury in comparison with the individually-treated groups [17].

FM19G11 was first identified as an inhibitor of HIFα protein expression and transcriptional activity under hypoxic conditions repressing a variety of key genes involved in stemness. Moreover, directed differentiation experiments demonstrated that FM19G11 favors oligodendrocyte differentiation blocked under hypoxia, possibly through the negative modulation of Sox2 (sex determining region Y-box 2) and Oct4 (octamer-binding transcription factor 4) expression and by allowing the epSPCs to differentiate under hypoxia [27]. However, under normoxic conditions, FM19G11 modifies the mitochondrial uncoupling process, by induction of UCP sensors, which induces glucose uptake by activation of AMPK (AMP-activated protein kinase), as well as AKT (Protein Kinase B) signaling pathways. The consequence of these molecular events is an increase of the self-renewal machinery of different stem cell populations, including the epSPCs. FM19G11 induces early glycolytic-related responses associated with PI3K/AKT/mTOR signaling induction [28,29]. Interestingly, when FM19G11 is infused during three days starting immediately after SCI, in the intrathecal space, it induces functional locomotion recovery one month after treatment, which is associated with an increase of vimentin expression and in the number of neuronal fibers in the injured area [30].

Here, we look for an enhanced effect to rescue neuronal activity for progressive motor function in severe SCI using a combination that includes cell therapy, epSPCi and the pharmacological treatment based on the local application of FM19G11.

2. Results

2.1. FM19G11 or epSPCi Improve Locomotion in Severe SCI with No Synergistic Effect

Individual treatments with FM19G11 by intrathecal administration [30] or epSPCi by intramedullary transplantation [24,25] improved locomotion when applied immediately after injury. Herein, in order to study a potential additive or synergistic effect among both treatments, a combination of both was assayed. The epSPCi, or growth medium in the control group, were transplanted by intramedullary injection at the injured area immediately after spinal cord contusion (Figure 1A, top pictures). Afterwards, the pharmacological treatment was performed by continual delivery of FM19G11 or DMSO (in the control group), using an osmotic pump, connected to a catheter, into the intrathecal space (Figure 1A, bottom pictures). All treated animals distributed into control, epSPCi, FM19G11 and FM19G11 + epSPCi groups were individually videotaped, and locomotor functional recovery was scored blind by two unbiased observers by using the 21-point Basso, Beattie, Bresnahan (BBB) scale. All three treated animals had a significant increase in the BBB scores after the fourth week, in comparison with the control group (control: 6.3 $\pm$ 0.26; epSPCi: 8.8 $\pm$ 0.4 *; FM19G11: 8 $\pm$ 0.6 *; FM19G11 + epSPCi: 9 $\pm$ 0.7 *; *, $p < 0.05$ vs. control). However, no significant differences were found among the three treatments (Figure 1B). Interestingly, epSPCi transplanted animals (epSPCi and FM19G11 + epSPCi) always showed better maximum scores in the BBB test at shorter times after SCI (Figure 1B). The frame captures of representative video tape recordings in the open field test, eight weeks after surgery, showed a typical plantar placement of the paw with weight support instance, consistently found in animals treated with the combination of treatments, as well as the weight support by dorsal stepping, consistently found in the epSPCi group. Plantar placement of the paw with no weight support in the stepping was also frequently found in the FM19G11-treated group. The control animals did not show any stepping, but occasionally sweeping, without showing any weight support (Figure 1C).

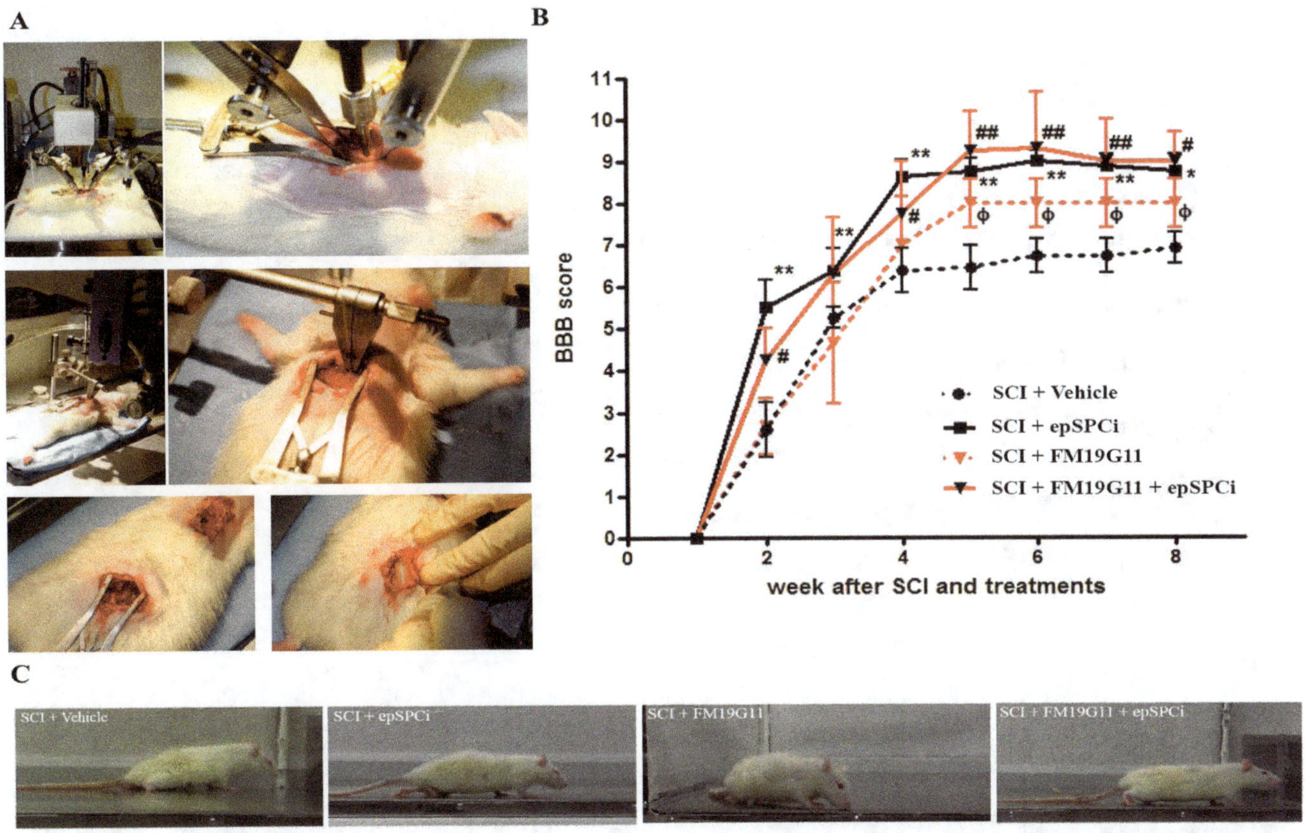

Figure 1. FM19G11, epSPCi or the combination of both improve locomotion in severe spinal cord injury (SCI) in comparison with the control group. (**A**) Surgery strategy to induce severe SCI by a 250-kdyn impact and acute transplantation by intramedullary injection of epSPCi and intrathecal catheterization for local and sustained delivery of FM19G11 using an osmotic pump; (**B**) functional locomotor analysis (BBB scores) over eight weeks post-treatment with vehicle, as a control, epSPCi, FM19G11 or FM19G11 + epSPCi; quantitative data are expressed as the mean ± S.E.M.; *, or #, or ϕ, $p < 0.05$, ** or ##, $p < 0.01$; (**C**) representative capture images from video recordings of one animal of every group for BBB analysis at the eighth week after SCI are shown as follows: SCI + vehicle (control), SCI + epSPCi, SCI + FM19G11, SCI + FM19G11 + epSPCi.

2.2. FM19G11 Intrathecal Administration after SCI Preserves Spinal Cord Tissue

The lost tissue due to the destructive secondary damage including the inflammatory reaction following the SCI was evaluated. As is indicated in the illustrative model (Figure 2A, top representation of the analyzed planes in the spinal cord), the quantification of the spinal cord width (Figure 2B) at the injury area (Figure 2C) at eight consecutive points along four mm of the epicenter of the lesion was performed. The spinal cord injury area was monitored via hematoxylin-eosin (H&E) histological analysis, eight weeks post-injury (Figure 2A, bottom panels). The comparative analysis among all the groups after quantification of the spinal cord width at the injury epicenter demonstrated that since larger tissue degeneration remained in the SCI site following control treatment or epSPCi transplantation alone, FM19G11- and FM19G11 + epSPCi-treated rats presented wider cords (Figure 2B). The quantification of the total spinal cord area at the epicenter of the injury, by taking into account the elliptic shape of the cord and including the width and the length average, showed the same result. The FM19G11 and FM19G11 + epSPCi groups presented higher total areas in comparison with the control or epSPCi groups, tending to recover a closer shape to the non-injured tissue (Figure 2C).

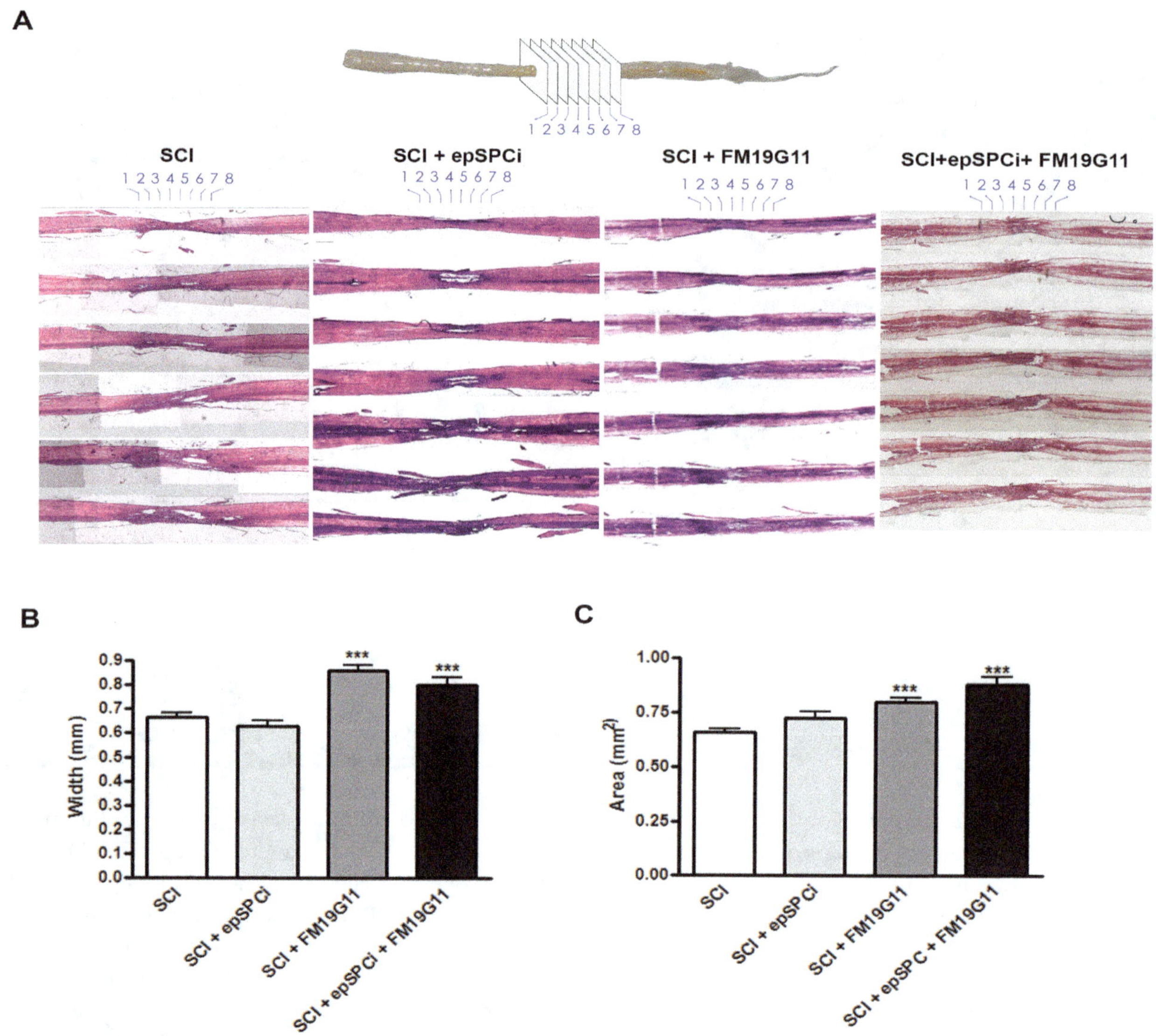

Figure 2. FM19G11 preserves spinal cord tissue. (**A**) Top panel: spinal cord model showing the eight selected points for the quantification of the width and the lesion area at the spinal cord injury epicenter; bottom panels: representative histological sections of hematoxylin/eosin staining for each experimental condition; Scale bar = 500 μM; (**B**) quantification of the whole width epicenter area, including all eight selected points; (**C**) quantification of the lesion area considering the elliptic shape of the spinal cord, the higher and smaller radius at each section. Quantitative data are expressed as the mean ± S.E.M; *** $p < 0.001$ in comparison with SCI (control).

2.3. *FM19G11 and epSPCi Combination Treatment Reduces the Scar Extension and Astrogliosis and Increases the Neuronal Fibers at the Injury Area*

The glial scar has been accepted to be delimited by the astrocytes expressing glial fibrillary acidic protein (GFAP) [7]; then, as we previously reported [17,25,30], we evaluated the extension of the glial scar by measuring the negative GFAP stained area at the epicenter of the injury (Figure 3A,B). We found that only the combinatory treatment, FM19G11 and epSPCi, decreased the extension of the astrocytic negative area in comparison with the control group or the individual treatments (Figure 3B), indicating a reduction of the glial scar formation, creating a more permissive neuronal environment. However, all treatments, FM19G11 or epSPCi or their combination, reduced the astrogliosis based on a lower GFAP positive staining at the epicenter of the lesion, surrounding the scar (Figure 3A,C). Further assessment at the glial scar area was performed by measuring the β-tubulin-III-positive staining for neuronal filament for those neurons crossing the glial scar. All treatments, epSPCi, FM19G11 and the combination of both, were found to always show a larger positive area for β-tubulin-III in comparison with the control group (Figure 3D), indicating an independent effect of the individual treatments on neuronal fiber preservation and the glial scar formation.

However, when the β-tubulin-III positive area was quantified at the total epicenter of the injury, including the rostral and caudal tissue surrounding the scar, only the animals that received the combination of treatments, FM19G11 + epSPCi, presented a significant result in comparison with the control group (Figure 3E).

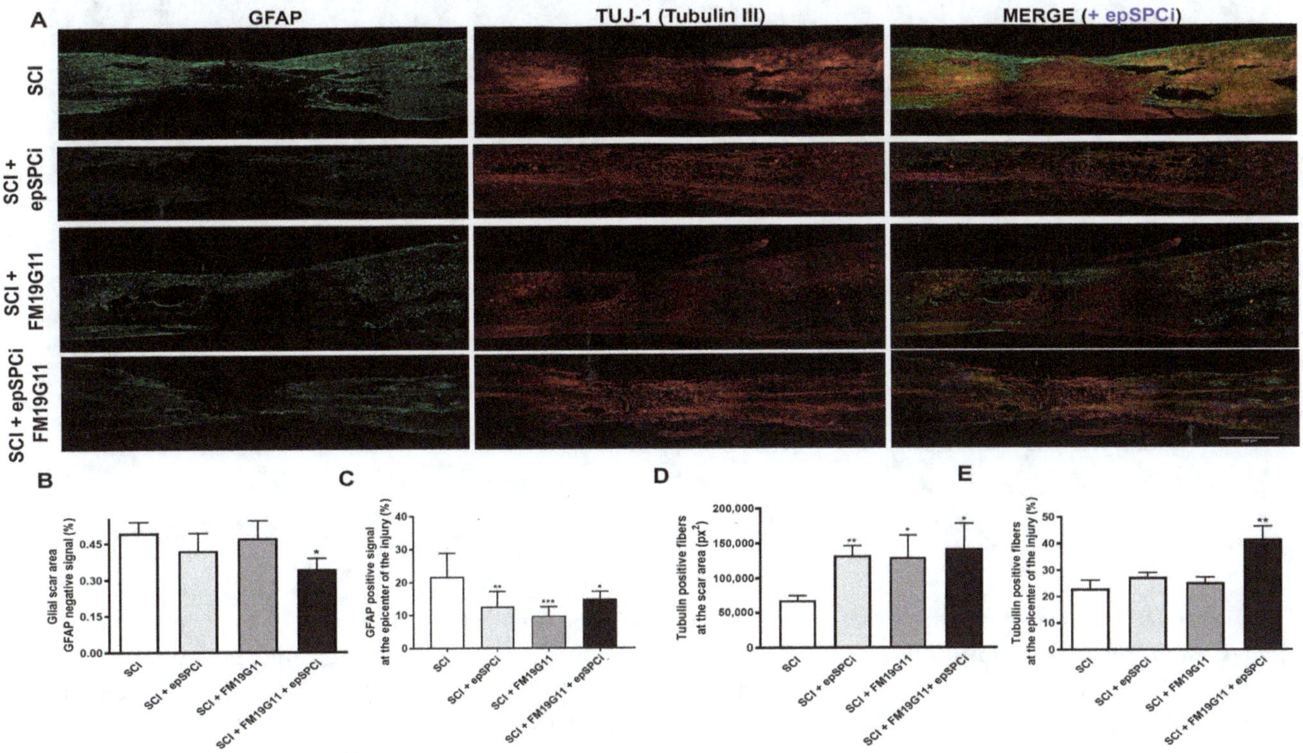

Figure 3. Combinatory treatment reduces the glial scar formation and preserves larger numbers of neuronal fibers. (**A**) Representative immunofluorescence images from glial fibrillary acidic protein (GFAP; **green**), β-tubulin-III (**red**) and merge including green fluorescence protein (GFP)-epSPCi in the transplanted groups (GFP, **blue**) with positive signals at the epicenter of the injury from spinal cord longitudinal sections in every experimental condition; Scale bar, 500 μm; (**B**) quantification of the negative area or (**C**) the positive signal at the injury site for GFAP expressed as a percentage of the total epicenter area, equivalent in length for all tested groups; (**D**) quantification of the positive signal for β-tubulin-III (tubulin) at the negative GFAP area or (**E**) covering all the injury area, expressed as a percentage of the total epicenter area, equivalent in length for all tested groups. Quantitative data are expressed as the mean ± S.E.M; * $p < 0.05$, ** $p < 0.01$, *** $p < 0.001$ in comparison with SCI (control).

2.4. FM19G11 and epSPCi Induce the Expression of GAP43 Expression, an Axon Growth Marker, and RIP, a Marker for Myelinated Oligodendrocytes at the Injury

GAP43, a known marker for axonal cone growth formation [31], was assayed to analyze the capacity of each treatment to favor neuronal plasticity. Encouragingly, eight weeks after injury and treatments, a significant induction of the GAP43 positive signal was detected along the neuronal fibers at the injured site by all treated groups in comparison with the non-treated animals (Figure 4A,B). The substantial increases in β-tubulin-III (Figure 3D,E) and GAP43 labeling for the combinatory treatment indeed suggest a more efficient relationship between the increased preservation in the number and quality of axon fibers. Interestingly, although no significant differences in the expression for the receptor interacting protein (RIP), a cell marker for mature oligodendrocytes by detecting 2′,3′-cyclic nucleotide 3′-phosphodiesterase [32], were detected when the control group was compared to any treatment (Figure 4C), the detected signal of GAP43 maintains a significant parallel expression with the mature and myelinated axons stained with RIP in the epSPCi transplanted groups (Figure 4D), as is also shown in the representative magnified images of double staining detection of GAP43 (red) and RIP (green) for each experimental condition (Figure 4A).

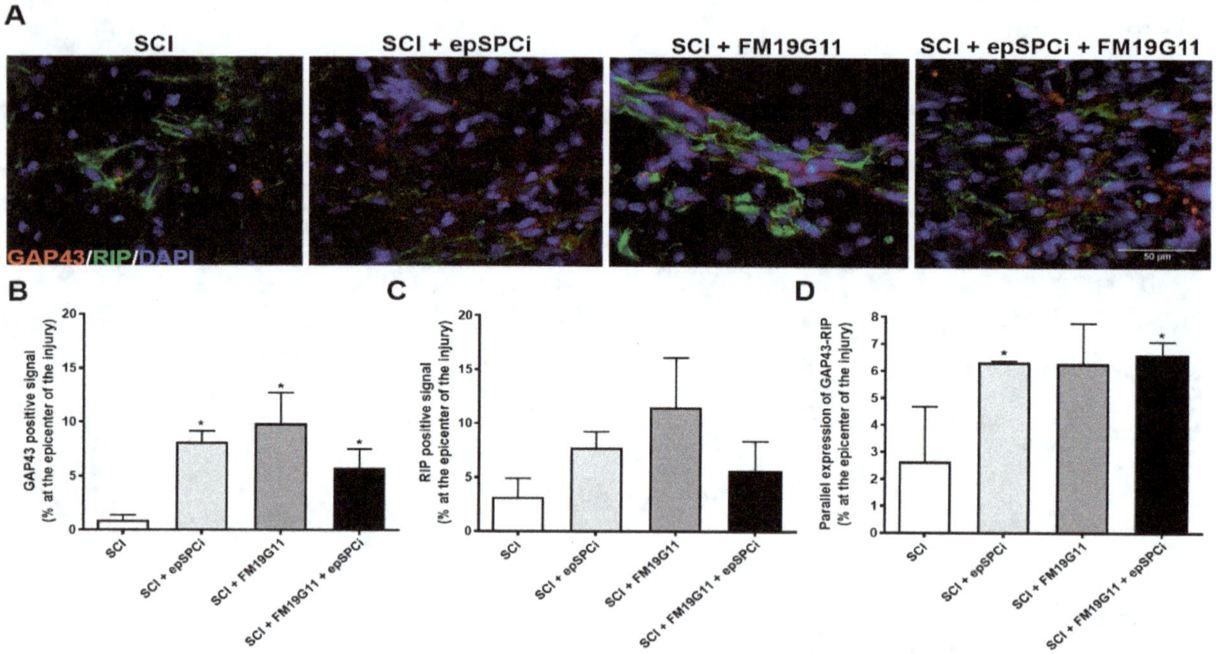

Figure 4. Treatment with FM19G11 plus epSPCi preserves larger numbers of neuronal fibers. (**A**) Representative immunofluorescence images at high magnification of receptor interacting protein (RIP, **green**) and GAP43 (**red**) expression at the epicenter of the injury are shown for every experimental condition (scale bar, 50 μm); (**B**) quantification of the GAP43 (growth cone marker); (**C**) RIP (mature oligodendrocyte marker) or (**D**) the parallel detection of the GAP43 and RIP-positive signal at the epicenter of the injury expressed as a percentage of the total epicenter area, equivalent in length for all tested groups. Quantitative data are expressed as the mean ± S.E.M. (ANOVA), * $p < 0.05$ in comparison with SCI (control).

2.5. FM19G11 Favors Oligodendrocyte Replacement

It is well established that after SCI, which causes extensive oligodendrocyte cell death [33], surviving oligodendrocyte progenitor cells (OPC) are the major source for oligodendrocyte replacement and remyelination [34]. It also has been shown that, over the first weeks post-injury, the OPCs differentiate into mature oligodendrocytes, particularly along the lesion borders, and contribute to the re-myelination process [35–37]. The detection of Olig1 expression, an early OPC marker [38], eight weeks after SCI, demonstrates a significant induction of this population by the FM19G11 treatment in combination with epSPCi transplantation (Figure 5A). However, at the time of sacrifice, no significant differences were found in the RIP population (Figure 4C), indicating a lack of maturation induction of the proliferating OPC by the treatments. FM19G11 was previously shown to allow the oligodendrocyte differentiation in vitro efficiently when it was delayed under hypoxia [27]. Here, we found that the presence of FM19G11 also improves the maturation of epSPCi into oligodendrocyte precursor cells measured as an increment of RIP expression at the protein level (Figure 5B) and NG2 expression at the protein (Figure 5C) and mRNA levels (Figure 5D) with a parallel decrease of the proliferative marker PCNA (proliferating cell nuclear antigen) or the stemness factor Sox2 (Figure 5C).

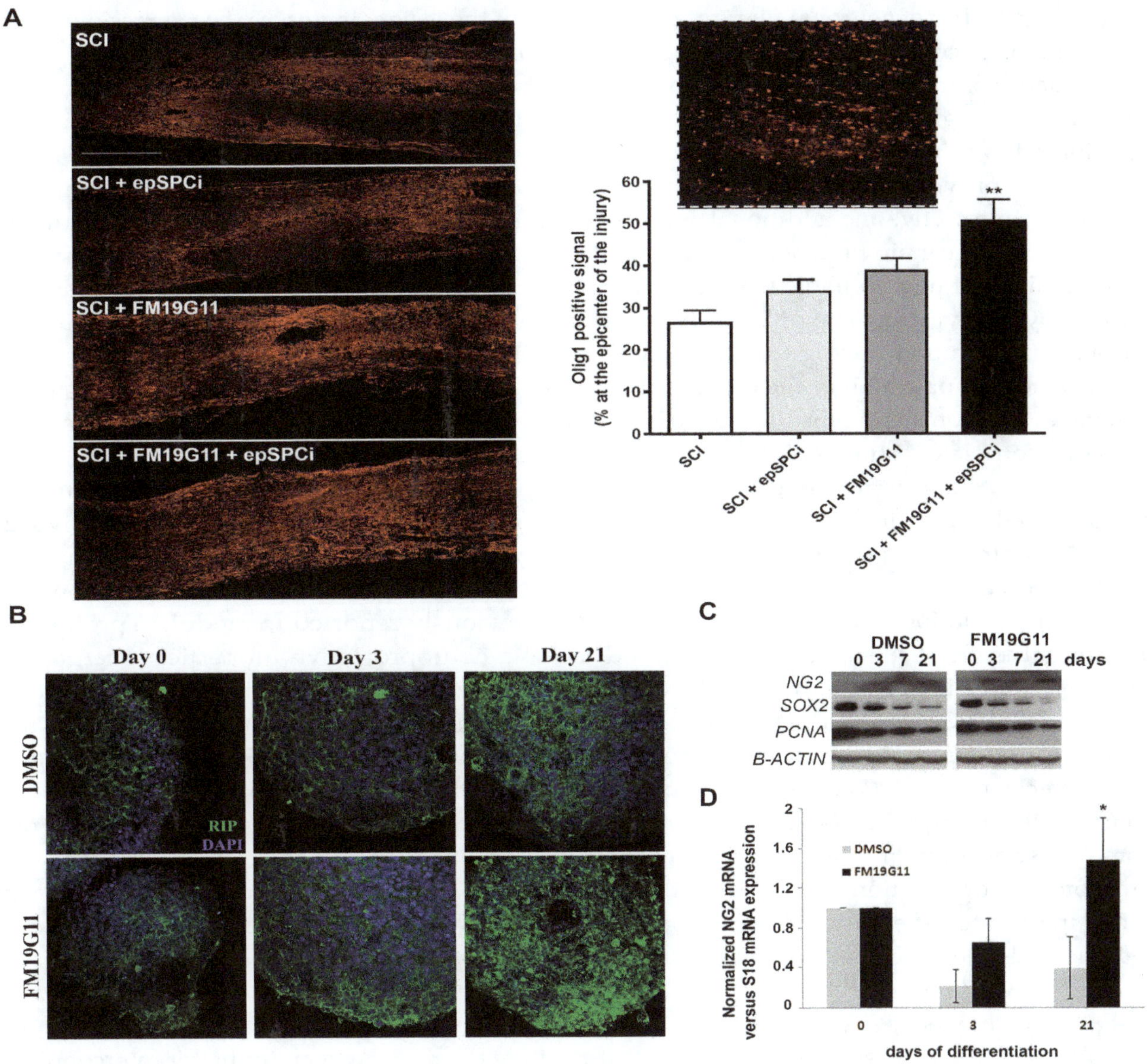

Figure 5. FM19G11 promotes in vivo and in vitro oligodendrocyte turnover. (**A**) (**left** panel) Representative immunofluorescent images of the Olig1-positive signal at the epicenter of the injury in every experimental condition (scale bar, 500 µm); (**right** panel) quantification of the positive signal for Olig1 expressed as a percentage of the total epicenter area, equivalent in length for all tested groups. Inset: high magnification of Olig1 immunostaining. Quantitative data are expressed as the mean ± S.E.M. ** $p < 0.01$ in comparison with SCI (control); (**B**) representative immunofluorescent images of RIP (mature oligodendrocyte marker) at different time points through the directed induced oligodendrocyte differentiation process of epSPCi in culture in the presence of FM19G11 or vehicle (DMSO) (scale bar, 500 µm); (**C**) western blotting of NG2, Sox2, PCNA and β-actin semi-quantitative expression and (**D**) quantitative RT-PCR analysis for the expression of NG2 (oligodendrocyte marker) at the different stages of the directed in vitro differentiation process into oligodendrocytes from epSPCi in the presence of FM19G11 or DMSO (vehicle), * $p < 0.05$ in comparison with DMSO.

3. Discussion

A combination of strategies with a synergistic effect of improved neuroprotection and neural plasticity may lead to significant improvements not yet achieved by unique treatments. Here, we show how the combinatory use of FM19G11 and epSPCi reduces glial scar formation, reduces astrogliosis, increases the number of neuronal fibers at the epicenter of the lesion, increases the expression markers for neuronal plasticity and induces oligodendrocyte turnover for potential re-myelination.

Traumatic contusion injury generates a rim of spared white matter tissue, with extensive neuronal degeneration and glial scar formation generating an incomplete lesion with a variable remaining demyelinated, but initially non-interrupted axons depending on the initial severity of the trauma, which, in fact, provides a more realistic experimental setting mimicking the clinical lesions to test potential neuroprotective and additional neurorestorative strategies. Extensive proliferation of different cell types occurs at certain time points, like oligodendrocyte, neural precursor cells and also astrocytes and microglia, in a more reliable way than the transection models [39]. Here, we induced a severe contusion by applying a force of 250 kdyn (kilo dyne) in rats of ~200 g, limiting the spontaneous functional regeneration during the first weeks after injury in comparison with moderate injuries and completely impairing it at the chronic stages (one month after injury), allowing the restorative functional evaluation among the different experimental groups in a shorter period than for instance in models of a complete section [40].

We recently showed that transplantation of epSPCi, the ependymal cells that represent the latent neural stem cell population in the adult spinal cord, activated and induced to proliferate in vivo after spinal cord injury [33] in combination with PA-curcumin significantly improves the locomotion in a chronic and sever traumatic SCI [17]. Here, we demonstrated the beneficial contribution to the epSPCi transplantation of the addition of FM19G11 previously reported to modulate proliferation and differentiation of this cell population and to have neuroprotective properties when applied immediately after injury [30]. When all treatments were compared, the cell transplanted groups, epSPCi and FM19G11 + epSPCi, showed faster functional rescue by measuring locomotor tasks, significantly different from the locomotor recover found in the vehicle- or the FM19G11-treated group. Neither vehicle- nor FM19G11-treated animals exhibited coordinated movement, but occasional weight support or plantar steps. The NPC progeny were found to be necessary to produce several neurotrophic factors that support neuronal survival after injury [41]. A2B5-positive glial cells have been shown to promote neuroprotection and repair of the injured spinal cord, promoting axonal sprouting when induced in vitro to differentiate into a more astroglial fate [42]. Accumulating evidence in the last decade defends the beneficial role of the astrocytes in response to SCI, giving support to the survival cells and allowing their processes [8]. We found, eight weeks after injury, a significant decrease of the GFAP-positive reactivity for astrocyte detection at the epicenter of the injury in response to all treatments, with an increase in the neurofilament-positive fibers. However, for better interconnection of both events, additional experimentation at a shorter time of analysis or specific deletion of the astrocytic population will be required to understand a potential associated mechanism of action.

The global detection of infiltrating macrophages, positive for CD68-ED1, eight weeks after injury, did not show significant differences in any of the tested conditions; however, it has been shown by others that the focal transplantation of NPCs decreases the relative proportion of classically-activated M1-like cells among the macrophage lineage cells infiltrating the injured cord [43], favoring the shift of the balance towards tissue remodelling/repair associated also with the M2-like cells and facilitating the recovery from spinal cord injury-induced secondary damage, undetected in a global analysis [44]. The lower astrogliosis activation found in all treated groups would additionally contribute to reduce the scar extension; the combined treatment exhibited in fact the best functional outcome with reduced spared tissue, where the combination with FM19G11 with an additional neuroprotective effect could contribute to favoring environmental homeostasis. It was very interesting that GAP43, previously described as a growth cone marker for growing axons, was induced in all treated animals at the scar area showing a similar effect as TUJ-1. Moreover, the growing axon ends positive for GAP43 were mostly accompanied by myelinated oligodendrocytes when the animals were treated with FM19G11, or with epSPCi, or both, supporting more effective neuronal plasticity in comparison with non-treated animals.

At the SCI area, the vascular network is lost with edema and disruption of the BSCB, extensively justifying the local application at the subarachnoid space of the pharmacological treatment. We previously showed that FM19G11 intrathecal administration immediately after SCI accelerates locomotor recovery in the rats one month after treatment. Indeed, the sustained administration of FM19G11 during one week showed a plausible neuroprotective role, preserving more neurofilament β-tubulin III-positive fibers in the injured area surrounded by an increased number of neural precursor vimentin-positive cells [30]. Here, we found that this neuroprotective effect by FM19G11 treatment was maintained, as was determined by the histological analysis, for two months. The analysis of both the in vitro and in vivo mechanism of action of FM19G11 reveals an important influence on the mitochondrial activity by early activation of UCP proteins, and therefore, the compound modifies oxidative metabolism at least in the epSPCi population by activation of the AKT/mTOR signaling pathway, which creates an adaptive response in the cells by increasing the GLUT-4 receptors [29,30] and probably improving the exocytosis and exchange program between cells and the tissue environment, which would contribute to the neuroprotective effect.

The promotion of OPC generation would contribute and accelerate the re-myelination process after SCI. Diverse clinical trials [45,46] based on previous successful pre-clinical studies [47–50] have tried to activate oligodendrocyte replacement for inducing re-myelination. FM19G11 was shown before to accelerate the maturation of OPC when the in vitro differentiation process was under the control of the related self-renewal transcriptional machinery in hypoxia [30]. Here, we show that FM19G11 can accelerate the differentiation and maturation of epSPCs in vitro derived from adult spinal cord also under normoxic conditions, showing a relevant effect of this compound in the reprogramming of the undifferentiated progenitors into mature lineages independently in certain micro-environmental conditions. FM19G11 modulates the expression of Sox2, Oct4 and Nanog depending on the oxygen tension to which the precursor cells are exposed [27,30]. Along the oligodendrocyte-directed differentiation process, FM19G11 more quickly decreased Sox2, Oct4 and PCNA undifferentiated and proliferative markers, respectively, in parallel with the increased expression of mature oligodendrocytes like RIP. Interestingly, FM19G11 was able to significantly induce the OPC population, revealed by the increased signal of Olig1, an early oligodendrocyte marker, showing an additive effect on the combinatory treatment with epSPCi. No significant co-localization of epSPCi and Olig1 was found; however, because all samples were studied at the time of sacrifice, two months after injury, a direct influence on the differentiation of the transplanted cells by FM19G11 cannot be discarded.

4. Materials and Methods

4.1. Ethical Statement Regarding the Use of Animals

Female 2-month-old Sprague Dawley rats (weighing ~200 g) from Charles River and SD-Tg(GFP)2BalRrrc from Rat Resource & Research Center (University of Missouri Columbia, Columbia, MO, USA) were bred at the Animal Experimentation Unit of the Research Institute Príncipe Felipe (Valencia, Spain). The experimental protocol included humanized endpoint criteria by using a score for body weight changes (>20%), body condition (lethargy, pain), autophagy or severe ulcerations and was previously approved by the Animal Care Committee of the Research Institute Principe Felipe (Valencia, Spain) with the protocols identified as 10-0181 and 09-0131 in accordance with the National Guide to the Care and Use of Experimental Animals (Real Decreto 1 December 2005).

4.2. EpSPCi Cell Culture

EpSPCi (eGFP+/+ for cell transplantation in vivo or eGFP$^{-/-}$ for in vitro assays) were isolated from adult female Sprague Dawley rats and SD-Tg(GFP)2BalRrrc five days after severe contusion of spinal cord (250 kdyn at T8–T9, see above) and cultured as previously described [25,51].

Oligodendrocyte precursor cell (OPC)-induced differentiation was performed as previously described [25] with slight modifications, including in the FM19G11 condition 500 nM of the compound

FM19G11 (refreshed every two days) or the corresponding amount of vehicle, DMSO in the control group. The differentiation procedure was performed until Day 21 on culture in order to induce the early oligodendrocyte precursors. Part of the OPCs was destined to immunostainings for RIP marker and the other part for total mRNA and protein isolation for quantitative PCR of NG2 and Western blotting detection of Oc4, Sox2 and PCNA. Three independent experiments were performed.

4.3. Spinal Cord Contusion, epSPCi Transplantation, Intrathecal Drug Administration and Functional Locomotor Analysis

SCI by contusion was performed as previously described [25]. Briefly, severe contusion (250 kdyn, "Infinite Horizon Impactor") at thoracic segment T8 was performed. For intramedullary transplantation, 10^6 in 10 μL of total volume epSPCi were transplanted by stereotaxis distributed into rostral and caudal regions at a distance of 2 mm from the lesion at a rate of 2 μL/min by using a 30 G Hamilton pipette filled with cell suspension and mounted on the microinjector. We waited 1 min between injections before moving the syringe to allow cell deposition into the medullar tissue. The compound FM19G11 or DMSO (as vehicle control) was administrated via intrathecal catheterization. Partial laminectomy at T13 allows introducing the catheter (Alzet Corp., Cupertino, CA, USA; previously filled with 0.9% saline solution) through a perforation in dura mater, up to the injured segments (T8). The osmotic pump, Model 1007D (Alzet Corp. Germany; previously filled with FM19G11 or DMSO and incubated overnight at 37 °C in a saline solution), delivers 0.5 μL per hour of a 9 mM FM19G11 solution or DMSO (vehicle) during 3 days.

The rats were pre-medicated with subcutaneous morphine (2.5 mg/kg) and Baytril (enrofloxacin, 5 mg/kg, Bayer, Leverkusen, Germany) and anesthetized with 2% isoflurane in a continuous oxygen flow of 1 L/min. All animals were subjected to post-surgery care and passive and active rehabilitation protocols as previously described [25]. Open-field locomotion was evaluated by two blinded observers by using the 21-point BBB locomotion scale after blind visualization of a minimum of 5 min of free walking in an open space once a week [52]. The animals were sacrificed after 8 weeks of evaluation.

4.4. Histology and Quantification of the Tissue Volume at the Injury Area

The animals were transcardially perfused with a 0.9% saline solution followed by 4% PFA in PBS and 2 days incubation time in 30% sucrose before inclusion in Tissue-Teck OCT (Sakura Finetek Barcelona, Spain). Sagittal cryosections of a 10-μm thickness were used for immunoassays. Every fifth section was collected for eosin and hematoxylin (E&H) staining to determine the anatomical structure and tissue volume calculations in the injured area. E&H-stained sections were scanned in a Pannoramic 250 Flash II scanner (3DHISTECH Ltd.; Budapest, Hungary), and images of approximately 20 mm^2 of medullar tissue (including the epicenter of the lesion) were acquired with the Pannoramic viewer software. The quantification of the spinal cord width was done at eight different points within the injured area. Using Adobe Photoshop® software (version CS2, San Jose, CA, USA), the images of every section, from dorsal to ventral areas, were placed consecutively, and 8 guidelines were traced vertically separated 0.5 mm along the epicenter of the injury. Spinal cord width was measured in every eighth point of every section following the guidelines using the scale bar for absolute quantification and normalization in mm.

The total thickness of the SC at the site of the lesion was quantified by including all the consecutive slides and multiplying them by the thickness of every cryosection (10 μm). Considering the elliptic-shape of the SC, the area quantification was calculated as follows:

$$\text{Area (mm}^2\text{)} = \text{higher radius (higher diameter/2)} \times \text{smaller radius (smaller diameter/2)} \times \pi$$

4.5. Immunocytochemistry and Immunohistochemistry

Cells or cryosectioned tissues (10 μm) were post-fixed with 4% paraformaldehyde at room temperature for 10 min. After permeabilization with PBS containing 0.5% Triton and 2% goat serum (blocking solution), the primary antibodies were incubated overnight at 4 °C. Cells or tissue sections were incubated with GAP43 (α-rabbit; Cat. ab128005 Abcam, Hong Kong, China), β-tubulin III (α-mouse; Cat. MO15052 Neuromics, Edina, MN, USA), GFAP (α-rabbit; Cat. Z0334 DAKO, Santa Clara, CA, USA), RIP (α-mouse; Cat. MAB1580 Chemicon, Pittsburgh, PA, USA) and OLIG1 (α-rabbit; Cat. AB5320 Chemicon). Primary antibodies were diluted 1:200 in blocking solution. After being rinsed three times with PBS, the cells or the tissue sections were incubated with Oregon Green-Alexa488, Alexa555 or Alexa647 dye-conjugated secondary antibodies for 1 h at room temperature. All cells and tissue sections were counterstained by incubation with DAPI for 5 min at room temperature followed by washing steps. Signals were visualized by both fluorescent microscopy (fluorescence microscope Leica DM6000B, Wetzlar, Germany) and confocal microscopy (confocal microscope Leica TCS-SP2-AOBS, Wetzlar, Germany). The quantification of immunostainings was performed using ImageJ software (Image J2, Madison, WI, USA).

4.6. Western Blot

epSPCi neurosphere-like cultures at the indicated points of the OPC differentiation process were lysed in 50 mM Tris-HCl, pH 7.5, 150 mM NaCl, 0.02% NaN3, 0.1 SDS, 1% NP40, 1 mM ethylene diamine tetra acetic acid (EDTA), 2 μg/mL leupeptin, 2 μg/mL aprotinin, 1 mM PMSF and 1 × Protease Inhibitor Cocktail (Roche Diagnostics, San Diego, CA, USA), stored on ice for 30 min and boiled for 10 min. Twenty five μg of each protein extract were subjected to sodium dodecyl sulfate (SDS) polyacrylamide gel electrophoresis (PAGE; MiniProtean®, Bio-Rad, Hercules, CA, USA) and blotted with antibodies overnight at 4 °C. Signal detection was performed with an enhanced chemiluminescence kit (ECL Plus Western blotting detection reagent from GE Healthcare, Piscataway Township, NJ, USA). Primary antibodies used were Sox2 (α-mouse; Cat. MAB2018. R&D System, Minneapolis, MN, USA), NG2 (α-mouse; Cat. MAB5384. Chemicon), PCNA (α-mouse; Cat. ab29. Abcam) and β-actin for the loading control (α-mouse; Cat. A5441 Sigma, Sant Louis, MO, USA). At least 3 biologically independent replicates were always performed; a representative Western blot is shown.

4.7. RNA Isolation and Quantitative RT-PCR

Total RNA of epSPCi at the indicated points of the OPC differentiation process was extracted by using the RNeasy Mini-kit (Qiagen, Hilden, Germany) according to the manufacturer's instructions. One microgram of total RNA was reverse-transcribed in a total reaction volume of 50 μL at 42 °C for 30 min using random hexamer primers. For quantitative analyses, we used LightCycler SYBR® Green I technology, and the relative expression of mRNA transcripts was analyzed by the ABI PRISM 5700 Sequence Detection System (Applied Biosystems, Foster City, CA, USA). As a template, we used 40 ng of cDNA to analyze the expression of target and housekeeping genes (18S) in separate tubes for each pair of primers. The sequences from 5′ to 3′of each pair of primers are: rNG2, forward primer: 5′-ATGCTTCTCAGCCCGGGACA-3′; reverse primer: 5′-GGTTGCGGCCATTGAGAATG-3′; r18S, forward primer: ggaagggcaccaccaggagt; reverse primer: tgcagccccggacatctaag. The comparative threshold cycle (Ct) method was used to calculate the relative expression as follows:

$$\Delta C_t\ (\Delta C_t = C_t\ (\text{test gene}) - C_t\ (\text{GAPDH}))$$

ΔC_t for FM19G11-treated samples was then subtracted from the ΔC_t for vehicle-treated samples, to generate $\Delta\Delta C_t$ ($\Delta\Delta C_t = \Delta C_t$ (*FM19G11*) $-$ ΔC_t (vehicle)). The mean of these $\Delta\Delta C_t$ measurements was used to calculate the fold change in gene expression ($2^{-\Delta\Delta Ct}$). Results were presented as the mean ± standard error.

4.8. Statistical Analysis

Student's *t*-test was performed for pair comparisons and one-way analysis of variance (ANOVA) for multiple value comparisons. All measurements in cell culture experiments were carried out in at least three different culture preparations, and the results were expressed as the mean ± SEM. Statistical analysis was performed using GraphPad Prism 4 Project software (San Diego, CA, USA). In all cases, $p < 0.05$ was considered significant.

5. Conclusions

Altogether, significant beneficial cellular changes at the histological level were found in the combinatory treatment with epSPCi and FM19G11 in the SCI acute rat model. The obtained results justify the combination of both strategies, cell transplantation and pharmacological treatment, as opposed to the use of the individual ones, for better success on locomotor improvements after SCI, although further investigation would be necessary to demonstrate plausible functional benefits by adjusting doses and/or treatment administrations for long-term treatment and analysis.

Acknowledgments: This work was supported by research grants from the Foundation Step by Step, the Spanish Ion Channel Initiative (CSD2008-00005), the Instituto Salud Carlos III (PI13/00319) and MINECO (MAT2015-66666-C3-2-R). The authors would like to thank Maravillas Mellado López for essential technical support. The authors would like to thank Richard Griffeth for manuscript editing and critical comments.

Author Contributions: Victoria Moreno-Manzano conceived of the idea and contribute to the materials. Slaven Erceg provided conceptual advice and contributed materials. Victoria Moreno-Manzano, Ana Alastrue-Agudo and Francisco Javier Rodriguez-Jimenez designed the research. Ana Alastrue-Agudo, Victoria Moreno-Manzano, Francisco Javier Rodriguez-Jimenez, Eric López Mocholi and Francesca De Giorgio performed the research. Victoria Moreno-Manzano, Ana Alastrue-Agudo and Francisco Javier Rodriguez-Jimenez analyzed the data. Victoria Moreno-Manzano wrote the manuscript.

Abbreviations

BBB	Basso, Beattie and Bresnahan
BSCB	Blood-spinal cord barrier
DMSO	Dimethyl sulfoxide
epSPC	Ependymal stem/progenitor cells
epSPCi	Ependymal stem/progenitor cells of the spinal cord after injury
GFAP	Glial fibrillary acidic protein
GFP	Green fluorescence protein
H&E	Hematoxylin-eosin
HIF	Hypoxia inducible factor
NPC	Neural precursor cell
OPC	Oligodendrocyte precursor cell
PFA	Paraformaldehyde
PBS	Phosphate buffer solution
RT-PCR	Reverse transcription-polymerase chain reaction
SC	Spinal cord
SCI	Spinal cord injury
UCP	Uncoupling protein

References

1. Hulsebosch, C.E. Recent advances in pathophysiology and treatment of spinal cord injury. *Adv. Physiol. Educ.* **2002**, *26*, 238–255. [CrossRef] [PubMed]
2. Robinson, J.; Lu, P. Optimization of trophic support for neural stem cell grafts in sites of spinal cord injury. *Exp. Neurol.* **2017**, *291*, 87–97. [CrossRef] [PubMed]

3. Negro, S.; Lessi, F.; Duregotti, E.; Aretini, P.; La Ferla, M.; Franceschi, S.; Menicagli, M.; Bergamin, E.; Radice, E.; Thelen, M.; et al. CXCL12alpha/SDF-1 from perisynaptic Schwann cells promotes regeneration of injured motor axon terminals. *EMBO Mol. Med.* **2017**, *9*, 1000–1010. [CrossRef] [PubMed]
4. Liu, Y.; Wang, X.; Li, W.; Zhang, Q.; Li, Y.; Zhang, Z.; Zhu, J.; Chen, B.; Williams, P.R.; Zhang, Y.; et al. A sensitized IGF1 treatment restores corticospinal axon-dependent functions. *Neuron* **2017**, *95*, 817–833. [CrossRef] [PubMed]
5. Sandler, A.N.; Tator, C.H. Review of the effect of spinal cord trama on the vessels and blood flow in the spinal cord. *J. Neurosurg.* **1976**, *45*, 638–646. [CrossRef] [PubMed]
6. Kitayama, M.; Ueno, M.; Itakura, T.; Yamashita, T. Activated microglia inhibit axonal growth through RGMa. *PLoS ONE* **2011**, *6*, e25234. [CrossRef] [PubMed]
7. Okada, S.; Hara, M.; Kobayakawa, K.; Matsumoto, Y.; Nakashima, Y. Astrocyte reactivity and astrogliosis after spinal cord injury. *Neurosci. Res.* **2017**, *126*, 39–43. [CrossRef] [PubMed]
8. Lukovic, D.; Stojkovic, M.; Moreno-Manzano, V.; Jendelova, P.; Sykova, E.; Bhattacharya, S.S.; Erceg, S. Concise review: Reactive astrocytes and stem cells in spinal cord injury: Good guys or bad guys? *Stem Cells* **2015**, *33*, 1036–1041. [CrossRef] [PubMed]
9. David, S.; Kroner, A. Repertoire of microglial and macrophage responses after spinal cord injury. *Nat. Rev. Neurosci.* **2011**, *12*, 388–399. [CrossRef] [PubMed]
10. Donnelly, D.J.; Popovich, P.G. Inflammation and its role in neuroprotection, axonal regeneration and functional recovery after spinal cord injury. *Exp. Neurol.* **2008**, *209*, 378–388. [CrossRef] [PubMed]
11. Gensel, J.C.; Zhang, B. Macrophage activation and its role in repair and pathology after spinal cord injury. *Brain Res.* **2015**, *1619*, 1–11. [CrossRef] [PubMed]
12. Ahuja, C.S.; Nori, S.; Tetreault, L.; Wilson, J.; Kwon, B.; Harrop, J.; Choi, D.; Fehlings, M.G. Traumatic spinal cord injury-repair and regeneration. *Neurosurgery* **2017**, *80*, S9–S22. [CrossRef] [PubMed]
13. Grossman, S.D.; Rosenberg, L.J.; Wrathall, J.R. Temporal-spatial pattern of acute neuronal and glial loss after spinal cord contusion. *Exp. Neurol.* **2001**, *168*, 273–282. [CrossRef] [PubMed]
14. Ahuja, C.S.; Fehlings, M. Concise review: Bridging the gap: Novel neuroregenerative and neuroprotective strategies in spinal cord injury. *Stem Cells Transl. Med.* **2016**, *5*, 914–924. [CrossRef] [PubMed]
15. Ronaghi, M.; Erceg, S.; Moreno-Manzano, V.; Stojkovic, M. Challenges of stem cell therapy for spinal cord injury: Human embryonic stem cells, endogenous neural stem cells, or induced pluripotent stem cells? *Stem Cells* **2010**, *28*, 93–99. [CrossRef] [PubMed]
16. Gazdic, M.; Volarevic, V.; Arsenijevic, A.; Erceg, S.; Moreno-Manzano, V.; Arsenijevic, N.; Stojkovic, M. Stem cells and labeling for spinal cord injury. *Int. J. Mol. Sci.* **2016**, *18*, 6. [CrossRef] [PubMed]
17. Requejo-Aguilar, R.; Alastrue-Agudo, A.; Cases-Villar, M.; Lopez-Mocholi, E.; England, R.; Vicent, M.J.; Moreno-Manzano, V. Combined polymer-curcumin conjugate and ependymal progenitor/stem cell treatment enhances spinal cord injury functional recovery. *Biomaterials* **2017**, *113*, 18–30. [CrossRef] [PubMed]
18. Jin, W.; Wang, J.; Zhu, T.; Yuan, B.; Ni, H.; Jiang, J.; Wang, H.; Liang, W. Anti-inflammatory effects of curcumin in experimental spinal cord injury in rats. *Inflamm. Res.* **2014**, *63*, 381–387. [CrossRef] [PubMed]
19. Ormond, D.R.; Shannon, C.; Oppenheim, J.; Zeman, R.; Das, K.; Murali, R.; Jhanwar-Uniyal, M. Stem cell therapy and curcumin synergistically enhance recovery from spinal cord injury. *PLoS ONE* **2014**, *9*, e88916. [CrossRef] [PubMed]
20. Sahin Kavakli, H.; Koca, C.; Alici, O. Antioxidant effects of curcumin in spinal cord injury in rats. *Ulus. Travma Acil Cerrahi Derg.* **2011**, *17*, 14–18. [CrossRef] [PubMed]
21. Wang, Y.F.; Zu, J.N.; Li, J.; Chen, C.; Xi, C.Y.; Yan, J.L. Curcumin promotes the spinal cord repair via inhibition of glial scar formation and inflammation. *Neurosci. Lett.* **2014**, *560*, 51–56. [CrossRef] [PubMed]
22. Yuan, J.; Zou, M.; Xiang, X.; Zhu, H.; Chu, W.; Liu, W.; Chen, F.; Lin, J. Curcumin improves neural function after spinal cord injury by the joint inhibition of the intracellular and extracellular components of glial scar. *J. Surg. Res.* **2015**, *195*, 235–245. [CrossRef] [PubMed]
23. Meletis, K.; Barnabe-Heider, F.; Carlen, M.; Evergren, E.; Tomilin, N.; Shupliakov, O.; Frisén, J. Spinal cord injury reveals multilineage differentiation of ependymal cells. *PLoS Biol.* **2008**, *6*, e182. [CrossRef] [PubMed]
24. Gomez-Villafuertes, R.; Rodriguez-Jimenez, F.J.; Alastrue-Agudo, A.; Stojkovic, M.; Miras-Portugal, M.T.; Moreno-Manzano, V. Purinergic receptors in spinal cord-derived ependymal stem/progenitor cells and their potential role in cell-based therapy for spinal cord injury. *Cell Transplant.* **2015**, *24*, 1493–1509. [CrossRef] [PubMed]

25. Moreno-Manzano, V.; Rodriguez-Jimenez, F.J.; Garcia-Rosello, M.; Lainez, S.; Erceg, S.; Calvo, M.T.; Ronaghi, M.; Lloret, M.; Planells-Cases, R.; Sánchez-Puelles, J.M. Activated spinal cord ependymal stem cells rescue neurological function. *Stem Cells* **2009**, *27*, 733–743. [CrossRef] [PubMed]
26. Thuret, S.; Moon, L.D.; Gage, F.H. Therapeutic interventions after spinal cord injury. *Nat. Rev. Neurosci.* **2006**, *7*, 628–643. [CrossRef] [PubMed]
27. Moreno-Manzano, V.; Rodriguez-Jimenez, F.J.; Acena-Bonilla, J.L.; Fustero-Lardies, S.; Erceg, S.; Dopazo, J.; Montaner, D.; Stojkovic, M.; Sánchez-Puelles, J.M. FM19G11, a new hypoxia-inducible factor (HIF) modulator, affects stem cell differentiation status. *J. Biol. Chem.* **2010**, *285*, 1333–1342. [CrossRef] [PubMed]
28. Rodriguez-Jimenez, F.J.; Moreno-Manzano, V.; Lucas-Dominguez, R.; Sanchez-Puelles, J.M. Hypoxia causes downregulation of mismatch repair system and genomic instability in stem cells. *Stem Cells* **2008**, *26*, 2052–2062. [CrossRef] [PubMed]
29. Rodriguez-Jimenez, F.J.; Moreno-Manzano, V.; Mateos-Gregorio, P.; Royo, I.; Erceg, S.; Murguia, J.R.; Sánchez-Puelles, J.M. FM19G11: A new modulator of HIF that links mTOR activation with the DNA damage checkpoint pathways. *Cell Cycle* **2010**, *9*, 2803–2813. [CrossRef] [PubMed]
30. Rodriguez-Jimnez, F.J.; Alastrue-Agudo, A.; Erceg, S.; Stojkovic, M.; Moreno-Manzano, V. FM19G11 favors spinal cord injury regeneration and stem cell self-renewal by mitochondrial uncoupling and glucose metabolism induction. *Stem Cells* **2012**, *30*, 2221–2233. [CrossRef] [PubMed]
31. Morita, S.; Miyata, S. Synaptic localization of growth-associated protein 43 in cultured hippocampal neurons during synaptogenesis. *Cell Biochem. Funct.* **2013**, *31*, 400–411. [CrossRef] [PubMed]
32. Watanabe, M.; Sakurai, Y.; Ichinose, T.; Aikawa, Y.; Kotani, M.; Itoh, K. Monoclonal antibody Rip specifically recognizes 2′,3′-cyclic nucleotide 3′-phosphodiesterase in oligodendrocytes. *J. Neurosci. Res.* **2006**, *84*, 525–533. [CrossRef] [PubMed]
33. Barnabe-Heider, F.; Goritz, C.; Sabelstrom, H.; Takebayashi, H.; Pfrieger, F.W.; Meletis, K.; Frisén, J. Origin of new glial cells in intact and injured adult spinal cord. *Cell Stem Cell* **2010**, *7*, 470–482. [CrossRef] [PubMed]
34. Hesp, Z.C.; Goldstein, E.Z.; Miranda, C.J.; Kaspar, B.K.; McTigue, D.M. Chronic oligodendrogenesis and remyelination after spinal cord injury in mice and rats. *J. Neurosci.* **2015**, *35*, 1274–1290. [CrossRef] [PubMed]
35. Sellers, D.L.; Maris, D.O.; Horner, P.J. Postinjury niches induce temporal shifts in progenitor fates to direct lesion repair after spinal cord injury. *J. Neurosci.* **2009**, *29*, 6722–6733. [CrossRef] [PubMed]
36. Gledhill, R.F.; Harrison, B.M.; McDonald, W.I. Demyelination and remyelination after acute spinal cord compression. *Exp. Neurol.* **1973**, *38*, 472–487. [CrossRef]
37. Harrison, B.M.; McDonald, W.I. Remyelination after transient experimental compression of the spinal cord. *Ann. Neurol.* **1977**, *1*, 542–551. [CrossRef] [PubMed]
38. Cheng, X.; Wang, Y.; He, Q.; Qiu, M.; Whittemore, S.R.; Cao, Q. Bone morphogenetic protein signaling and olig1/2 interact to regulate the differentiation and maturation of adult oligodendrocyte precursor cells. *Stem Cells* **2007**, *25*, 3204–3214. [CrossRef] [PubMed]
39. McDonough, A.; Martinez-Cerdeno, V. Endogenous proliferation after spinal cord injury in animal models. *Stem Cells Int.* **2012**, *2012*, 387513. [CrossRef] [PubMed]
40. Lukovic, D.; Moreno-Manzano, V.; Lopez-Mocholi, E.; Rodriguez-Jimenez, F.J.; Jendelova, P.; Sykova, E.; Oria, M.; Stojkovic, M.; Erceg, S. Complete rat spinal cord transection as a faithful model of spinal cord injury for translational cell transplantation. *Sci. Rep.* **2015**, *5*, 9640. [CrossRef] [PubMed]
41. Stenudd, M.; Sabelstrom, H.; Frisen, J. Role of endogenous neural stem cells in spinal cord injury and repair. *JAMA Neurol.* **2015**, *72*, 235–237. [CrossRef] [PubMed]
42. Davies, J.E.; Proschel, C.; Zhang, N.; Noble, M.; Mayer-Proschel, M.; Davies, S.J. Transplanted astrocytes derived from BMP- or CNTF-treated glial-restricted precursors have opposite effects on recovery and allodynia after spinal cord injury. *J. Biol.* **2008**, *7*, 24. [CrossRef] [PubMed]
43. Cusimano, M.; Biziato, D.; Brambilla, E.; Donega, M.; Alfaro-Cervello, C.; Snider, S.; Salani, G.; Pucci, F.; Comi, G.; Garcia-Verdugo, J.M. Transplanted neural stem/precursor cells instruct phagocytes and reduce secondary tissue damage in the injured spinal cord. *Brain J. Neurol.* **2012**, *135 Pt 2*, 447–460. [CrossRef] [PubMed]
44. Gensel, J.C.; Kopper, T.J.; Zhang, B.; Orr, M.B.; Bailey, W.M. Predictive screening of M1 and M2 macrophages reveals the immunomodulatory effectiveness of post spinal cord injury azithromycin treatment. *Sci. Rep.* **2017**, *7*, 40144. [CrossRef] [PubMed]

45. Mekhail, M.; Almazan, G.; Tabrizian, M. Oligodendrocyte-protection and remyelination post-spinal cord injuries: A review. *Prog. Neurobiol.* **2012**, *96*, 322–339. [CrossRef] [PubMed]
46. Plemel, J.R.; Keough, M.B.; Duncan, G.J.; Sparling, J.S.; Yong, V.W.; Stys, P.K.; Tetzlaff, W. Remyelination after spinal cord injury: Is it a target for repair? *Prog. Neurobiol.* **2014**, *117*, 54–72. [CrossRef] [PubMed]
47. Karimi-Abdolrezaee, S.; Eftekharpour, E.; Wang, J.; Morshead, C.M.; Fehlings, M.G. Delayed transplantation of adult neural precursor cells promotes remyelination and functional neurological recovery after spinal cord injury. *J. Neurosci.* **2006**, *26*, 3377–3389. [CrossRef] [PubMed]
48. Cao, Q.; He, Q.; Wang, Y.; Cheng, X.; Howard, R.M.; Zhang, Y.; DeVries, W.H.; Shields, C.B.; Magnuson, D.S.; Xu, X.M. Transplantation of ciliary neurotrophic factor-expressing adult oligodendrocyte precursor cells promotes remyelination and functional recovery after spinal cord injury. *J. Neurosci.* **2010**, *30*, 2989–3001. [CrossRef] [PubMed]
49. Plemel, J.R.; Chojnacki, A.; Sparling, J.S.; Liu, J.; Plunet, W.; Duncan, G.J.; Park, S.E.; Weiss, S.; Tetzlaff, W. Platelet-derived growth factor-responsive neural precursors give rise to myelinating oligodendrocytes after transplantation into the spinal cords of contused rats and dysmyelinated mice. *Glia* **2011**, *59*, 1891–1910. [CrossRef] [PubMed]
50. Sun, Y.; Xu, C.C.; Li, J.; Guan, X.Y.; Gao, L.; Ma, L.X.; Li, R.X.; Peng, Y.W.; Zhu, G.P. Transplantation of oligodendrocyte precursor cells improves locomotion deficits in rats with spinal cord irradiation injury. *PLoS ONE* **2013**, *8*, e57534. [CrossRef] [PubMed]
51. Rodriguez-Jimenez, F.J.; Alastrue, A.; Stojkovic, M.; Erceg, S.; Moreno-Manzano, V. Connexin 50 modulates Sox2 expression in spinal-cord-derived ependymal stem/progenitor cells. *Cell Tissue Res.* **2016**, *365*, 295–307. [CrossRef] [PubMed]
52. Basso, D.M.; Beattie, M.S.; Bresnahan, J.C. A sensitive and reliable locomotor rating scale for open field testing in rats. *J. Neurotrauma* **1995**, *12*, 1–21. [CrossRef] [PubMed]

8

Stress-Activated Protein Kinases in Spinal Cord Injury: Focus on Roles of p38

Yoshitoshi Kasuya [1,2,*], Hiroki Umezawa [1,2,3] and Masahiko Hatano [1]

1 Department of Biomedical Science, Graduate School of Medicine, Chiba University, Chiba City, Chiba 260-8670, Japan; h-umepan@hotmail.co.jp (H.U.); hatanom@faculty.chiba-u.jp (M.H.)
2 Department of Biochemistry and Molecular Pharmacology, Graduate School of Medicine, Chiba University, Chiba City, Chiba 260-8670, Japan
3 Department of Respirology, Graduate School of Medicine, Chiba University, Chiba City, Chiba 260-8670, Japan
* Correspondence: kasuya@faculty.chiba-u.jp

Abstract: Spinal cord injury (SCI) consists of three phases—acute, secondary, and chronic damages—and limiting the development of secondary damage possibly improves functional recovery after SCI. A major component of the secondary phase of SCI is regarded as inflammation-triggered events: induction of cytokines, edema, microglial activation, apoptosis of cells including oligodendrocytes and neurons, demyelination, formation of the astrocytic scar, and so on. Two major stress-activated protein kinases (SAPKs)—c-Jun N-terminal kinase (JNK) and p38 mitogen-activated protein kinase (p38 MAPK)—are activated in various types of cells in response to cellular stresses such as apoptotic stimuli and inflammatory waves. In animal models of SCI, inhibition of either JNK or p38 has been shown to promote neuroprotection-associated functional recovery. Here, we provide an overview on the roles of SAPKs in SCI and, in particular, the pathological role of p38 will be discussed as a promising target for therapeutic intervention in SCI.

Keywords: spinal cord injury; stress-activated protein kinases; c-Jun N-terminal kinase; p38 mitogen-activated protein kinase

---

1. Introduction

Traumatic spinal cord injury (SCI) is a severe, devastating disease which often results in sensorimotor dysfunction, largely due to the poor regenerative capacity of neuronal cells in the adult mammalian central nervous system (CNS) [1]. Following the initial physical injury, the lesion proceeds to receive secondary waves of complex neuroinflammatory events that cause additional tissue destruction and functional impairments [2,3]. Under the secondary phase of SCI, however, gradual functional recovery is observed in not only several animal models but also humans to some extent, and is inversely proportional to the initial damage intensity of the SC [4]. In developing beneficial drugs for SCI, it is therefore clinically reasonable to target the secondary damages involving inflammation, blood–cerebrospinal fluid (CSF) barrier disruption, glial scar formation, cell death of neurons and oligodendrocytes, lipid peroxidation, and glutamate excitotoxicity. Indeed, many studies have recently focused on pharmacological interventions targeting the secondary damage symptoms. To strengthen the reliability of therapeutic candidates for SCI, however, the exact molecular mechanism underlying the secondary damage symptoms and the pivotal signaling pathway mediating each symptom should be evaluated precisely.

The stress-activated protein kinase (SAPK) group of mitogen-activated protein kinases (MAPKs) includes two members of the c-Jun NH2-terminal kinase (JNK) and p38 MAPK families, which are activated in response to environmental stresses such as inflammatory stimuli by cytokines and Toll-like receptor (TLR) ligands, oxidative stress, trophic factor withdrawal, osmolarity shock, ultraviolet (UV) irradiation, chemotherapeutic drugs, and so on [5,6]. The JNK family (JNK1, JNK2, and JNK3) are encoded by three separate but closely related genes. JNK1 and JNK2 are expressed ubiquitously in adult tissues, whereas the expression of JNK3 is primarily observed in brain, heart, and testis. Ten different JNK isoforms are produced by alternative splicing of the *Jnk* transcripts: JNK1α1, JNK1β1, JNK2α1, JNK2β1, and JNK3α1 have a molecular weight of 46 kDa; and JNK1α2, JNK1β2, JNK2α2, JNK2β2, and JNK3α2 have a molecular weight of 54 kDa with an extended C-terminus [7]. Their relative contributions to the overall JNK activity remain to be elucidated. JNKs are activated by dual phosphorylation of the TPY motif within their activation loop by two upstream MAPK kinases (MAP2Ks)—MKK4 and MKK7—which are activated by various MAPKK kinases (MAP3Ks), MEKKs, Mixed-lineage kinases (MLKs), apoptosis signal-regulating kinase 1 (ASK1), thousand-and-one amino acid kinase 2 (TAO2), TNF receptor-associated factor 2- and NCK-interacting protein kinase (TNIK), and dual leucine zipper-bearing kinase (DLK) [8].

On the other hand, the p38 family consists of four isoforms (α, β, γ, and δ) arising from separate genes. p38α and -β are ubiquitously expressed in adult tissues, whereas expression of p38γ is predominant in skeletal muscle and p38δ shows high expression levels in the kidney and lung [9,10]. As an alternative form of p38β that was initially identified, p38β2 with an internal deletion of 8 amino acids has been reported. p38β2 showed much higher sensitivity to extracellular stimuli and p38 inhibitor than does p38β, which shows a level similar to that of p38α. In particular, p38β2 but not p38β phosphorylated various substrates (as p38α does) in response to sorbitol [11]. Therefore, p38β means p38β2 at present. Among p38 isoforms, the best characterized isoform is p38α, the physiological and pathological roles of which have been well investigated [5,12]. In this review, we therefore mostly refer to p38α as p38, unless otherwise indicated. p38 MAPKs are activated by dual phosphorylation of the TGY motif within their activation loop by two upstream MAP2K—MKK3 and MKK6—which are activated by various MAP3Ks, MEKKs, MLKs, ASK1, TAO2, TGF-β-activated kinase 1 (TAK1), and Tumor progression locus 2 (TPL2). Consequently, JNK and p38 pathways share a number of upstream MAP3Ks although the two pathways are not redundant. In addition to this canonical activation pathway composed of three stepwise modules, specific binding of TAK1-binding protein 1 (TAB1) to p38α and TCR/ζ chain-associated protein kinase (ZAP70)-mediated phosphorylation of Tyr^{323} in the C-terminal domain of p38 MAPKs (except p38δ) are described as new p38 activation pathways via upregulating autophosphorylation of p38 MAPKs [13,14].

Overview of the SAPK activation pathway is shown in Figure 1A. SAPKs activated through a typical kinase cascade promote a variety of cellular responses. In this review, we introduce increasing evidence concerning pathological functions of JNK and p38 in SCI. In particular, we will discuss the potential of targeting the p38 pathway as a disease-modifying therapy in SCI.

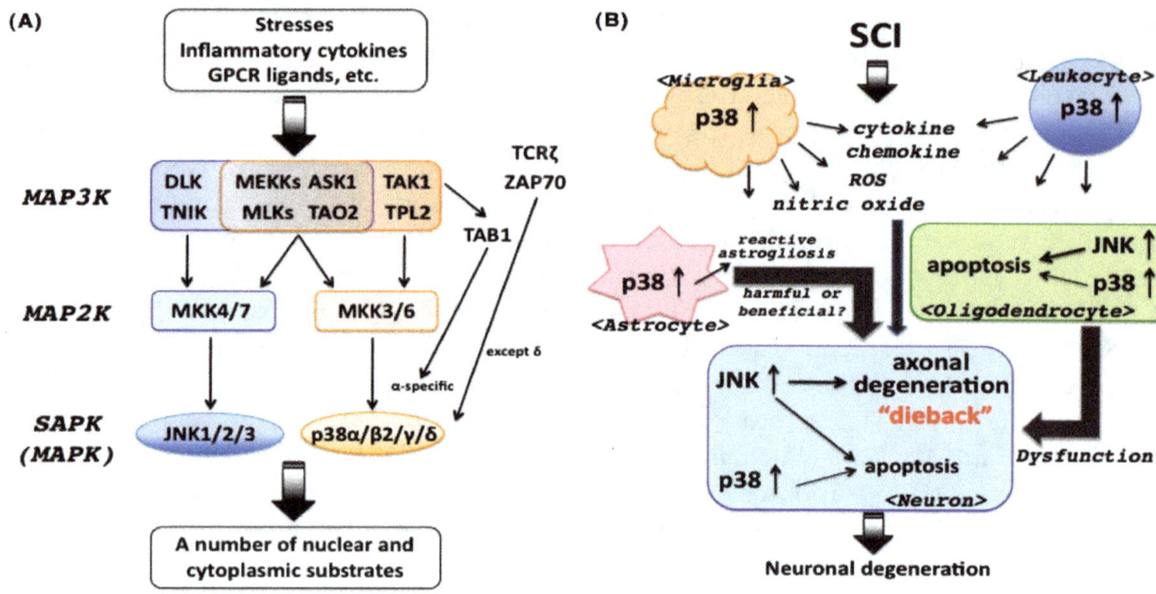

Figure 1. (**A**) Overview of the stress-activated protein kinase (SAPK) pathway. SAPKs, c-Jun N-terminal kinases (JNKs), and p38 mitogen-activated protein kinases (MAPKs) are activated in response to a variety of cellular stresses through a three-step pathway (MAP3K/MAP2K/MAPK). In addition to this canonical pathway, several pathways for p38 activation have been demonstrated. (**B**) Overview of the SAPK-mediated neuronal degeneration after spinal cord injury (SCI). JNK contributes to neuronal degeneration in a direct manner and also induces neuronal dysfunction in an indirect manner through oligodendrocytic cell-death-associated demyelination. p38 predominantly orchestrates SCI-triggered inflammatory responses such as activation of microglia, production of inflammatory and neurotoxic mediators from infiltrated leukocytes and activated microglia, and reactive astrogliosis. Reactive astrogliosis shows bidirectional effects on neuronal regeneration after SCI.

2. SAPKs in the CNS

In the CNS, JNK1 and JNK2 are expressed in various types of cells. On the other hand, the expression of JNK3 is predominantly observed in neuronal cells. The most highly expressed transcript of JNK isoform in the adult rodent brain is *Jnk3* mRNA followed by *Jnk2* mRNA and then *Jnk1* mRNA [15,16]. The cellular and behavioral phenotypes observed in *JNK* isoform- and compound *JNK* isoforms-knockout mice models clearly suggest crucial roles of JNKs in the CNS as follows: (i) *Jnk3*-knockout mice exhibit a marked reduction in kainate-induced neuronal apoptosis in the hippocampus secondary to seizure response, and in dopaminergic cell loss in the Parkinson's disease model mice using 1-methyl-4-phenyl-1,2,4,6-tetrahydropyridine (MPTP) [17–19]; (ii) *Jnk2*-knockout mice show a decrease in dopaminergic cell loss in the MPTP Parkinson's disease model [18]; (iii) *Jnk1/Jnk2*-double-knockout mice show an embryonic lethality at E11.5 because of severe dysregulation of apoptosis in the hindbrain at E9.0 [20]; (iv) *Jnk1/Jnk2/Jnk3*-triple-knockout neuronal cells (primary cultured neurons from $Jnk1^{LoxP/LoxP}Jnk2^{-/-}Jnk3^{-/-}$ mice were infected with *Ad-cre* to establish deficiency of the *JNKs*) exhibit marked life span extension during culture in vitro [21]. Therefore, JNK is the central player at least in neuronal apoptosis, which tempts us to consider that JNKs are able to contribute to the development of various neural diseases. Here, "knockout" represents a traditional gene knockout, unless otherwise indicated.

In contrast to the cases of *JNK*-knockout mice, deficiency of each p38 isoform gene does not result in defects in the CNS. *p38α*-knockout mice result in embryonic lethality due to dysfunction of erythropoiesis and placental organogenesis [22,23]. A deficiency of the *p38β* gene is functionally compensated by p38 in both activation of downstream kinases and TNF-α-mediated inflammatory diseases [24]. *p38γ*-knockout mice exhibit loss of myogenic precursor cells that are primarily responsible for skeletal muscle growth and regeneration [25]. *p38δ*-knockout mice exhibit a marked resistance to skin tumor development induced by chemical agents [26]. However, increasing evidence indicates that at least p38α is expressed in neurons, astrocytes, oligodendrocytes, and microglia and controls their cell fate and functions [12,27–30]. For instance, it has been proposed that amyloid β-peptide (Aβ)-induced disruption of N-cadherin-based synaptic contact results in p38 activation, which in turn phosphorylates Tau leading to neuronal apoptosis. This phenomenon is one of the neurodegenerative processes in Alzheimer's disease (AD) [31]. Likewise, p38 as well as JNK are activated and play roles in the innate and adaptive immune responses, and various p38 inhibitors have been energetically developed and are in clinical trials as potential anti-inflammatory drugs [5] (Clinicaltrials.gov, https://clinicaltrials.gov/). In inflammation-associated disorders of the CNS, p38 may therefore be a valid therapeutic target. In fact, several reports including our study have demonstrated that p38α contributes to the pathogenesis of experimental autoimmune encephalomyelitis (EAE, a model for multiple sclerosis) mainly via mobilizing the Th17/IL-17 axis [32–36]. Notably, p38 inhibitors ameliorate the progression of EAE if administered even after the onset of clinical symptoms [35,36]. In AD, moreover, the intense signal of p38 activation was observed in the brain area where neuritic β-amyloid plaques were accumulated. It has been also demonstrated that p38 plays a crucial role in amyloid precursor protein-induced production of neurotoxic cytokines (e.g., TNF-α and IL-1β) in microglia [37]. It is noteworthy that p38α inhibition ameliorates the overproduction of proinflammatory cytokines associated with neuronal dysfunction and behavioral deficits in the Aβ-infused AD-relevant animal model [38].

3. Involvement of JNK in the Pathogenesis of SCI

Early evidence has demonstrated that contusion SCI activates the ASK1/JNK-p38 signaling axis in both neurons and oligodendrocytes proceeding to apoptosis [39]. These events were followed by further study using tiptoe-walking Yoshimura (TWY) mice that developed aging-associated spontaneous calcification in the cervical ligament, thereby causing chronic mechanical compression of the spinal cords. [40]. In those reports, the activation of ASK1-JNK and -p38 pathways was observed in apoptotic sign-bearing neurons and oligodendrocytes, suggesting that JNK and p38 contribute to neuronal and oligodendrocytic apoptosis in SCI at least phenomenologically.

The JNK-mediated apoptosis of oligodendrocytes in SCI has been precisely investigated [41]. The injury-activated JNK3 phosphorylated myeloid cell leukemia sequence-1 (Mcl-1) and facilitated the degradation of Mcl-1 by ubiquitination in oligodendrocytes, which in turn induced apoptosis-associated release of cytochrome C from mitochondria. This JNK-mediated oligodendrocytic apoptosis was canceled by a disruption of the *Jnk3* gene. Interestingly, the peak activation ratio of JNK3 was 500-fold higher than those of JNK1/2 in the SC after hemisection injury, and JNK activation monitored by phosphorylation of c-Jun was typically detected in neurons as well. Nevertheless, the number of apoptotic neuron somas ($TUNEL^+/NeuN^+$) was not significantly different between *Jnk3*-knockout mice and wild-type (WT) littermates, suggesting several possibilities as follows: (i) low activation of JNK1 or JNK2 functionally contributes to neuronal cell death after SCI; (ii) JNK3 may induce not apoptosis but another type of cell death—autophagic death—after SCI; (iii) JNK3 may not directly regulate apoptosis of neurons but may play a role in transporting the damage signal under nerve degeneration or regeneration like the case in the previous report [42]. The last notion was supported by a subsequent study.

Superior cervical ganglion 10 (SCG10), an axonal-maintenance factor, has phosphorylation sites (Ser63 and Ser73) specific for JNK and is at least partly regulated by the phosphorylation-triggered degradation program. In healthy axons, SCG10 protein may undergo rapid JNK-dependent degradation versus replenishment by axonal transport from cell bodies. Once axons were injured, loss of function of the replenishment in concert with continuous JNK-dependent degradation might result in a marked loss of SCG10 selectively in distal axon segments, which accelerates axonal fragmentation leading to anterograde axonal degeneration [43]. Hence, the JNK/SCG10 axis may contribute to Wallerian degeneration, one of the typical pathological aspects in SCI. Furthermore, the involvement of JNK in retrograde axonal degeneration—so-called "dieback"—has been clearly demonstrated [44]. The SCI-upregulated phospho-JNK was observed in the dorsal corticospinal tract (CST) fibers labeled with biotinylated dextran amine (BDA) in the gray matter rostral to the lesion site, where amyloid-β precursor protein, a marker for axonal degradation, was apparently accumulated. This SCI-induced axonal dieback was markedly suppressed by continuous intrathecal administration of a JNK inhibitor, SP600125, which was replicated in both *JNK1*-knockout and *JNK3*-knockout mice. Likewise, hindlimb locomotor recovery after SCI was improved in SP600125-treated WT, *JNK1*-knockout, and *JNK3*-knockout mice, suggesting that at least JNK1 and JNK3 positively regulate axonal dieback limiting locomotor recovery after SCI. It has been also demonstrated that the improvement of functional recovery after SCI is performed by D-JNKI1—the cell-permeable peptide inhibitor against JNK [45]. Notably, a single intraperitoneal injection of D-JNKI1 showed beneficial effects on SCI, which may be valuable as a minimally invasive strategy for clinical application of JNK inhibition.

In contrast to the axonal degeneration activity of JNK in SCI, a lot of previous reports have demonstrated that JNKs might play important roles in axonal guidance and neurite growth [8]. During the axonal regeneration process, JNK activity is necessary for neuritogenesis and sustained neurite elongation [46]. These findings strongly suggest that JNK elicits neuroregenerative function as well, tempting us to think whether the anti-JNK strategy prevents spontaneous axonal regeneration after SCI. JNK inhibition by D-JNKI1 did not reduce long-term sprouting of the serotonergic fibers in the glial scar after SCI [45]. In this case, the single administration of D-JNKI1 was performed 6 h after SCI, under the experimental condition in which D-JNKI1 might not affect the relatively late-onset sprouting. On the other hand, continuous administration with SP600125 did not interfere with axonal branches extending from the CST into the gray matter far rostral to the lesion and, more likely, preserved the axonal branches sprouting in the rostral part close to the lesion epicenter more frequently compared with vehicle-treated control mice [44]. The reason why SP600125 efficiently leads to axonal regeneration after SCI is not clear. As a plausible explanation, SCI-induced JNK activation under the axonal degeneration process may be stronger than that under the axonal regeneration process, because a significant activation of JNK in the SC is observed at 1–3 days post-injury [44]. However, further investigation as to whether JNK inhibition especially during the axonal regeneration process worsens functional recovery after SCI is informative in considering the adverse effect of JNK inhibitors.

Taken together, JNK activity (at least in neurons and oligodendrocytes) can contribute to the pathogenesis of SCI. In addition, several reports have described that JNK activity in endothelial cells and astrocytes may be involved in the breakdown of the blood–CSF barrier and neuropathic pain, respectively, after SCI [45,47]. Although JNK is closely related to innate and adaptive immunity in various pathological situations, neither activation of microglial cells nor infiltration of myeloperoxidase-positive neutrophils were affected under the condition in which JNK inhibitors improved locomotor recovery after SCI [5,45,48]. Further precise studies are required, but JNK may not primarily orchestrate inflammatory events in the secondary damage of SCI.

4. Involvement of p38 in the Pathogenesis of SCI

4.1. p38 as a Central Player in Inflammatory Responses

In the secondary phase of SCI, infiltrated leukocytes and activated glial cells exacerbate tissue damage by releasing proinflammatory cytokines/chemokines, proteases, and reactive oxygen intermediates, though they exhibit certain beneficial aspects as well in some cases. The post-traumatic inflammatory responses may contribute to axonal degeneration, neuronal and oligodendrocytic cell death, and scar formation, and finally result in the impairment of neuronal function [49]. A number of studies have described that proinflammatory cytokines such as IL-6, TNF-α and IL-1β are potent mediators for the pathogenesis of SCI at the early stage of secondary damage [50]. Initially, p38 has been identified as a target protein for cytokine-suppressive anti-inflammatory drugs (CSAIDs) as well as a lipopolysaccharide (LPS)/TLR-activated kinase and shown to contribute to mRNA stabilization of IL-1β and TNF-α [51,52]. In addition to the function of transducing extracellular signals to the transcriptional machinery through regulating transcriptional factors (e.g., activating transcription factor 2 (ATF2), myocyte-specific enhance factor 2C/A, cAMP response element binding protein (CREB) and CEBP-homologous protein) as substrates of p38, p38 has been found to play an important role in both translation and stability of inflammatory mRNAs. For instance, AU-rich elements (AREs) found in the 3′-untranslated region of TNF-α mRNAs are binding sites for various factors regulating mRNA decay. The downstream kinase of p38, MAPK-activated protein kinase 2 (MK2 also known as MAPKAPK2), interferes with the interaction between AREs and the binding factors and thereby stabilizes TNF-α mRNA [53]. Expression of IL-6, which provokes activation and infiltration of leukocytes as one of its pleiotropic functions in SCI, is controlled by the mechanism of p38/MK2-induced mRNA stabilization as well [54]. Therefore, p38 can mobilize major SCI-related proinflammatory cytokines in the post-traumatic inflammatory process.

Using genetically manipulated mice and p38 inhibitors, it has been well documented that p38 plays important roles in various steps of inflammatory responses as follows: (i) p38 in macrophages stimulated with different TLR ligands regulates the expression of proinflammatory factors (e.g., inducible nitric oxide synthase (iNOS), cyclooxygenase 2, IL-6 and TNF-α) via gene regulatory mechanisms at both transcriptional and post-transcriptional levels [5,55]; (ii) p38 is required for the LPS-, TNF-, or UV-B-induced maturation of monocyte-derived dendritic cells (DCs) [5]; (iii) p38 is involved in production of interferon (IFN)-γ and Th1 differentiation of $CD4^+$ T cells under stimulation with antigen and/or cytokines [5,56]; (iv) p38 upregulates the translational regulation of cytokine production in NKT cells through activating the MAPK-interacting serine/threonine kinase (Mnk)-eukaryotic translation initiation factor 4E (eIF4E) pathway, a downstream target of p38 [57]; (v) p38 is involved in DC-driven Th17 differentiation, Th17 proliferation, and regulation of IL-17 expression in Th17 [33,34]. As for IL-17 expression in Th17 cells, both the transcriptional regulation via ATF2/CREB activated by p38α and the translational regulation via the p38α/Mnk-eIF4E pathway have been proposed [35,36]. In conjunction with the fact that inhibition of p38 efficiently blocks the highly pathogenic avian influenza virus (HPAIV)-induced "cytokine storm", the p38 pathway can regulate inflammatory responses as a central player [58].

4.2. Spatial Activation of p38 after SCI

In addition to neurons and oligodendrocytes, activation of p38 was observed in activated microglia/macrophages, infiltrated neutrophils, and reactive astrocytes forming a glial scar after SCI [39,40,59,60]. Several reports have described the mechanism of p38-mediated SCI development. In a complete transection model of SCI, activation of p38 induced the expression of iNOS in activated microglia/macrophages and then caused a decrease in $NeuN^+$ cells. The loss of neuronal cells was effectively inhibited by either a p38 inhibitor, SB203580, or N(ω)-nitro-L-arginine methyl ester, suggesting that the p38/NO signaling axis mediates the microglial cell-induced neurotoxicity after SCI [59]. In the SC after contusion injury, induction of IL-1β expression and p38 phosphorylation was observed prior to neuronal apoptosis identified as the $TUNEL^+$/active caspase-3^+ somas in the gray matter. An inhibitor of the IL-1β pathway, IL-1Ra suppressed phosphorylation of p38, indicating that p38 functions downstream of IL-1R1. Likewise, the neuronal apoptosis was sensitive to both IL-1Ra and SB203580, suggesting that the IL-1β/p38 signaling axis is involved in neuronal apoptosis after SCI [61].

4.3. Correlation between p38 Pathway Inhibition and Functional Recovery after SCI

4.3.1. p38 Inhibitors

Initially, SB203580 was reported to prevent damage to hindlimb function after SCI [62]. In contrast, a subsequent study has shown that SB203580 could not improve functional recovery after SCI [60]. The two reports are controversial in spite of employing a similar contusion SCI model and the same administration protocol (continuous intrathecal administration). The difference in intensity of SC damage between the two cases might influence the beneficial effect of p38 inhibition on SCI. In the former report, moreover, the treatment with SB203580 did not affect inflammatory responses in the lesion area, indicating that the anti-inflammatory potential of p38 inhibition may not work as a primary therapeutic effect on SCI.

Then, we have recently validated whether p38α is a potential therapeutic target in SCI. A single-copy disruption of *p38α* gene (p38$\alpha^{+/-}$, p38$\alpha^{-/-}$ is embryonic lethal as described above) reduced the tissue degenerative events (e.g., induction of various cytokines/chemokines, leukocytic infiltration, apoptosis of oligodendrocytes, loss of neuronal cells, and reactive astrogliosis) and augmented the tissue regenerative events (e.g., recruitment of oligodendrocyte progenitor cells, compaction of microglia/macrophages, and axonal regrowth), thereby causing a better functional recovery following lateral hemisection SCI. In our investigation, hence, genetic inhibition of p38α markedly suppressed at least the SCI-induced inflammatory responses: an increase in infiltration of both T lymphocytes and monocytes/macrophages into the lesion epicenter, and upregulation of inflammatory-related proteins (e.g., C-X-C motif chemokine 12, macrophage inflammatory protein (MIP)-1α, MIP-2, and matrix metalloproteinase 9) in the SC. These findings strongly suggest that the decrease of leukocytic infiltration associated with the suppression in expression of inflammatory-related proteins may contribute to the reduced development of SCI in p38$\alpha^{+/-}$ mice and further that inhibition of p38 can ameliorate SCI-associated inflammatory responses. In addition, the analysis using Texas Red-BDA, an anterograde tracer, showed that axonal regeneration after SCI was accelerated or enhanced in the caudal part of the SC in p38$\alpha^{+/-}$ mice compared with WT mice. Notably, SB239063, a p38 inhibitor that is transferable across the blood–CSF barrier, significantly improved functional recovery after SCI in WT mice if orally administered once a day at 1–3 days post-injury [63]. An overview of the SAPK-associated pathological outcome, especially the neuronal degenerative process in SCI, is shown in Figure 1B.

4.3.2. Minocycline

Minocycline, known as a second-generation tetracycline, is an interesting candidate in the treatment of traumatic CNS injuries and neurodegenerative diseases because it possesses neuroprotective and anti-inflammatory properties. A number of reports have proposed that minocycline-evoked anti-inflammatory and anti-apoptotic actions could be mediated through inhibition of p38 as follows: (i) low doses of minocycline protected neurons in mixed spinal cord cultures from *N*-methyl-D aspartate excitotoxicity by inhibiting the p38-promoted microglial activation [64]; (ii) minocycline protected cerebellar granule neurons from NO-induced cell death via reduction of p38 activity [65]; (iii) minocycline ameliorated carrageenan-induced inflammation-associated hyperalgesia through inhibiting p38 activation in spinal microglia [66]. In fact, it has been shown that the minocycline-p38 inhibition loop improves functional recovery after SCI mainly by decreasing cell death of oligodendrocytes [67]. In that report, minocycline inhibited oligodendrocytic apoptosis via reduction of the p38 activity-dependent pro-nerve growth factor (proNGF) production in microglia, leading to the improvement of functional recovery after SCI.

NGF can promote cell death via stimulation of p75 neurotrophin receptor (p75^{NTR}) in addition to the well-known function of neuronal differentiation/survival via tyrosine receptor kinase A (TrkA). Likewise, proNGF, the unprocessed NGF precursor, can bind p75^{NTR} preferentially over TrkA, and the expression of p75^{NTR} is specifically upregulated in oligodendrocytes after

SCI. Thus, the proNGF/p75^{NTR} signaling axis-induced apoptosis may occur predominantly in oligodendrocytes after SCI [68].

In another report, gene array analysis of mRNA from the SCs of rats with SCI showed the expression of p38β2 was typically and specifically downregulated by treatment with minocycline, the phenomenon of which is of interest [69]. In regards to the LPS-induced neurotoxicity secondary to the proinflammatory cytokine production in microglia, however, p38β but not p38α is dispensable in the brain, which is similar to the case of peripheral inflammation mentioned above [24,70]. Furthermore, neuron-selective microRNAs (miRs)—miR-124 and miR-128—selectively deplete p38α but not p38β in neurons, which results in loss of function of the p38/Mnk-eIF4E pathway in neurons. Thus, p38β cannot compensate p38α loss at least in the translational machinery mediated by the Mnk-eIF4E pathway [71]. Further investigation is required for the pathophysiological significance of minocycline treatment-specific downregulation of p38β2.

Currently, an interventional clinical trial, MASC (Minocycline in Acute Spinal Cord Injury) in phase III, is in progress with minocycline for patients with SCI (clinicaltrials.gov, registration number NCT01828203). The indication expansion for minocycline is much expected [72].

4.3.3. Plant-Derived Agents

Some plant-derived agents showing a beneficial effect on SCI can inhibit the p38 pathway. Curcumin, a yellow polyphenol derived from the *Curcuma longa* plant, is commonly used as a spice and also has a variety of medicinal properties including anti-inflammatory, analgesic, anti-oxidant, and antiseptic activity. It has been clearly demonstrated that curcumin enhances locomotor and sensory recovery after SCI at least partly through inhibiting the nuclear factor κ-light-chain-enhancer of activated B cells (NF-κB) pathway [73].

NF-κB elicits pleiotropic functions by regulating the transcription of various genes such as cytokines/chemokines, adhesion molecules, proinflammatory transcription factors, proinflammatory enzymes, and so on. In addition, it is well described that NF-κB is activated downstream of TLR and cytokine receptors like p38 is. In the CNS, the basal activity of NF-κB in glial cells is low but highly inducible in response to the change of neural environment, which may play a crucial role in brain inflammation [74]. In fact, transgenic mice with astrocyte-specific loss of function of NF-κB activity show a dramatic improvement of functional recovery after contusive SCI [75]. Therefore, NF-κB activity at least in glial cells contributes to the pathogenesis of SCI. Subsequently, it has been demonstrated that curcumin ameliorates secondary damage (e.g., production of IL-6, TNF-α, IL-1β, and nitric oxide) presumably through inhibiting both the TAK1/MKK6/p38 pathway and the NF-κB pathway, which may contribute to the improvement of locomotor recovery after SCI [76].

Geraniol (an acyclic monoterpene alcohol) is primarily found in rose oil, palmarosa oil, and citronella oil and commonly used in flavors and perfumes due to its rose-like scent. Geraniol has various properties including antibacterial, immune regulation, insecticidal, and antitumor activities. It has been demonstrated that Geraniol ameliorates secondary damage (e.g., edema, induction of proinflammatory cytokines, oxidative stress, and neural apoptosis) and improves locomotor recovery after SCI. As the main signaling mechanism of action, geraniol was shown to inhibit the SCI-upregulated expression of NF-κB and p38 [77]. Through a similar mechanism, improvement of locomotor recovery after SCI was observed in rats treated with asiaticoside, a terpenoid component extracted form *Centella asiatica* [78].

4.4. p38 as a Promising Target for Therapeutic Intervention in SCI?

Accumulating evidence with animal models suggests that p38 plays a crucial role in the pathogenesis of SCI and that p38 is expected as a clinical target for the treatment of SCI. However, p38 signaling has a wide spectrum of biological activities beyond the inflammatory/stress responses in the CNS [12]. In addition, the obvious resistance of p38$\alpha^{+/-}$ mice to various pathological inputs raises the question whether a full inhibition of p38 results in improvement of clinical symptoms [36,63,79–82].

This notion may be partly supported by the fact that highly concentrated application of SB203580 loses its beneficial effect on SCI [62]. Likewise, mitogen- and stress-activated kinases (MSKs) 1 and 2 that are activated downstream of p38 play important roles in macrophages as follows: production of the anti-inflammatory cytokine, IL-10; production of IL-1Ra; and an increase in transcription of dual-specificity protein phosphatase 1 (DUSP1 also known as MAPK phosphatase-1) leading to dephosphorylation/inactivation of p38. Thus, the p38/MSK signaling axis can function as the negative feedback loop in p38-mediated inflammatory responses [83]. Furthermore, p38 inhibitor-based therapeutic investigation is sometimes limited because of its specificity [84]. Therefore, further precise investigation is needed, focusing on the exact spatial and temporal activation of p38 which positively or negatively contributes to the functional outcome after SCI. As a result, p38 inhibition will be received as a therapeutic option without adverse effects.

5. Closing Remarks

Here, we gave an overview on roles of SAPKs in SCI and, in particular, discussed the potential of targeting the p38 pathway as a disease-modifying therapy in SCI. In addition to its role in the development of neuronal degeneration after SCI, p38 may contribute to SCI-associated neuropathic pain development and maintenance. After spinal nerve ligation (SNL) that is commonly used as a neuropathic pain model, p38 was markedly activated predominantly in spinal microglia, and its activity was maintained over 3 weeks [85]. The relationships between nerve-injury-induced microglial activation and pain sensitization are well characterized [86] Therefore, p38 may represent a potent clinical target for neuropathic pain management after SCI. In fact, the therapeutic effect of SB681323, a p38 inhibitor, on neuropathic pain following nerve trauma was studied in a past clinical trial (clinicaltrials.gov, registration number NCT00390845). It has been reported that nearly 80% of patients with SCI are seriously affected by pain and unpleasant sensations [87]. The development of emerging strategies for both functional recovery and neuropathic pain management after SCI is regarded as a clinically and socially urgent matter.

Acknowledgments: This work was supported in part by Grants-in-Aid for Scientific Research ((B), 24390137 to Yoshitoshi Kasuya) from the Ministry of Education, Science, Sports and Culture of Japan.

Author Contributions: Yoshitoshi Kasuya, Hiroki Umezawa and Masahiko Hatano wrote the manuscript.

Abbreviations

Aβ	Amyloid β
AD	Alzheimer's disease
ARE	AU-rich element
ASK1	Apoptosis signal-regulating kinase 1
ATF2	Activating transcription factor 2
BDA	Biotinylated dextran amine
CNS	Central nervous system
CREB	cAMP response element binding protein
CSAID	Cytokine-suppressive anti-inflammatory drug
CSF	Cerebrospinal fluid
CST	Corticospinal tract
DCs	Dendritic cells
DLK	Dual leucine zipper-bearing kinase
EAE	Experimental autoimmune encephalomyelitis
eIF4E	Eukaryotic translation initiation factor 4E
HPAIV	Highly pathogenic avian influenza virus
IL	Interleukin
IFN-γ	Interferon-γ
iNOS	Inducible nitric oxide synthase

JNK	c-Jun *N*-terminal kinase
LPS	Lipopolysaccharide
MAPK	Mitogen-activated protein kinase
MAP2K	MAPK kinase
MAP3K	MAPKK kinase
Mcl-1	Myeloid cell leukemia sequence-1
miR	MicroRNA
MIP	Macrophage inflammatory protein
MK2	MAPK-activated protein kinase 2
MLK	Mixed lineage kinase
Mnk	MAPK-interacting serine/threonine kinase
MPTP	1-Methyl-4-phenyl-1,2,4,6-tetrahydropyridine
MSK	Mitogen- and stress-activated kinase
NF-κB	Nuclear factor κ-light-chain-enhancer of activated B cells
NGF	Nerve growth factor
$p75^{NTR}$	p75 Neurotrophin receptor
SAPK	Stress-activated protein kinase
SCI	Spinal cord injury
SCG10	Superior cervical ganglion 10
TAB1	TAK1-binding protein 1
TAK1	TGF-β-activated kinase 1
TAO2	Thousand-and-one amino acid kinase 2
TGF-β	Transforming growth factor-β
Th	T-helper
TNF-α	Tumor necrosis factor-α
TNIK	TNF receptor-associated factor 2- and NCK-interacting protein kinase
TLR	Toll-like receptor
TPL2	Tumor progression locus 2
TrkA	Tyrosine receptor kinase A
TWY	Tiptoe-walking Yoshimura
UV	Ultraviolet
ZAP70	ζ chain-associated protein kinase

References

1. Horner, P.J.; Gage, F.H. Regenerating the damaged central nervous system. *Nature* **2000**, *407*, 963–970. [CrossRef] [PubMed]
2. Hilton, B.J.; Moulson, A.J.; Tetzlaff, W. Neuroprotection and secondary damage following spinal cord injury: Concepts and methods. *Neurosci. Lett.* **2017**, *652*, 3–10. [CrossRef] [PubMed]
3. Zhou, X.; He, X.; Ren, Y. Function of microglia and macrophages in secondary damage after spinal cord injury. *Neural Regen. Res.* **2014**, *9*, 1787–1795. [CrossRef] [PubMed]
4. Becker, D.; Sadowsky, C.L.; McDonald, J.W. Restoring function after spinal cord injury. *Neurologist* **2003**, *9*, 1–15. [CrossRef] [PubMed]
5. Rincón, M.; Davis, R.J. Regulation of the immune response by stress-activated protein kinases. *Immunol. Rev.* **2009**, *228*, 212–224. [CrossRef] [PubMed]
6. Le-Niculescu, H.; Bonfoco, E.; Kasuya, Y.; Claret, F.-X.; Green, D.R.; Karin, M. Withdrawal of survival factors results in activation of the JNK pathway in neuronal cells leading to Fas ligand induction and cell death. *Mol. Cell. Biol.* **1999**, *19*, 751–763. [CrossRef] [PubMed]
7. Gupta, S.; Barrett, T.; Whitmarsh, A.J.; Cavanagh, J.; Sluss, H.K.; Dérijard, B.; Davis, R.J. Selective interaction of JNK protein kinase isoforms with transcription factors. *EMBO J.* **1996**, *15*, 2760–2770. [PubMed]

8. Coffey, E.T. Nuclear and cytosolic JNK signalling in neurons. *Nat. Rev. Neurosci.* **2014**, *15*, 285–299. [CrossRef] [PubMed]
9. Li, Z.; Young, J.; Ulevitch, R.J.; Han, J. The primary structure of p38γ: A new member of p38 group of MAP kinases. *Biochem. Biophys. Res. Commun.* **1996**, *228*, 334–340. [CrossRef] [PubMed]
10. Jiang, Y.; Chen, C.; Li, Z.; Guo, W.; Gegner, J.A.; Lin, S.; Han, J. Characterization of the structure and function of the fourth member of p38 group mitogen-activated protein kinases, p38δ. *J. Biol. Chem.* **1997**, *272*, 30122–30128. [CrossRef] [PubMed]
11. Kumar, S.; McDonnell, P.C.; Gum, R.J.; Hand, A.T.; Lee, J.C.; Young, P.R. Novel homologues of CSBP/p38 MAP kinase: Activation, substrate specificity and sensitivity to inhibition by pyridinyl imidazoles. *Biochem. Biophys. Res. Commun.* **1997**, *235*, 533–538. [CrossRef] [PubMed]
12. Takeda, K.; Ichijo, H. Neuronal p38 MAPK signalling: An emerging regulator of cell fate and function in the nervous system. *Genes Cells* **2002**, *7*, 1099–1111. [CrossRef] [PubMed]
13. Ge, B.; Gram, H.; Di Padova, F.; Huang, B.; New, L.; Ulevitch, R.J.; Luo, Y.; Han, J. MAPKK-Independent Activation of p38α Mediated by TAB1-Dependent Autophosphorylation of p38α. *Science* **2002**, *295*, 1291–1294. [CrossRef] [PubMed]
14. Salvador, J.M.; Mittelstadt, P.R.; Guszczynski, T.; Copeland, T.D.; Yamaguchi, H.; Appella, E.; Fornace, A.J., Jr.; Ashwell, J.D. Alternative p38 activation pathway mediated by T cell receptor-proximal tyrosine kinases. *Nat. Immunol.* **2005**, *6*, 390–395. [CrossRef] [PubMed]
15. Carboni, L.; Carletti, R.; Tacconi, S.; Corti, C.; Ferraguti, F. Differential expression of SAPK isoforms in the rat brain. An in situ hybridisation study in the adult rat brain and during post-natal development. *Mol. Brain Res.* **1998**, *60*, 57–68. [CrossRef]
16. Lein, E.S.; Hawrylycz, M.J.; Ao, N.; Ayres, M.; Bensinger, A.; Bernard, A.; Boe, A.F.; Boguski, M.S.; Brockway, K.S.; Byrnes, E.J.; et al. Genome-wide atlas of gene expression in the adult mouse brain. *Nature* **2007**, *445*, 168–176. [CrossRef] [PubMed]
17. Yang, D.D.; Kuan, C.; Whitmarsh, A.J.; Rinócn, M.; Zheng, T.S.; Davis, R.J.; Rakic, P.; Flavell, R.A. Absence of excitotoxicity-induced apoptosis in the hippocampus of mice lacking the Jnk3 gene. *Nature* **1997**, *389*, 865–870. [CrossRef] [PubMed]
18. Hunot, S.; Vila, M.; Teismann, P.; Davis, R.J.; Hirsch, E.C.; Przedborski, S.; Rakic, P.; Flavell, R.A. JNK-mediated induction of cyclooxygenase 2 is required for neurodegeneration in a mouse model of Parkinson's disease. *Proc. Natl. Acad. Sci. USA* **2004**, *101*, 665–670. [CrossRef] [PubMed]
19. Brecht, S.; Kirchhof, R.; Chromik, A.; Willesen, M.; Nicolaus, T.; Raivich, G.; Wessig, J.; Waetzig, V.; Goetz, M.; Claussen, M.; et al. Specific pathophysiological functions of JNK isoforms in the brain. *Eur. J. Neurosci.* **2005**, *21*, 363–377. [CrossRef] [PubMed]
20. Kuan, C.Y.; Yang, D.D.; Samanta Roy, D.R.; Davis, R.J.; Rakic, P.; Flavell, R.A. The Jnk1 and Jnk2 protein kinases are required for regional specific apoptosis during early brain development. *Neuron* **1999**, *22*, 667–676. [CrossRef]
21. Xu, P.; Das, M.; Reilly, J.; Davis, R.J. JNK regulates FoxO-dependent autophagy in neurons. *Genes Dev.* **2011**, *25*, 310–322. [CrossRef] [PubMed]
22. Tamura, K.; Sudo, T.; Senftleben, U.; Dadak, A.M.; Johnson, R.; Karin, M. Requirement for p38α in erythropoietin expression: A role for stress kinases in erythropoiesis. *Cell* **2000**, *102*, 221–231. [CrossRef]
23. Adams, R.H.; Porras, A.; Alonso, G.; Jones, M.; Vintersten, K.; Panelli, S.; Valladares, A.; Perez, L.; Klein, R.; Nebreda, A.R. Essential role of p38α MAP kinase in placental but not embryonic cardiovascular development. *Mol. Cell* **2000**, *6*, 109–116. [CrossRef]
24. Beardmore, V.A.; Hinton, H.J.; Eftychi, C.; Apostolaki, M.; Armaka, M.; Darragh, J.; McIlrath, J.; Carr, J.M.; Armit, L.J.; Clacher, C.; et al. Generation and characterization of p38β (MAPK11) gene-targeted mice. *Mol. Cell. Biol.* **2005**, *25*, 10454–10464. [CrossRef] [PubMed]
25. Gillespie, M.A.; Le Grand, F.; Scimè, A.; Kuang, S.; von Maltzahn, J.; Seale, V.; Cuenda, A.; Ranish, J.A.; Rudnicki, M.A. p38-γ-dependent gene silencing restricts entry into the myogenic differentiation program. *J. Cell Biol.* **2009**, *187*, 991–1005. [CrossRef] [PubMed]
26. Schindler, E.M.; Hindes, A.; Gribben, E.L.; Burns, C.J.; Yin, Y.; Lin, M.; Owen, R.J.; Longmore, G.D.; Kissling, G.E.; Arthur, J.S.C.; et al. p38δ mitogen-activated protein kinase is essential for skin tumor development in mice. *Cancer Res.* **2004**, *69*, 4648–4655. [CrossRef] [PubMed]

27. Bu, X.; Huang, P.; Qi, Z.; Zhang, N.; Han, S.; Fang, L.; Li, J. Cell type-specific activation of p38 MAPK in the brain regions of hypoxic preconditioned mice. *Neurochem. Int.* **2007**, *51*, 459–466. [CrossRef] [PubMed]
28. Maruyama, M.; Sudo, T.; Kasuya, Y.; Siga, T.; Hu, B.; Osada, H. Immunolocalization of p38 MAPK in mouse brain. *Brain Res.* **2000**, *887*, 350–358. [CrossRef]
29. Bruchas, M.R.; Macey, T.A.; Lowe, J.D.; Chavkin, C. Kappa opioid receptor activation of p38 MAPK is GRK3- and arrestin-dependent in neurons and astrocytes. *J. Biol. Chem.* **2006**, *281*, 18081–18089. [CrossRef] [PubMed]
30. Choudhury, G.R.; Ryou, M.; Poteet, E.; Wen, Y.; He, R.; Sun, F.; Yuan, F.; Jin, K.; Yang, S. Involvement of p38 MAPK in reactive astrogliosisinduced by ischemic stroke. *Brain Res.* **2014**, *1551*, 45–58. [CrossRef] [PubMed]
31. Ando, K.; Uemura, K.; Kuzuya, A.; Maesako, M.; Asada-Utsugi, M.; Kubota, M.; Aoyagi, N.; Yoshioka, K.; Okawa, K.; Inoue, H.; et al. N-cadherin regulates p38 MAPK signaling via association with JNK-associated leucine zipper protein: Implications for neurodegeneration in Alzheimer disease. *J. Biol. Chem.* **2011**, *286*, 7619–7628. [CrossRef] [PubMed]
32. Guo, X.; Harada, C.; Namekata, K.; Matsuzawa, A.; Camps, M.; Ji, H.; Swinnen, D.; Jorand-Lebrun, C.; Muzerelle, M.; Vitte, P.A.; et al. Regulation of the severity of neuroinflammation and demyelination by TLR-ASK1-p38 pathway. *EMBO Mol. Med.* **2010**, *12*, 504–515. [CrossRef] [PubMed]
33. Huang, G.; Wang, Y.; Vogel, P.; Kanneganti, T.-D.; Otsu, K.; Chi, H. Signaling via the kinase p38α programs dendritic cells to drive TH17 differentiation and autoimmune inflammation. *Nat. Immunol.* **2012**, *13*, 152–161. [CrossRef] [PubMed]
34. Jirmanova, L.; Torchia, M.L.G.; Sarma, N.D.; Mittelstadt, P.R.; Ashwell, J.D. Lack of the T-cell-specific alternative p38 activation pathway reduces autoimmunity and inflammation. *Blood* **2011**, *118*, 3280–3289. [CrossRef] [PubMed]
35. Noubade, R.; Krementsov, D.N.; Rio, R.; Thornton, T.; Nagaleekar, V.; Saligrama, N.; Spitzack, A.; Spach, K.; Sabio, G.; Davis, R.J.; et al. Activation of p38 MAPK in CD4 T cells controls IL-17 production and autoimmune encephalomyelitis. *Blood* **2011**, *118*, 3290–3300. [CrossRef] [PubMed]
36. Namiki, K.; Matsunaga, H.; Yoshioka, K.; Tanaka, K.; Murata, K.; Ishida, J.; Sakairi, A.; Kim, J.; Tokuhara, N.; Shibakawa, N.; et al. Mechanism for p38α-mediated experimental autoimmune encephalomyelitis. *J. Biol. Chem.* **2012**, *287*, 24228–24238. [CrossRef] [PubMed]
37. Munoz, L.; Ammit, A.J. Targeting p38 MAPK pathway for the treatment of Alzheimer's disease. *Neuropharmacology* **2010**, *58*, 561–568. [CrossRef] [PubMed]
38. Munoz, L.; Ranaivo, H.R.; Roy, S.M.; Hu, W.; Craft, J.M.; McNamara, L.K.; Chico, L.W.; Van Eldik, L.J.; Watterson, D.M. A novel p38α MAPK inhibitor suppresses brain proinflammatory cytokine up-regulation and attenuates synaptic dysfunction and behavioral deficits in an Alzheimer's disease mouse model. *J. Neuroinflamm.* **2007**, *4*, 21. [CrossRef] [PubMed]
39. Nakahara, S.; Yone, K.; Sakou, T.; Wada, S.; Nagamine, T.; Niiyama, T.; Ichijo, H. Induction of apoptosis signal regulating kinase 1 (ASK1) after spinal cord injury in rats: Possible involvement of ASK1-JNK and -p38 pathways in neuronal apoptosis. *J. Neuropathol. Exp. Neurol.* **1999**, *58*, 442–450. [CrossRef] [PubMed]
40. Takenouchi, T.; Setoguchi, T.; Yone, K.; Komiy, S. Expression of apoptosis signal-regulating kinase 1 in mouse spinal cord under chronic mechanical compression: Possible involvement of the stress-activated mitogen-activated protein kinase pathways in spinal cord cell apoptosis. *Spine* **2008**, *33*, 1943–1950. [CrossRef] [PubMed]
41. Li, Q.M.; Tep, C.; Yune, T.Y.; Zhou, X.Z.; Uchida, T.; Lu, K.P.; Yoon, S.O. Opposite regulation of oligodendrocyte apoptosis by JNK3 and Pin1 after spinal cord injury. *J. Neurosci.* **2007**, *27*, 8395–8404. [CrossRef] [PubMed]
42. Cavalli, V.; Kujala, P.; Klumperman, J.; Goldstein, L.S.B. Sunday Driver links axonal transport to damage signaling. *J. Cell Biol.* **2005**, *168*, 775–787. [CrossRef] [PubMed]
43. Shin, J.E.; Miller, B.R.; Babetto, E.; Cho, Y.; Sasaki, Y.; Qayum, S.; Russler, E.V.; Cavalli, V.; Milbrandt, J.; DiAntonio, A. SCG10 is a JNK target in the axonal degeneration pathway. *Proc. Natl. Acad. Sci. USA* **2012**, *109*, E3696–E3705. [CrossRef] [PubMed]
44. Yoshimura, K.; Ueno, M.; Lee, S.; Nakamura, Y.; Sato, A.; Yoshimura, K.; Kishima, H.; Yoshimine, T.; Yamashita, T. C-Jun N-terminal kinase induces axonal degeneration and limits motor recovery after spinal cord injury in mice. *Neurosci. Res.* **2011**, *71*, 266–277. [CrossRef] [PubMed]

45. Repici, M.; Chen, X.; Morel, M.-P.; Doulazmi, M.; Sclip, A.; Cannaya, V.; Veglianese, P.; Kraftsik, R.; Mariani, J.; Borsello, T.; et al. Specific inhibition of the JNK pathway promotes locomotor recovery and neuroprotection after mouse spinal cord injury. *Neurobiol. Dis.* **2012**, *46*, 710–721. [CrossRef] [PubMed]
46. Barnat, M.; Enslen, H.; Propst, F.; Davis, R.J.; Soares, S.; Nothias, F. Distinct roles of c-Jun N-terminal kinase isoforms in neurite initiation and elongation during axonal regeneration. *J. Neurosci.* **2010**, *30*, 7804–7816. [CrossRef] [PubMed]
47. Lee, J.Y.; Choi, D.C.; Oh, T.H.; Yune, T.Y. Analgesic effect of acupuncture is mediated via inhibition of JNK activation in astrocytes after spinal cord injury. *PLoS ONE* **2013**, *8*, e73948. [CrossRef] [PubMed]
48. Martini, A.C.; Forner, S.; Koepp, J.; Rae, G.A. Inhibition of spinal c-Jun-NH2-terminal kinase (JNK) improves locomotor activity of spinal cord injured rats. *Neurosci. Lett.* **2016**, *621*, 54–61. [CrossRef] [PubMed]
49. Beattie, M.S. Inflammation and apoptosis: Linked therapeutic targets in spinal cord injury. *Trends Mol. Med.* **2004**, *10*, 580–583. [CrossRef] [PubMed]
50. Okada, S. The pathophysiological role of acute inflammation after spinal cord injury. *Inflamm. Regen.* **2016**, *36*, 20. [CrossRef] [PubMed]
51. Lee, J.C.; Laydon, J.T.; McDonnell, P.C.; Gallagher, T.F.; Kumar, S.; Green, D.; McNulty, D.; Blumenthal, M.J.; Heys, J.R.; Landvatter, S.W.; et al. A protein kinase involved in the regulation of inflammatory cytokine biosynthesis. *Nature* **1994**, *372*, 739–746. [CrossRef] [PubMed]
52. Han, J.; Lee, J.D.; Bibbs, L.; Ulevitch, R.J. A MAP kinase targeted by endotoxin and hyperosmolarity in mammalian cells. *Science* **1994**, *265*, 808–811. [CrossRef] [PubMed]
53. Dean, J.L.E.; Sully, G.; Clark, A.R.; Saklatvala, J. The involvement of AU-rich element-binding proteins in p38 mitogen-activated protein kinase pathway-mediated mRNA stabilization. *Cell. Signal.* **2004**, *16*, 1113–1121. [CrossRef] [PubMed]
54. Zhao, W.; Liu, M.; Kirkwood, K.L. p38α stabilizes interleukin-6 mRNA via multipleAU-rich elements. *J. Biol. Chem.* **2008**, *283*, 1778–1785. [CrossRef] [PubMed]
55. Kang, Y.J.; Chen, J.; Otsuka, M.; Mols, J.; Ren, S.; Wang, Y.; Han, J. Macrophage deletion of p38α partially impairs lipopolysaccharide-induced cellular activation. *J. Immunol.* **2008**, *180*, 5075–5082. [CrossRef] [PubMed]
56. Krementsov, D.N.; Thornton, T.M.; Teuscher, C.; Rinócn, M. The emerging role of p38 mitogen-activated protein kinase in multiple sclerosis and its models. *Mol. Cell. Biol.* **2013**, *33*, 3728–3734. [CrossRef] [PubMed]
57. Nagaleekar, V.K.; Sabio, G.; Aktan, I.; Chant, A.; Howe, I.W.; Thornton, T.M.; Benoit, P.J.; Davis, R.J.; Rincon, M.; Boyson, J.E. Translational control of NKT cell cytokine production by p38 MAPK. *J. Immunol.* **2011**, *186*, 4140–4146. [CrossRef] [PubMed]
58. Börgeling, Y.; Schmolke, M.; Viemann, D.; Nordhoff, C.; Roth, J.; Ludwig, S. Inhibition of p38 mitogen-activated protein kinase impairs influenza virus-induced primary and secondary host gene responses and protects mice from lethal H5N1 infection. *J. Biol. Chem.* **2014**, *289*, 13–27. [CrossRef] [PubMed]
59. Xu, Z.; Wang, B.R.; Wang, X.; Kuang, F.; Duan, X.L.; Jiao, X.Y.; Ju, G. ERK1/2 and p38 mitogen-activated protein kinase mediate iNOS-induced spinal neuron degeneration after acute traumatic spinal cord injury. *Life Sci.* **2006**, *79*, 1895–1905. [CrossRef] [PubMed]
60. Stirling, D.P.; Liu, J.; Plunet, W.; Steeves, J.D.; Tetzlaff, W. SB203580, a p38 mitogen-activated protein kinase inihbitor, fails to improve functional outcome following a moderate spinal cord injury in rat. *Neuroscience* **2008**, *155*, 128–137. [CrossRef] [PubMed]
61. Wang, X.J.; Kong, K.M.; Qi, W.L.; Ye, W.L.; Song, P.S. Interleukin-1 beta induction of neuron apoptosis depends on p38 mitogen-activated protein kinase activity after spinal cord injury. *Acta Pharmacol. Sin.* **2005**, *26*, 934–942. [CrossRef] [PubMed]
62. Horiuchi, H.; Ogata, T.; Morino, T.; Chuai, M.; Yamamoto, H. Continuous intrathecal infusion of SB203580, a selective inhibitor of p38 mitogen-activated protein kinase, reduces the damage of hind-limb function after thoracic spinal cord injury in rat. *Neurosci. Res.* **2003**, *47*, 209–217. [CrossRef]
63. Umezawa, H.; Naito, Y.; Tanaka, K.; Yoshioka, K.; Suzuki, K.; Sudo, T.; Hagihara, M.; Hatano, M.; Tatsumi, K.; Kasuya, Y. Genetic and pharmacological inhibition of p38α improves locomotor recovery after spinal cord injury. *Front. Pharmacol.* **2017**, *8*, 72. [CrossRef] [PubMed]
64. Tikka, T.M.; Koistinaho, J.E. Minocycline provides neuroprotection against **N**-methyl-d-aspartate neurotoxicity by inhibiting microglia. *J. Immunol.* **2001**, *166*, 7527–7533. [CrossRef] [PubMed]

65. Lin, S.; Zhang, Y.; Dodel, R.; Farlow, M.R.; Paul, S.M.; Du, Y. Minocycline blocks nitric oxide-induced neurotoxicity by inhibition p38 MAP kinase in rat cerebellar granule neurons. *Neurosci. Lett.* **2011**, *315*, 61–64. [CrossRef]
66. Hua, X.; Svensson, C.I.; Matsui, T.; Fitzsimmons, B.; Yaksh, T.L.; Webb, M. Intrathecal minocycline attenuates peripheral inflammationinduced hyperalgesia by inhibiting p38 MAPK in spinal microglia. *Eur. J. Neurosci.* **2005**, *22*, 2431–2440. [CrossRef] [PubMed]
67. Yune, T.Y.; Lee, J.Y.; Jung, G.Y.; Kim, S.J.; Jiang, M.H.; Kim, Y.C.; Oh, Y.J.; Markelonis, G.J.; Oh, T.H. Minocycline alleviates death of oligodendrocytes by inhibiting pro-nerve growth factor production in microglia after spinal cord injury. *J. Neurosci.* **2007**, *27*, 7751–7761. [CrossRef] [PubMed]
68. Beattie, M.S.; Harrington, A.W.; Lee, R.; Kim, J.Y.; Boyce, S.L.; Longo, F.M.; Bresnahan, J.C.; Hempstead, B.L.; Yoon, S.O. ProNGF induces p75-mediated death of oligodendrocytes following spinal cord injury. *Neuron* **2002**, *36*, 375–386. [CrossRef]
69. Stirling, D.P.; Koochesfahani, K.M.; Steeves, J.D.; Tetzlaff, W. Minocycline as a neuroprotective agent. *Neuroscientist* **2005**, *11*, 308–322. [CrossRef] [PubMed]
70. Xing, B.; Bachstetter, A.D.; Van Eldik, L.J. Deficiency in p38β MAPK fails to inhibit cytokine production or protect neurons against inflammatory insult in in vitro and in vivo mouse models. *PLoS ONE* **2015**, *8*, e56852. [CrossRef] [PubMed]
71. Lawson, S.K.; Dobrikova, E.Y.; Shveygert, M.; Gromeier, M. p38α mitogen-activated protein kinase depletion and repression of signal transduction to translation machinery by miR-124 and -128 in neurons. *Mol. Cell. Biol.* **2013**, *33*, 127–135. [CrossRef] [PubMed]
72. Casha, S.; Zygun, D.; McGowan, M.D.; Bains, I.; Yong, V.W.; Hurlbert, R.J. Results of a phase II placebo-controlled randomized trial of minocycline in acute spinal cord injury. *Brain* **2012**, *135*, 1224–1236. [CrossRef] [PubMed]
73. Urdzikova, L.M.; Karova, K.; Ruzicka, J.; Kloudova, A.; Shannon, C.; Dubisova, J.; Murali, R.; Kubinova, S.; Sykova, E.; Jhanwar-Uniyal, M.; et al. The anti-inflammatory compound curcumin enhances locomotor and sensory recovery after spinal cord injury in rats by immunomodulation. *Int. J. Mol. Sci.* **2016**, *17*, 49. [CrossRef] [PubMed]
74. Shih, R.; Wang, C.; Yang, C. NF-kappaB signaling pathways in neurological inflammation. *Front. Mol. Neurosci.* **2015**, *8*, 77. [CrossRef] [PubMed]
75. Brambilla, R.; Bracchi-Ricard, V.; Hu, W.; Frydel, B.; Bramwell, A.; Karmally, S.; Green, E.J.; Bethea, J.R. Inhibition of astroglial nuclear factor κB reduces inflammation and improves functional recovery after spinal cord injury. *J. Exp. Med.* **2005**, *202*, 145–156. [CrossRef]
76. Zhang, N.; Wei, G.; Ye, J.; Yang, L.; Hong, Y.; Liu, G.; Zhong, H.; Cai, X. Effect of curcumin on acute spinal cord injury in mice via inhibition of inflammation and TAK1 pathway. *Pharmacol. Rep.* **2017**, *69*, 1001–1006. [CrossRef] [PubMed]
77. Wang, J.; Su, B.; Zhu, H.; Chen, C.; Zhao, G. Protective effect of geraniol inhibits inflammatory response, oxidative stress and apoptosis in traumatic injury of the spinal cord through modulation of NF-κB and p38 MAPK. *Exp. Ther. Med.* **2016**, *12*, 3607–3613. [CrossRef] [PubMed]
78. Luo, Y.; Fu, C.; Wang, Z.; Zhang, Z.; Wang, H.; Liu, Y. Asiaticoside attenuates the effects of spinal cord injury through antioxidant and anti-inflammatory effects, and inhibition of the p38-MAPK mechanism. *Mol. Med. Rep.* **2015**, *12*, 8294–8300. [CrossRef] [PubMed]
79. Takanami-Ohnishi, Y.; Amano, S.; Kimura, S.; Asada, S.; Utani, A.; Maruyama, M.; Osada, H.; Tsunoda, H.; Irukayama-Tomobe, Y.; Goto, K.; et al. Essential role of p38 mitogen-activated protein kinase in contact hypersensitivity. *J. Biol. Chem.* **2002**, *277*, 37896–37903. [CrossRef] [PubMed]
80. Matsuo, Y.; Amano, S.; Furuya, M.; Namiki, K.; Sakurai, K.; Nishiyama, M.; Sudo, T.; Tatsumi, K.; Kuriyama, T.; Kimura, S.; et al. Involvement of p38α mitogen-activated protein kinase in lung metastasis of tumor cells. *J. Biol. Chem.* **2006**, *281*, 36767–36775. [CrossRef] [PubMed]
81. Namiki, K.; Nakamura, A.; Furuya, M.; Mizuhashi, S.; Matsuo, Y.; Tokuhara, N.; Sudo, T.; Hama, H.; Kuwaki, T.; Yano, S.; et al. Involvement of p38α in kainate-induced seizure and neuronal cell damage. *J. Recept. Signal Transduct.* **2007**, *27*, 99–111. [CrossRef] [PubMed]
82. Yoshioka, K.; Namiki, K.; Sudo, T.; Kasuya, Y. p38α controls self-renewal and fate decision of neurosphere-forming cells in adult hippocampus. *FEBS Open Bio* **2015**, *5*, 437–444. [CrossRef] [PubMed]

83. Bachstetter, A.D.; Van Eldik, L.J. The p38 MAP kinase family as regulators of proinflammatory cytokine production in degenerative diseases of the CNS. *Aging Dis.* **2010**, *1*, 199–211. [PubMed]
84. Godl, K.; Wissing, J.; Kurtenbach, A.; Habenberger, P.; Blencke, S.; Gutbrod, H.; Salassidis, K.; Stein-Gerlach, M.; Missio, A.; Cotton, M. An efficient proteomics method to identify the cellular targets of protein kinase inhibitors. *Proc. Natl. Acad. Sci. USA* **2003**, *100*, 15434–15439. [CrossRef] [PubMed]
85. Jin, S.X.; Zhuang, Z.Y.; Woolf, C.J.; Ji, R.R. p38 mitogen-activated protein kinase is activated after a spinal nerve ligation in spinal cord microglia and dorsal root ganglion neurons and contributes to the generation of neuropathic pain. *J. Neurosci.* **2003**, *23*, 4017–4022. [PubMed]
86. Ji, R.R.; Suter, M.R. p38 MAPK, microglial signaling, and neuropathic pain. *Mol. Pain* **2007**, *3*, 33. [CrossRef] [PubMed]
87. Finnerup, N.B.; Johannesen, I.L.; Sindrup, S.H.; Bach, F.W.; Jensen, T.S. Pain and dysesthesia in patients with spinal cord injury: A postal survey. *Spinal Cord* **2001**, *39*, 256–262. [CrossRef] [PubMed]

9

Perineuronal Nets in Spinal Motoneurones: Chondroitin Sulphate Proteoglycan around Alpha Motoneurones

Sian F. Irvine [1] and Jessica C. F. Kwok [1,2,*]

1 School of Biomedical Sciences, University of Leeds, Leeds LS2 9JT, UK; bs11sfi@leeds.ac.uk
2 Centre of Reconstructive Neurosciences, Institute of Experimental Medicine, The Czech Academy of Sciences, Prague 4, Czech Republic
* Correspondence: J.Kwok@leeds.ac.uk

Abstract: Perineuronal nets (PNNs) are extracellular matrix structures surrounding neuronal sub-populations throughout the central nervous system, regulating plasticity. Enzymatically removing PNNs successfully enhances plasticity and thus functional recovery, particularly in spinal cord injury models. While PNNs within various brain regions are well studied, much of the composition and associated populations in the spinal cord is yet unknown. We aim to investigate the populations of PNN neurones involved in this functional motor recovery. Immunohistochemistry for choline acetyltransferase (labelling motoneurones), PNNs using *Wisteria floribunda* agglutinin (WFA) and chondroitin sulphate proteoglycans (CSPGs), including aggrecan, was performed to characterise the molecular heterogeneity of PNNs in rat spinal motoneurones (Mns). CSPG-positive PNNs surrounded ~70–80% of Mns. Using WFA, only ~60% of the CSPG-positive PNNs co-localised with WFA in the spinal Mns, while ~15–30% of Mns showed CSPG-positive but WFA-negative PNNs. Selective labelling revealed that aggrecan encircled ~90% of alpha Mns. The results indicate that (1) aggrecan labels spinal PNNs better than WFA, and (2) there are differences in PNN composition and their associated neuronal populations between the spinal cord and cortex. Insights into the role of PNNs and their molecular heterogeneity in the spinal motor pools could aid in designing targeted strategies to enhance functional recovery post-injury.

Keywords: perineuronal nets; spinal cord; alpha motoneurone; gamma motoneurone; chondroitin sulphate proteoglycans

---

1. Introduction

Perineuronal nets (PNNs) are dense specialised extracellular matrix (ECM) structures that surround neuronal sub-populations throughout the central nervous system (CNS). First described by Golgi as reticular structures in the late 1800s [1], PNNs have since been implicated in pathologies of various neurological disorders, including Alzheimer's disease, epilepsy and schizophrenia [2–5], as well as in traumatic CNS injuries [6], particularly spinal cord injury (SCI) models [7,8]. A key role of PNNs is their involvement in the termination of developmental plasticity, where they form an interdigitating mesh with mature somatic and dendritic contacts to confer synaptic stabilisation [9–11].

PNNs are composed of a compact arrangement of a variety of neural ECM proteoglycans and proteins [12,13]. These components primarily consist of chondroitin sulphate proteoglycans (CSPGs) including the hyaluronan (HA) binding CSPGs called lecticans, bound upon a long HA backbone and stabilised by the HA and proteoglycan link proteins (HAPLNs) and tenascin-R [14]. Upon this basic PNN structure, the binding of other CSPGs (such as phosphacan) are thought to provide much of the heterogeneity of PNNs [15]. CSPGs are composed of chondroitin sulphate glycosaminoglycan

(CS-GAG) chains attached to a core protein that differentiates the various CSPGs from one another [15]. CS-GAGs confer a further vast degree of heterogeneity through variation of expression, chain length and sulphation patterns, even to the same core protein [16,17].

Although many studies have investigated the molecular heterogeneity of PNNs in distinct neuronal populations in regions of the brain [18–21], much of the composition and associated populations in the spinal cord is relatively unknown. Similar to the brain [22], in the spinal cord many of the known cells enwrapped by PNNs are fast-spiking inhibitory parvalbumin (PV)-positive interneurones (approximately half) [23,24], and have also been associated with calbindin-positive Renshaw cells [22]. However, in contrast to the brain, reports suggest that PNNs in the spinal cord also surround cells with large neuronal cell bodies, particularly within the ventral horn likely representing motoneurones (Mns) [22,25–27]. Mns are a heterogeneous population of neurones with the main subclasses, alpha and gamma Mns, innervating contractile extrafusal fibres and proprioceptive intrafusal fibres within the motor unit, respectively [28].

Enzymatic removal of PNNs using chondroitinase ABC (ChABC) after CNS injury has been shown in multiple models, predominately SCI, to reopen a window of plasticity to promote improvements in motor functions [7,8]. Regeneration of descending tracts can contribute to this functional recovery [29,30]; however, the extent and mechanism of changes in local spinal circuitry attributing to this recovery remains unclear. Additionally, studies also implicate exercise and rehabilitative training to activity-dependant modulation of PNNs in the ventral motor pools [31,32], suggesting a relationship between PNNs and Mns that is important for normal motor functions.

This study therefore aims to investigate the normal expression and molecular composition of PNNs in the spinal motor pools; the population of PNN-associated neurones in the spinal cord likely to be involved in functional motor recovery after SCI, and to identify the best PNN marker for this population. Immunohistochemical staining was performed using antibodies against choline acetyltransferase (ChAT), a marker of spinal Mns [33], alongside labelling for primary PNN components, including various CSPGs and the acclaimed "universal" PNN marker *Wisteria floribunda* agglutinin (WFA), to elucidate the composition of PNNs associated with spinal motor circuitry. Selective staining for the primary functional Mn subclasses was combined with PNN labelling to categorise PNN expression within the motor pool. It was found that distinct populations of Mns were surrounded by PNNs labelled by various CSPGs yet lacking WFA, indicating a difference between the composition of PNNs and associated neuronal cell types in the brain and spinal cord. PNNs were found to surround the majority of alpha Mns, suggesting that these are the main populations affected by ChABC-mediated recovery after SCI.

2. Results

We aim to determine the molecular heterogeneity of PNNs in the spinal cord, with a particular focus to the Mns in the ventral horn. Spinal cord sections from three different spinal levels, cervical, thoracic and lumbar, were used to compare the spatial differences of PNNs. Alongside ChAT staining, we also stained for WFA, a common PNN marker [6,7,10,34], and for CSPGs including aggrecan (ACAN), brevican (BCAN), neurocan (NCAN), versican (VCAN) and phosphacan (PTPRZ).

2.1. *WFA-Positive PNNs Only Partially Overlap with Other CSPGs in the Ventral Motor Pools*

2.1.1. ACAN

ACAN is a CSPG in the lectican family and is widely considered to be a major component in PNNs [2,35,36]. Immunohistochemical staining of ACAN core protein illustrated clear expression of PNNs surrounding ventral Mns labelled with ChAT (Figure 1J–L). ACAN-positive PNNs surrounded approximately 85% of ChAT-positive Mns in all levels of the spinal cord investigated (Figure 1A–C). In comparison, WFA-positive PNNs enwrapped significantly fewer Mns (approximately 68% of the ChAT-positive Mns) than ACAN-positive PNNs (cervical $p < 0.001$, thoracic $p < 0.05$ and lumbar $p < 0.01$;

$n = 4$), illustrating that WFA does not label all PNNs in the ventral motor pools. Compounding this, the total number of ACAN-positive PNNs surrounding Mns was significantly greater than the number of ACAN+/WFA+ PNNs (cervical $p < 0.001$, thoracic $p < 0.05$, lumbar $p < 0.01$; $n = 4$). ACAN and WFA PNN populations appeared to overlap (Figure 1D–I). Further breakdown of PNN type revealed that, at each level, all PNNs that are positive for WFA co-localised with ACAN (n.s.; $p = 1$). No investigated PNNs were WFA-positive and ACAN-negative. The results demonstrate that ACAN labels a larger population of PNN-positive Mns, and suggest that it is a better marker for PNN in the spinal cord.

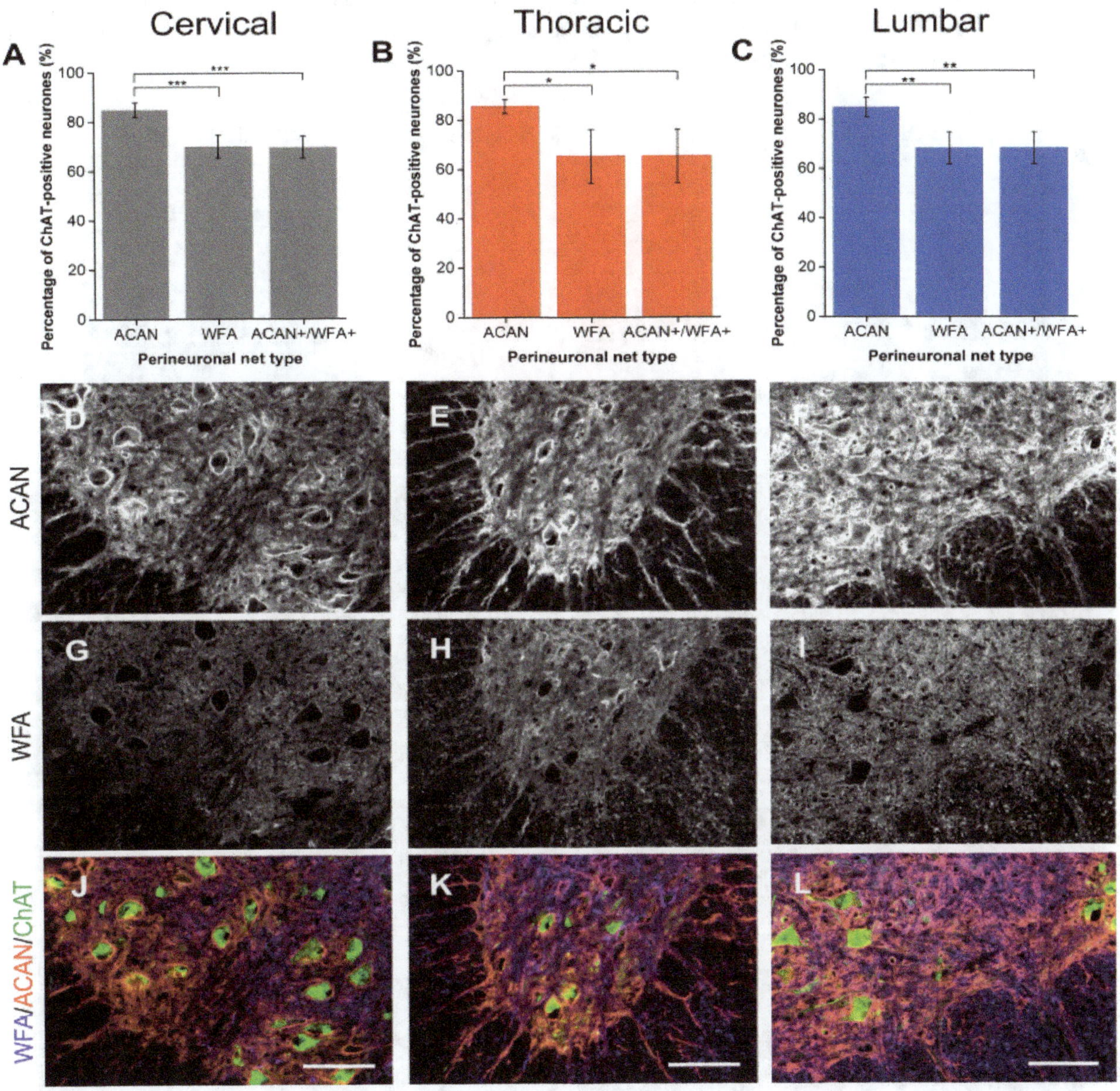

Figure 1. Comparison of perineuronal nets (PNNs) in the spinal ventral motor pools labelled by *Wisteria floribunda* agglutinin (WFA) and aggrecan (ACAN). (**A–C**) Bar graphs showing percentage of ChAT-positive motoneurones (Mns) in the ventral motor pools surrounded by ACAN-positive and WFA-positive PNNs and their co-localisation (ACAN+/WFA+) in cervical (**A**), thoracic (**B**) and lumbar (**C**) rat spinal cord. Error bars ± SD; $n = 4$. Statistics one-way ANOVA; significance levels: * $p < 0.05$, ** $p < 0.01$, *** $p < 0.001$. Confocal images showing ACAN-positive (**D–F**) and WFA-positive (**G–I**) PNNs surrounding ChAT-positive Mns (**J–L**) in the cervical, thoracic and lumbar spinal cord, respectively. Scale bars, 100 μm.

2.1.2. BCAN

BCAN is a lectican CSPG found specifically in the CNS with growing evidence of its importance in regulating the plastic properties of PNNs [37]. Co-staining with ChAT-positive neurones in the ventral horn revealed a high degree of localisation, with approximately 88% of Mns encircled by BCAN-positive PNNs (Figure 2A–C). Similar to ACAN, WFA-positive PNNs appeared to denote some but not all of the BCAN-positive PNN-ensheathed Mns, labelling approximately 30% fewer Mns than BCAN (all levels $p < 0.001$; $n = 5$). BCAN+/WFA+ PNNs in the motor pools appeared to represent a proportion that is significantly less that the total BCAN-positive PNN population (all levels $p < 0.001$; $n = 5$). Additional categorisation again revealed that all WFA-positive PNNs in the motor pool co-localised with BCAN-positive PNNs.

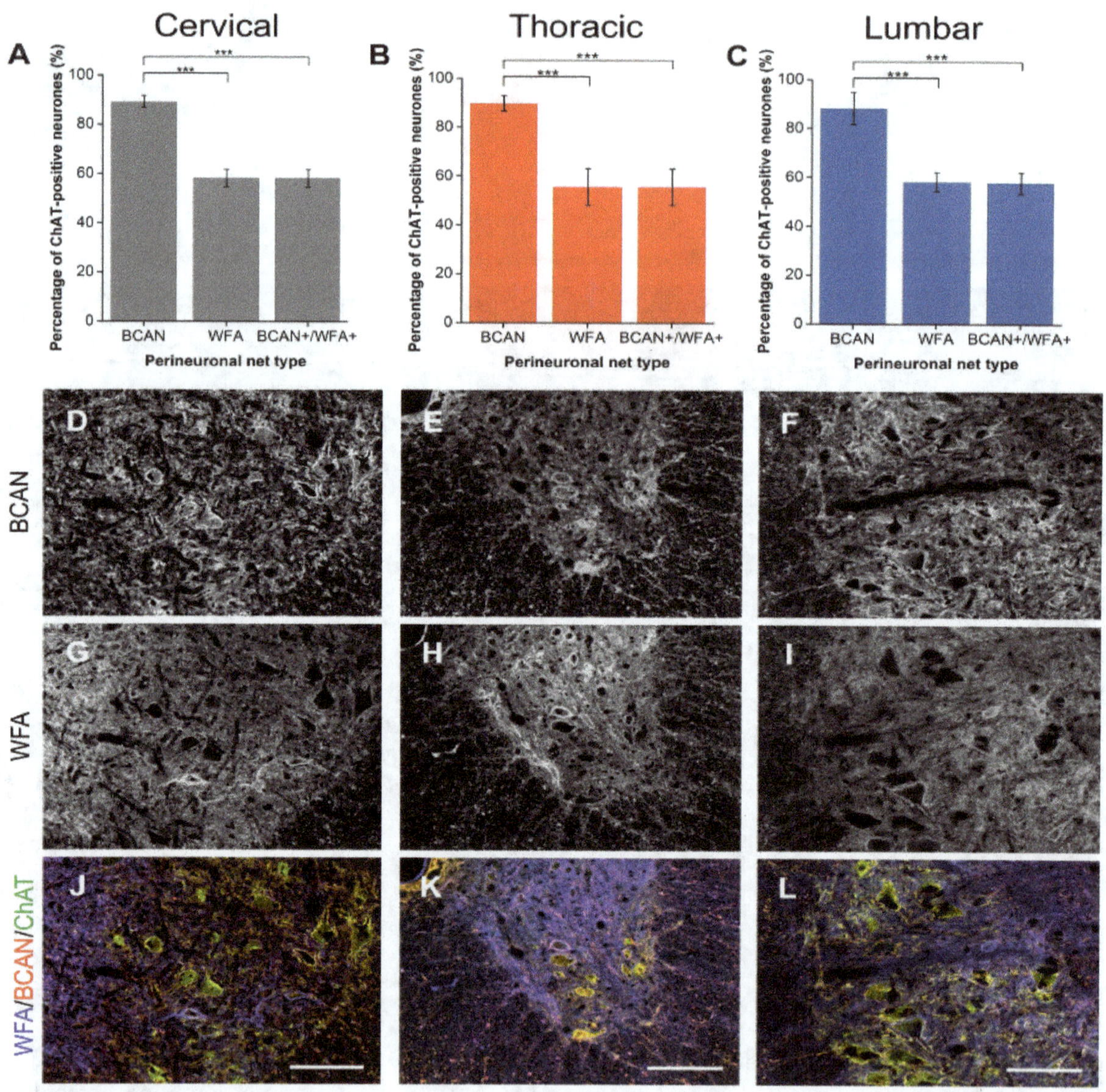

Figure 2. Comparison of perineuronal nets (PNNs) in the spinal ventral motor pools labelled by *Wisteria floribunda* agglutinin (WFA) and brevican (BCAN). (**A–C**) Bar graphs showing percentage of ChAT-positive motoneurones (Mns) in the ventral motor pools surrounded by BCAN-positive and WFA-positive PNNs and their co-localisation (BCAN+/WFA+) in cervical (**A**), thoracic (**B**) and lumbar (**C**) rat spinal cord. Error bars ± SD; $n = 5$. Statistics one-way ANOVA; significance levels: *** $p < 0.001$. Confocal images showing BCAN-positive (**D–F**) and WFA-positive (**G–I**) PNNs surrounding ChAT-positive Mns (**J–L**) in the cervical, thoracic and lumbar spinal cord, respectively. Scale bars, 100 μm.

2.1.3. NCAN

NCAN is a nervous system-specific lectican, like BCAN, known to be present in PNNs in the spinal cord [18,22,38]. In the ventral horn, NCAN staining revealed PNNs encircling approximately 87% of Mns (Figure 3A–C). Echoing the trend with ACAN and BCAN, WFA-positive PNNs enveloped 28% fewer Mns than NCAN (all levels $p < 0.001$; $n = 5$). Significantly, only approximately two-thirds of these NCAN-positive PNNs co-localised with WFA (all levels $p < 0.001$; $n = 5$). No WFA-positive PNNs lacking NCAN co-staining were observed, signifying that all WFA co-localised with NCAN.

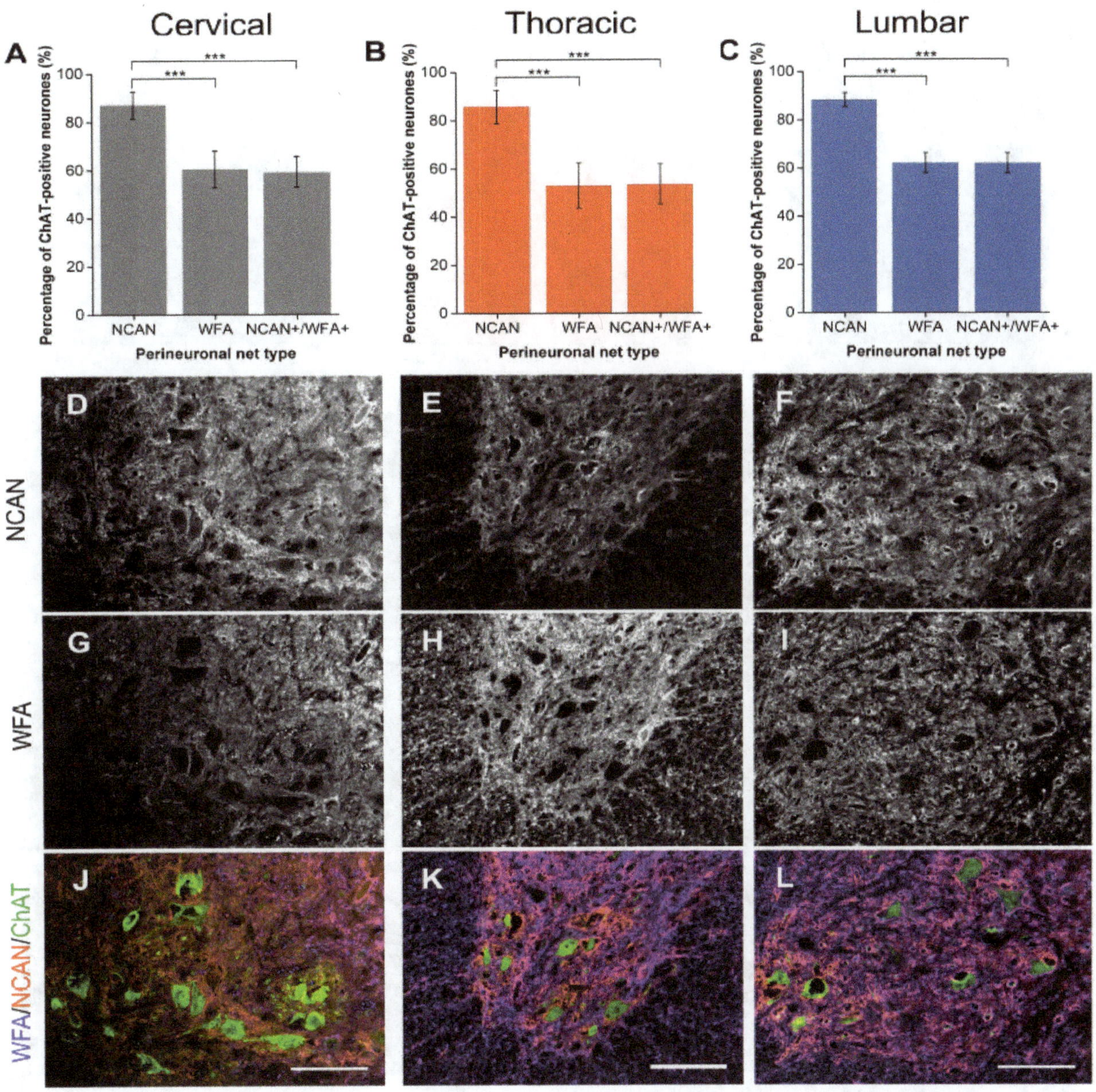

Figure 3. Comparison of perineuronal nets (PNNs) in the spinal ventral motor pools labelled by *Wisteria floribunda* agglutinin (WFA) and neurocan (NCAN). (**A–C**) Bar graphs showing percentage of ChAT-positive motoneurones (Mns) in the ventral motor pools surrounded by NCAN-positive and WFA-positive PNNs and their co-localisation (NCAN+WFA+) in cervical (**A**), thoracic (**B**) and lumbar (**C**) rat spinal cord. Error bars ± SD; $n = 5$. Statistics: one-way ANOVA; significance levels: *** $p < 0.001$. Confocal images showing NCAN-positive (**D–F**) and WFA-positive (**G–I**) PNNs surrounding ChAT-positive Mns (**J–L**) in the cervical, thoracic and lumbar spinal cord, respectively. Scale bars, 100 μm.

2.1.4. VCAN

VCAN staining revealed intense diffuse ECM expression in both the white and gray matter of the spinal cord due to its expression in the nodes of Ranvier [18,39,40]. VCAN did not show strong PNN staining in laminae other than the ventral horn. In the ventral horn, VCAN-positive PNNs surrounded approximately 82% of Mns at all spinal levels (Figure 4A–C). WFA and VCAN populations of PNNs showed a clear overlap at all spinal levels (Figure 4D–L). However, all WFA-positive PNNs co-localised with VCAN with a significant population of VCAN-positive PNNs WFA-negative (all levels $p < 0.001$; $n = 4$).

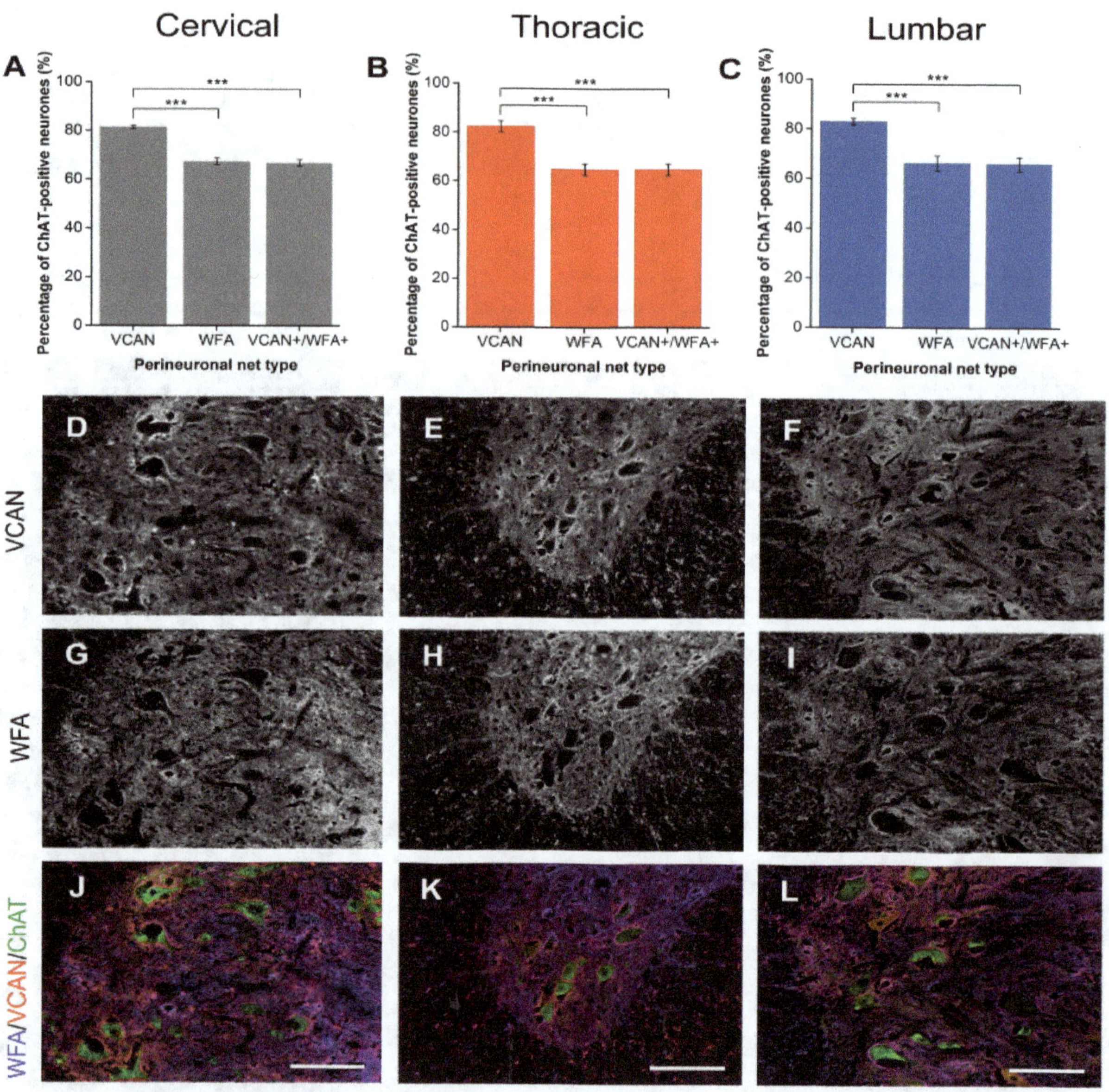

Figure 4. Comparison of perineuronal nets (PNNs) in the spinal ventral motor pools labelled by *Wisteria floribunda* agglutinin (WFA) and versican (VCAN). (A-C) Bar graphs showing percentage of ChAT-positive motoneurones (Mns) in the ventral motor pools surrounded by VCAN-positive and WFA-positive PNNs and their co-localisation (VCAN+/WFA+) in cervical (**A**), thoracic (**B**) and lumbar (**C**) rat spinal cord. Error bars ± SD, $n = 4$. Statistics: one-way ANOVA; significance levels: * $p < 0.05$, ** $p < 0.01$, *** $p < 0.001$. Confocal images showing VCAN-positive (**D–F**) and WFA-positive (**G–I**) PNNs surrounding ChAT-positive Mns (**J–L**) in the cervical, thoracic and lumbar spinal cord, respectively. Scale bars, 100 μm.

2.1.5. PTPRZ

Phosphacan or PTPRZ is a non-HA binding CSPG that represents the extracellular domain of protein tyrosine phosphatase receptor zeta (PTPRZ) modified by glial cells [41,42] and has been found to be present in WFA-positive PNNs in the cerebral cortex [18,22,43]. Immunohistochemistry showed that PTPRZ is also found in PNNs in the ventral motor pool, surrounding approximately 76% of Mns in all levels of the cord studied (Figure 5A–C). However, in all levels of the spinal cord investigated, PTPRZ-positive PNNssurrounded 15% more Mns than WFA (all levels $p < 0.01$; $n = 4$), reiterating the trend shown by the lecticans above. Approximately 82% of PTPRZ-positive PNNs were also labelled by WFA, representing a significantly lower proportion of the total observed PTPRZ-positive PNNs in the motor pool (all level $p < 0.05$; $n = 4$).

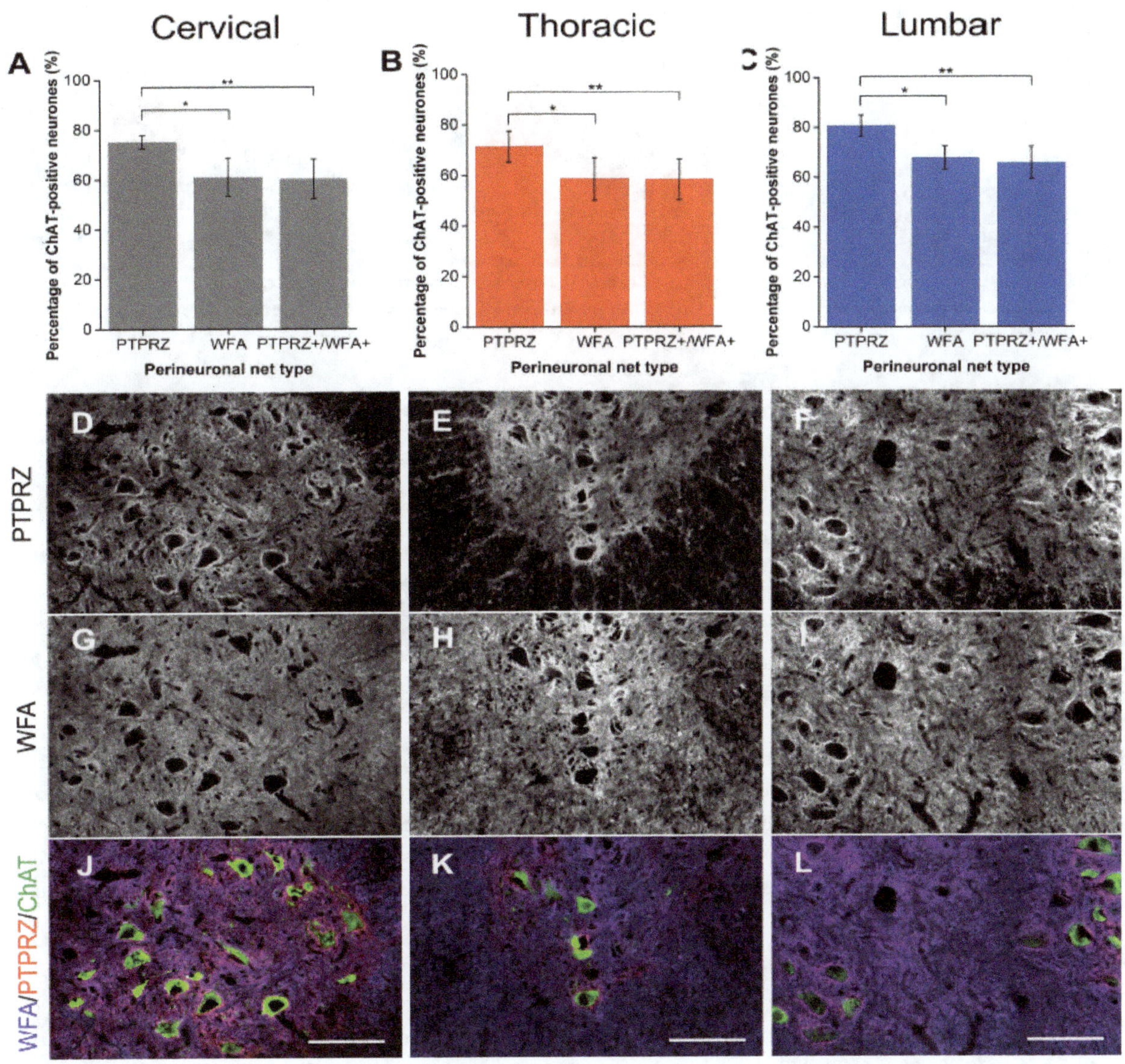

Figure 5. Comparison of perineuronal nets (PNNs) in the spinal ventral motor pools labelled by *Wisteria floribunda* agglutinin (WFA) and phosphacan (PTPRZ). (**A**–**C**) Bar graphs showing percentage of ChAT-positive motoneurones (Mns) in the ventral motor pools surrounded by PTPRZ-positive and WFA-positive PNNs and their co-localisation (PTPRZ+/WFA+) in cervical (**A**), thoracic (**B**) and lumbar (**C**) rat spinal cord. Error bars ± SD; $n = 4$. Statistics: one-way ANOVA; significance levels: * $p < 0.05$, ** $p < 0.01$. Confocal images showing PTPRZ-positive (**D**–**F**) and WFA-positive (**G**–**I**) PNNs surrounding ChAT-positive Mns (**J**–**L**) in the cervical, thoracic and lumbar spinal cord, respectively. Scale bars, 100 μm.

2.2. Distinct Populations of CSPG-Positive yet WFA-Negative PNNs in the Motor Pools

For each CSPG investigated, a significant percentage of Mns were surrounded by PNNs that were CSPG-positive yet WFA-negative (all levels, all CSPGs $p < 0.001$). The percentage of Mns with WFA-negative PNNs varied with CSPG investigated (Figure 6). While ACAN+/WFA−, VCAN+/WFA− and PTPRZ+/WFA− PNNs encircled roughly 15% of Mns (Figure 6A,D,E), a higher percentage of Mns (approximately 30%) appeared to be surrounded by BCAN+/WFA− and NCAN+/WFA− PNNs (Figure 6B,C). Overall, the results suggest that in the ventral motor pools, WFA does not denote all PNNs, and instead distinct populations of Mns with CSPG-positive, WFA-negative PNNs exist.

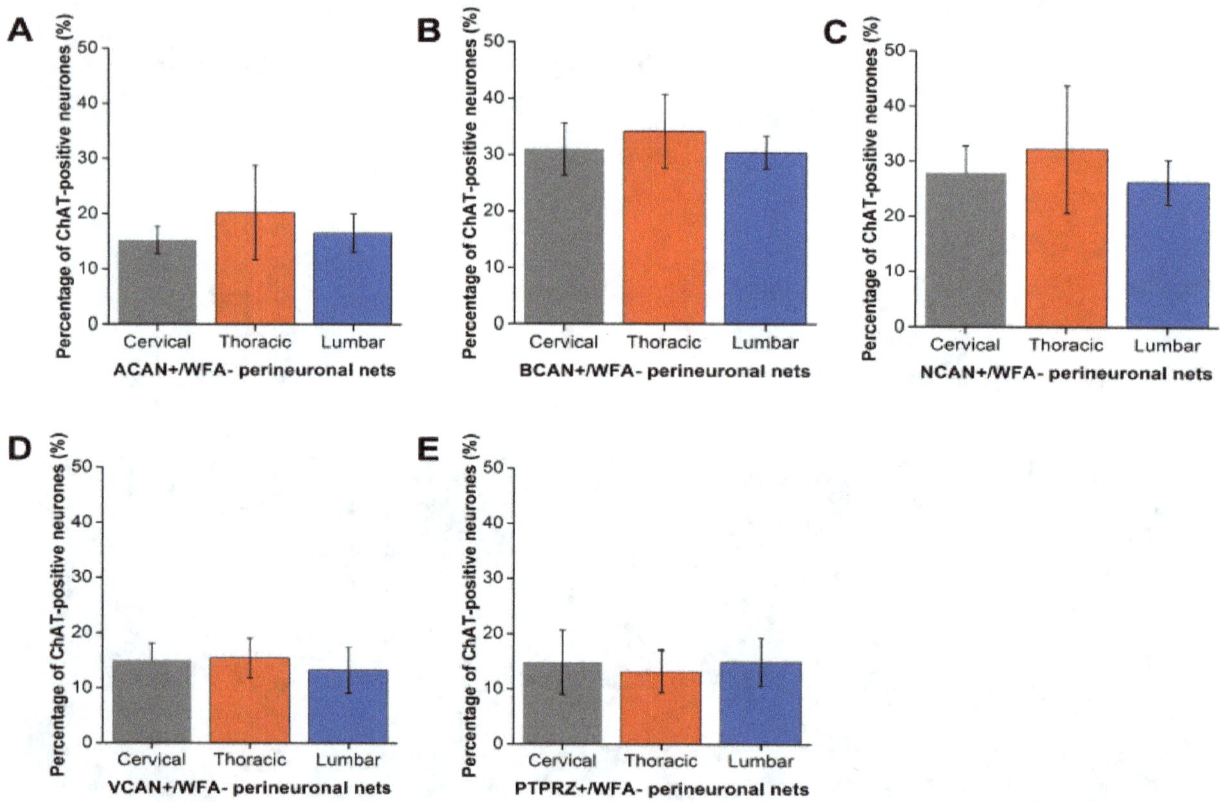

Figure 6. A proportion of perineuronal nets (PNNs) in the spinal motor pools were negative for *Wisteria floribunda* agglutinin (WFA). Percentage of ChAT-positive motoneurones in the ventral motor pools in the cervical, thoracic and lumbar spinal cord surrounded by CSPG-positive, WFA-negative PNNs. (**A**) Aggrecan (ACAN, $n = 4$); (**B**) brevican (BCAN, $n = 5$); (**C**) neurocan (NCAN, $n = 5$); (**D**) versican (VCAN, $n = 4$); and (**E**) phosphacan (PTPRZ, $n = 4$). Error bars ± SD. Statistics one-way ANOVA; n.s.

2.3. Alpha Mns Are Preferentially Surrounded by PNNs

Using NeuN and ChAT co-labelling, Mns in the spinal ventral motor pools were selectively labelled as either alpha (NeuN-positive) or gamma (NeuN-negative) [31,44]. It was observed that approximately 70–80% of ChAT-positive Mns were NeuN-positive (Figures 7 and 8), signifying thealpha Mn population. Firstly, as the universal marker for PNNs, WFA was used to determine the number of PNNs surrounding each Mn subtype. Similarly to the results above, WFA-positive PNNs surrounded approximately 60% of all Mns with approximately 98% of these PNNs surrounding NeuN-positive Mns (alphas; Figure 7A–C). In other words, a significant proportion of alpha Mns (~72%) were associated with WFA-positive PNNs (cervical and lumbar $p < 0.001$, thoracic $p < 0.05$; $n = 3$). As previous findings illustrated that in the ventral motor pools, WFA did not label all Mns, ACAN was also used to identify PNNs around Mn subtype. Again, most PNNs (95%) surrounded alpha Mns (Figure 8A–C). ACAN-positive PNNs encircled roughly 90% of alpha Mns, suggesting that PNN-positive Mns and alpha Mns are the same population.

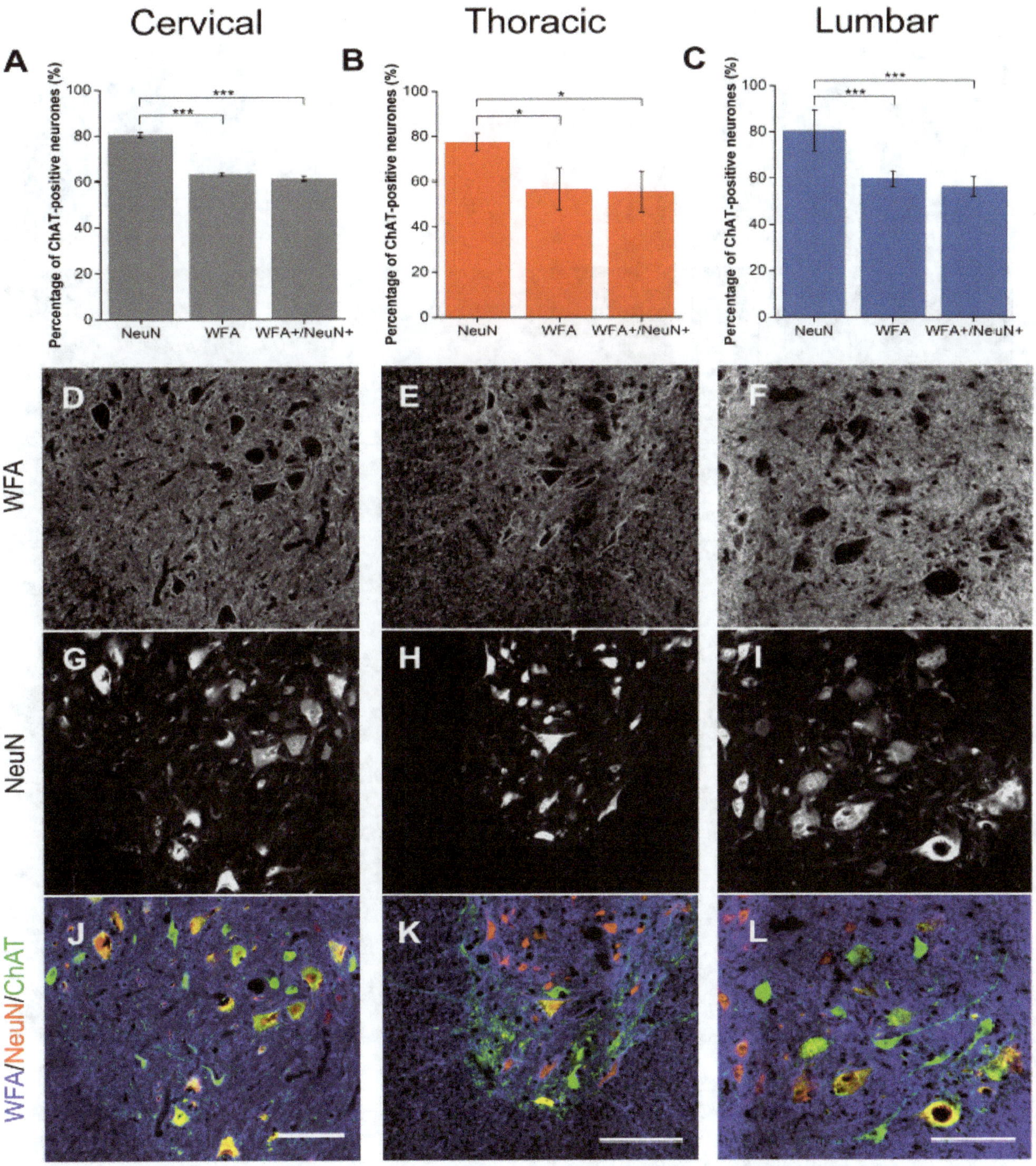

Figure 7. *Wisteria floribunda* agglutinin (WFA)-positive PNNs surrounded some but not all alpha motoneurones (Mns). (**A**–**C**) Bar graphs showing percentage of ChAT-positive Mns in the ventral motor pools surrounded by NeuN, WFA-positive PNNs and their co-localisation (WFA+/NeuN+) in cervical (**A**), thoracic (**B**) and lumbar (**C**) rat spinal cord. NeuN and ChAT co-localisation denotes alpha Mns. Error bars ± SD; $n = 3$. Statistics: one-way ANOVA; significance levels: * $p < 0.05$, *** $p < 0.001$. Confocal images showing WFA-positive PNNs (**D**–**F**) surrounding NeuN-positive (**G**–**I**) PNNs and ChAT-positive Mns (**J**–**L**) in the cervical, thoracic and lumbar spinal cord, respectively. Scale bars, 100 µm.

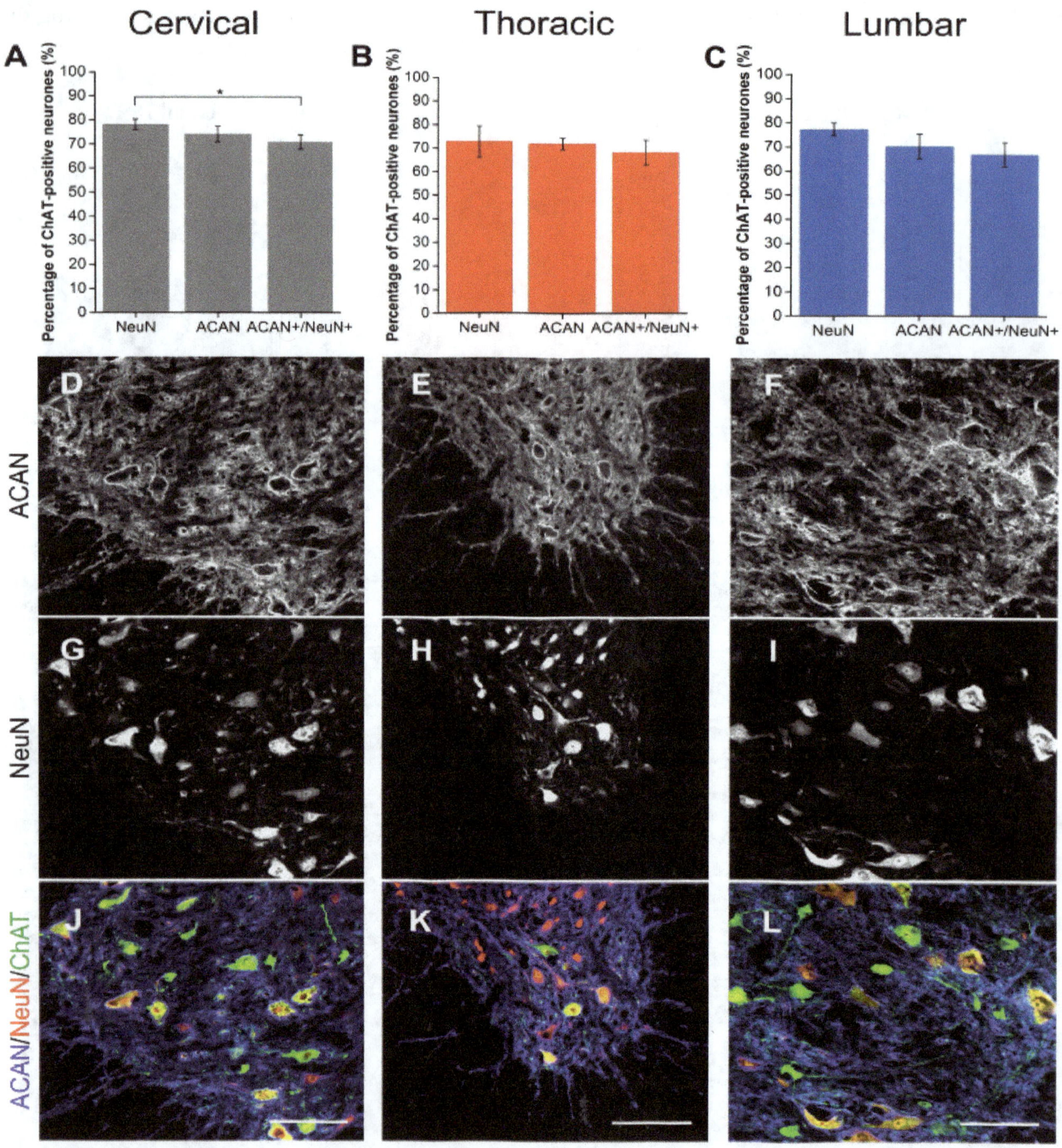

Figure 8. Aggrecan (ACAN)-positive PNNs surrounded most alpha motoneurones (Mns). (**A–C**) Bar graphs showing percentage of ChAT-positive Mns in the ventral motor pools surrounded by NeuN, ACAN-positive PNNs and their co-localisation (ACAN+/NeuN+) in cervical (**A**), thoracic (**B**) and lumbar (**C**) rat spinal cord. NeuN and ChAT co-localisation denotes alpha Mns. Error bars ± SD; $n = 3$. Statistics: one-way ANOVA; significance levels: * $p < 0.05$. Confocal images showing ACAN-positive PNNs (**D–F**) surrounding NeuN-positive (**G–I**) PNNs and ChAT-positive Mns (**J–L**) in the cervical, thoracic and lumbar spinal cord, respectively. Scale bars, 100 μm.

3. Discussion

As removal of PNNs in the spinal cord after injury enhances motor recovery, we looked to investigate the expression of PNNs and their heterogeneity in spinal Mns; the final order neurones for the control of voluntary movement. This is the first article to systemically and quantitatively compare the differences of CSPG- or WFA-positive PNN Mns in the ventral motor pools. Mns were identified using an antibody against ChAT to label cholinergic neurones alongside markers for PNN components and the acclaimed universal PNN marker WFA in comparison. We demonstrated that a high proportion of Mns in the ventral spinal cord were surrounded by PNNs, particularly alpha Mns. Unexpectedly, the universal marker for PNNs, WFA, did not label all of the PNNs with distinct populations of Mns surrounded by CSPG-positive yet WFA-negative PNNs. This suggests that, in contrast to the brain, WFA does not label the majority of PNN neurones in the ventral spinal cord and that studies using WFA in the spinal cord may be underestimating the number of PNNs.

3.1. PNNs in the Spinal Ventral Motor Pools

Previous studies have described ventral Mns as the most conspicuous neuronal population in the spinal cord to be surrounded by PNNs and this appears to be conserved across mammalian species [25,31,32,45,46]. Despite this, few studies have actually investigated the proportion of PNNs in the ventral motor pools and those that do use varying markers to determine this. Comparable to our own methods, using ChAT as a specific Mn marker, a similar proportion of ventral Mns was observed to be surrounded by PNNs to that found in our study (~80%) has been reported in non-human primates (75%), using WFA [45], and in human (71%) spinal cord, using ACAN [46]. In rats, however, this distribution has been investigated with the general neuronal marker (NeuN) using size and ventral location to identify Mns alongside WFA lectin staining to characterise PNN expression, resulting in estimates of only 30% of Mns associated with PNNs [25]. This is likely to underestimate for two reasons: (1) without a Mn-specific neuronal marker small sized Mns, including NeuN-negative gamma Mns [44,47], would have been absent from these counts, and (2) WFA does not appear to label all PNNs in the rat spinal cord. Indeed, our findings suggest that PNNs are present in almost 80% of the ChAT-positive Mns.

Although others have implicated that PNNs only surround large cell-bodied Mns in the motor pools, i.e., alpha Mns and not gamma Mns [25,31], we are the first to systematically categorise the proportion of specific Mn-subtypes associated with PNNs at different levels of the spinal cord. Despite contributing to the same goal of voluntary muscle control, alpha and gamma Mns represent distinct populations of Mns within the ventral motor pools, differing in both electrical and molecular properties [28,44,48,49]. These differences also include the innervation of different muscle targets, with alpha Mns responsible for force generation though contraction of extrafusal fibres whereas gamma Mns innervate the intrafusal fibres regulating muscle spindle sensitivity. The high proportion of enveloped alpha Mns revealed likely reflects the importance of the role of PNNs in providing synaptic stabilisation of inputs from the specific spinal circuitry and consequent contractile innervation of key muscle groups. After SCI, the stabilisation of synaptic plasticity conferred by PNNs instead becomes another mechanism inhibiting regenerative attempts and compensatory rearrangements of spared fibres. We suggest that ChABC-mediated removal of PNNs in SCI models is therefore able to induce a high degree of enhanced plasticity of synaptic connections to the abovementioned populations of alpha Mns contributing to the observed improvement of most functional motor recovery studies.

3.2. Differences in PNNs between the Brain and Spinal Cord

It is generally assumed that PNNs in the brain and the spinal cord are the same. While in the brain, WFA does not always co-localise with ACAN as previously discussed, other CSPG-positive PNNs always co-localise with WFA. Here, we demonstrate differences in the composition of PNNs between the brain and spinal cord, where ACAN and other CSPGs denote subclasses of Mns in the spinal cord lacking WFA. This study recommends that future staining for PNNs associated with the spinal motor pools, particularly SCI studies utilising therapies that modify PNNs such as ChABC, should seek alternatives to WFA to avoid underestimating total PNN number.

Additionally, brain PNNs are well known to target small fast-spiking inhibitory interneurones playing a modulatory role in the brain [50]. In sharp contrast, the associated neuronal populations studied here are large cell bodied neurones acting as the primary endpoint of neural control of the somatic motor system. Other neuronal cell types such as calbindin-positive Renshaw cells in the ventral spinal cord are surrounded by PNNs [22], further implicating the role of PNNs in stabilisation of connections within the spinal motor circuitry. In a recent systematic review of the CNS, motor regions, including the cerebellum and spinal cord, were more likely to have a higher proportion of neurones surrounded by PNNs than sensory structures [45]. It is possible that PNNs may have different roles in different parts of the nervous system or with different neuronal populations.

3.3. Composition of PNNs in the Spinal Motor Pools

Staining with the lectin WFA and antibodies for various CSPG core proteins revealed two distinct types of distributions throughout the grey matter: diffuse extracellular staining and a bright 'halo' of pericellular expression identifying the PNNs. The overall distributions of immunoreactivities for the CSPGs investigated and ChAT were generally similar to previous descriptions [18,22,25,33]. We showed that all of the CSPGs investigated were present in PNNs surrounding spinal Mns. These were also found to be present to varying degrees, indicating heterogeneity of PNNs in the motor pools.

ACAN in particular has been previously reported to be present in PNNs surrounding Mns [22,51,52], as well as BCAN, NCAN, VCAN and PTPRZ. It is estimated that VCAN begins to appear in PNNs around the Mns from postnatal day 8 [53]. Studies in the brain and spinal cord show that ACAN is present in all PNNs and generally co-localises with WFA expression [12,18,25]. However, consistent with all CSPGs investigated, WFA does not appear to show all PNN-associated neurones in the ventral motor pools. As WFA is supposed to bind to the CS-GAG sugar *N*-acetylgalactosamine (GalNAc) [50], it should bind to all CSPGs and therefore denote all PNNs. However, binding of WFA has previously been shown to be dependent on the presence of ACAN [12] and recently other studies in various regions of the brain, including the hippocampus, have reported PNNs with ACAN labelling but no WFA binding [21,54]. In the spinal cord, we observed a lack of WFA in ACAN-positive PNNs to a similar degree to that observed in the CA1 area of the hippocampus [21], appearing to denote distinct populations of Mns. As there is a vast degree of heterogeneity of CS-GAGs within CSPGs, further research is required to determine the conditions of WFA binding. It is possible that the molecular composition of CSPGs within PNNs may confer functional subclasses of Mns.

The expression of many PNN components such as ACAN, BCAN and tenascin-R show differences in expression between various brain regions [55]. In particular, BCAN is usually found at the para-nodal regions and has been shown to regulate the localisation of potassium channels and AMPA receptors [37]. The mechanism of how brevican performs these functions remains to be determined. Expression of CSPGs in PNNs across the spinal laminae has also been shown to display differential expression [22,25]. PNNs are a dynamic network of ECM components. Activity-dependant modulation has been demonstrated where the thickness of PNNs surrounding spinal Mns increases in response to exercise or rehabilitative training [31,32]. This is likely conveyed through dynamic regulation of CSPGs and/or CS-GAGs within the PNNs. There is a growing concept that the properties of the ECM have an important influence in both healthy and pathological states. Though it is beyond the scope of this study, it is hoped that further research into the heterogeneity of PNNs in CNS regions may help to unravel the functionality of these ECM components and their alterations in disease states.

3.4. Further Research and Conclusions

Despite the clinical relevance of PNNs targeted for CNS repair and regeneration, particularly in locomotor recovery models of SCI, the functional relationship between PNNs and the motor system is still mostly unexplored. Further research is required to look at the normal functional properties of PNNs surrounding Mns. Additionally, the molecular heterogeneity of PNNs displayed in spinal Mns may indicate a functional role. However, understanding how the varying molecular heterogeneity of PNNs affects CNS functions is a topic still in its infancy.

Though this study begins to address a research gap surrounding the properties of PNNs in the spinal cord, much characterisation remains to be done. While ChABC has been an invaluable investigative tool for understanding the role of PNNs in promoting plasticity and functional recovery after SCI, there are clinical limitations to its therapeutic use. It is hoped that insights into the properties of PNNs and their role in the spinal cord could aid the generation of alternative and non-invasive strategies for targeted PNN removal to enhance functional recovery post-injury.

4. Materials and Methods

4.1. Animals

Female Lister Hooded rats (200–250 g; $n = 5$) were obtained from Charles River Laboratories (Canterbury, UK) and were housed in groups in Central Biomedical Services (University of Leeds) in a temperature controlled environment (20 ± 1 °C), with a 12 h light/dark cycle (lights on at 07:00). Access to food and water was *ad libitum*. All procedures and experiments complied with the UK Animals (Scientific Procedures) Act 1986.

4.2. Tissue Preparation

Animals were given an overdose of sodium pentobarbital (Pentoject; Henry Schein; 200 mg/kg; intraperitoneal injection) to deeply anaesthetise without halting cardiac function. A transcardial perfusion [56] was then performed using sodium phosphate buffer (PB; 0.12 M sodium phosphate monobasic; 0.1 M NaOH; pH 7.4) followed by 4% paraformaldehyde (PFA; in PB; pH 7.4) for tissue fixation. The spinal cord was dissected out, post-fixed in PFA (4%; 4 °C) overnight and cryoprotected in 30% sucrose solution (30% v/w sucrose in PB; 4 °C) until tissue saturation. The appropriate cervical (C3-T1), mid-thoracic and lumbar (L1-6) spinal cord segments were removed and frozen in optimum temperature medium (OCT; Leica FSC 22 Frozen Section Media; Leica Biosystems) before storage at −80 °C until sectioning. Tissue was cut using a cryostat (Leica CM1850; Leica Biosystems) into 40 µm transverse sections. Sections were serially collected into 48-well plates containing physiological buffer solution (PBS; 0.13 M NaCl, 0.7 M sodium phosphate dibasic, 0.003 M sodium phosphate monobasic; pH 7.4) to remove the OCT before being transferred to 30% sucrose solution for storage at 4 °C.

4.3. Staining Procedures

Immunohistochemical techniques were used to label for cells in the spinal cord containing ChAT and the PNNs surrounding subsets of these cells labelled by biotinylated *Wisteria floribunda* agglutinin (bio-WFA) and CSPG components, including ACAN, BCAN and NCAN (Table 1). ChAT was used for Mn identification [57] whilst WFA is universally used as a marker for PNNs [10,12].

At room temperature (RT), free-floating sections were washed three times for 5 min each in Tris-buffered saline (TBS; 0.1 M tris base, 0.15 M NaCl; pH 7.4) to remove sucrose residue. Tissue was then blocked in 0.3% TBST (1× TBS solution and 0.3% v/v Triton X-100) and 3% normal donkey serum (NDS; v/v) for two hours. The sections were then transferred to co-incubate at 4 °C in blocking buffer (3% NDS in 0.3% TBST; pH 7.4) containing the following primary antibodies: anti-ChAT (goat; Millipore; 1:500; 48 h), biotin-conjugated *Wisteria floribunda* agglutinin (bio-WFA; Sigma; 1:150; 24 h) and either ACAN (rabbit; Millipore; 1:250; 24 h), BCAN (mouse; DSHB; 1:500; 24 h), NCAN (mouse; DSHB; 1:100; 24 h), VCAN (mouse; DSHB; 1:100; 24 h) or PTPRZ (mouse; DSHB; 1:80; 24 h) (Table 1).

Table 1. Immunohistochemical detection of extracellular matrix components and neuronal markers, including concentration (conc.) of antibody used.

Detected Component	Marker	Host	Antibody Conc.	Source	Characterisation
CSPGs					
Aggrecan (mouse ACAN core protein)	Anti-ACAN	Rabbit polyclonal IgG	500 μg/mL	Millipore #AB1031	WB[2] (Lendvai et al., 2013 & Sutkus et al., 2014)
Brevican (BCAN; mouse cell-line derived recombinant human Brevican)	Anti-BCAN	Sheep polyclonal IgG	1 mg/mL	R&D Systems #AF4009	WB[2] (R&D Systems data sheet)
Neurocan (NCAN; N-terminal epitope)	Anti-NCAN	Mouse monoclonal IgG	369 μg/mL	DSHB[1] #1F6	WB[2] (Asher et al., 2000 & Deepa et al., 2006)
Versican (VCAN; hyaluronate-binding region)	Anti-VCAN	Mouse monoclonal IgG	169 μg/mL	DSHB[1] #12C5	WB[2] (Asher et al., 2002 & Deepa et al., 2006)
Phosphacan (PTPRZ)	Anti- PTPRZ	Mouse monoclonal IgG	165 μg/mL	DSHB[1] #3F8	WB[2] (Deepa et al., 2006 & Vitellaro-Zuccarello et al., 2006)
Lectins					
N-acetylgalactosamine (GalNAc)	Biotinylated *Wisteria floribunda* agglutinin (WFA)	N/A	2 mg/mL	Sigma #L1766	Koppe et al., 1996
Neuronal markers					
Choline acetyltransferase (ChAT)	Anti-ChAT	Goat polyclonal IgG	-	Millipore #AB144P	-
Neuron-specific nuclear protein (NeuN)	Anti-NeuN	Mouse monoclonal IgG	1 mg/mL	Millipore #MAB377	WB[2] (Jin et al., 2003)

[1] DSHB, Developmental Studies Hybridoma Bank, University of Iowa, USA. [2] WB, Western blotting.

Immunostaining was routinely carried out using tissue from different animals and differing spinal segments. The combinations carried out in this study used the formula: ChAT—Bio-WFA—CSPG marker using various antibodies from Table 1, including for the lecticans ACAN, BCAN, NCAN and VCAN. To differentiate between alpha and gamma Mns [31,44], ChAT was co-stained with anti-NeuN (mouse; Millipore; 1:500; 24 h). Antibodies requiring 24-h incubation were added and mixed well 48 h into a 72-h incubation with ChAT, using the protocols as above. To visualise each primary antibody staining, the tissue was then co-incubated with the appropriate species of fluorescent-conjugated secondary antibodies (1:500; 2 h; RT; Table 2).

Table 2. Fluorescent-conjugated secondary antibodies (2 mg/mL) used for immuno-detection of primary antibodies.

Antibody	Host	Source
Alexa fluor 488	chicken anti-goat IgG	Invitrogen #A21467
Alexa fluor 568	donkey anti-mouse IgG	Invitrogen #A31571
Alexa fluor 568	donkey anti-rabbit IgG	Invitrogen #A10042
Alexa fluor 568	donkey anti-sheep IgG	Invitrogen #A21099
Alexa fluor 647	*Streptavidin*-conjugated	Invitrogen #S32357

4.4. Image Acquisition and Quantification Methods

The fluorophores used to label the spinal cord sections were visualised using a Zeiss LSM 880 (upright) confocal microscope and were used to generate tile scans of the entire spinal cord transverse section at 20× magnification (1.03 μs per pixel, averaging: 4). ChAT-positive cells and co-localisation with WFA-positive PNNs and other CSPG-positive PNNs were counted using the Cell Counter plugin (Kurt de Vos; https://imagej.nih.gov/ij/plugins/cell-counter.html) in the software FIJI [58]. Mns were identified by location within the ventral horn of ChAT-positive cellular staining. All ChAT-positive cells were individually counted and sequentially analysed for presence of PNN staining. PNNs were only counted around ChAT-positive neurones and were identified by the presence of intense staining as a bright 'halo' directly adjacent to the perimeter of ChAT-positive cells. Positive PNN staining was categorised into three classes: (1) only WFA-positive, (2) only positive for the appropriate CSPG stain or (3) WFA-positive and CSPG-positive. For differentiation of alpha and gamma Mns, cells co-localising both ChAT and NeuN staining where taken as alpha Mns whereas the absence of NeuN denoted gamma Mns [44,59].

4.5. Experimental Design and Statistical Analysis

A minimum of three sections per spinal level (cervical, thoracic or lumbar) per animal (n = 5) were stained and imaged, maintaining the same confocal microscopy settings per staining procedure. All counts per section were normalised by the number of ChAT-positive cells before averaging per animal. All data sets were analysed with OriginPro 2016 scientific graphing and data analysis software (OriginLab, Northampton, MA, USA), where results were statistically significant given that $p < 0.05$. To test the influence of spinal cord level on PNN expression and for differences between PNN types, results were pooled and analysed using one-way ANOVA, with Bonferroni correction for between-groups multiple comparison.

Acknowledgments: This work was financed by grants from the Wings for Life Foundation, The University of Leeds 110 Years Scholarship and the European Union-the Operational Programme Research, Development and Education in the framework of the project "Centre of Reconstructive Neuroscience", registration number CZ.02.1.01/0.0./0.0/15_003/0000419. The authors declare no competing financial interests.

Author Contributions: Jessica C. F. Kwok and Sian F. Irvine conceived and designed the experiments; Sian F. Irvine performed the experiments and analysed the data; Jessica C. F. Kwok contributed reagents/materials/analysis tools; Sian F. Irvine wrote the paper with amendments by Jessica C. F. Kwok.

Abbreviations

ACAN	Aggrecan core protein
BCAN	Brevican core protein
ChAT	Choline acetyltransferase
ChABC	Chondroitinase ABC
CNS	Central nervous system
CS-GAG	Chondroitin sulphate glycosaminoglycan
CSPGs	Chondroitin sulphate proteoglycans
ECM	Extracellular matrix
GalNAc	*N*-acetylgalactosamine
HA	Hyaluronic acid/hyaluronan
Mn	Motoneurone
NeuN	Neuron-specific nuclear protein
NCAN	Neurocan core protein
PTPRZ	Phosphacan/protein tyrosine phosphatase receptor zeta
PNN	Perineuronal net
Mn	Motoneurone
SCI	Spinal cord injury
VCAN	Versican core protein
WFA	*Wisteria floribunda* agglutinin

References

1. Celio, M.R.; Spreafico, R.; De Biasi, S.; Vitellaro-Zuccarello, L. Perineuronal nets: Past and present. *Trends Neurosci.* **1998**, *21*, 510–515. [CrossRef]
2. Suttkus, A.; Rohn, S.; Weigel, S.; Glöckner, P.; Arendt, T.; Morawski, M. Aggrecan, link protein and tenascin-R are essential components of the perineuronal net to protect neurons against iron-induced oxidative stress. *Cell Death Dis.* **2014**, *5*. [CrossRef] [PubMed]
3. Cabungcal, J.-H.H.; Steullet, P.; Morishita, H.; Kraftsik, R.; Cuenod, M.; Hensch, T.K.; Do, K.Q. Perineuronal nets protect fast-spiking interneurons against oxidative stress. *Proc. Natl. Acad. Sci. USA* **2013**, *110*, 9130–9135. [CrossRef] [PubMed]
4. Pantazopoulos, H.; Berretta, S. In Sickness and in Health: Perineuronal Nets and Synaptic Plasticity in Psychiatric Disorders. *Neural Plast.* **2016**, *2016*, 9847696. [CrossRef] [PubMed]
5. McRae, P.A.; Porter, B.E. The perineuronal net component of the extracellular matrix in plasticity and epilepsy. *Neurochem. Int.* **2012**, *61*, 963–972. [CrossRef] [PubMed]
6. Moon, L.D.F.; Asher, R.A.; Rhodes, K.E.; Fawcett, J.W. Regeneration of CNS axons back to their target following treatment of adult rat brain with chondroitinase ABC. *Nat. Neurosci.* **2001**, *4*, 465–466. [CrossRef] [PubMed]
7. Bradbury, E.J.; Moon, L.D.; Popat, R.J.; King, V.R.; Bennett, G.S.; Patel, P.N.; Fawcett, J.W.; McMahon, S.B. Chondroitinase ABC promotes functional recovery after spinal cord injury. *Nature* **2002**, *416*, 636–640. [CrossRef] [PubMed]
8. García-Alías, G.; Barkhuysen, S.; Buckle, M.; Fawcett, J.W. Chondroitinase ABC treatment opens a window of opportunity for task-specific rehabilitation. *Nat. Neurosci.* **2009**, *12*, 1145–1151. [CrossRef] [PubMed]
9. Carulli, D.; Pizzorusso, T.; Kwok, J.C.; Putignano, E.; Poli, A.; Forostyak, S.; Andrews, M.R.; Deepa, S.S.; Glant, T.T.; Fawcett, J.W. Animals lacking link protein have attenuated perineuronal nets and persistent plasticity. *Brain* **2010**, *133*, 2331–2347. [CrossRef] [PubMed]
10. Pizzorusso, T.; Medini, P.; Berardi, N.; Chierzi, S.; Fawcett, J.W.; Maffei, L. Reactivation of ocular dominance plasticity in the adult visual cortex. *Science* **2002**, *298*, 1248–1251. [CrossRef] [PubMed]
11. Tsien, R.Y. Very long-term memories may be stored in the pattern of holes in the perineuronal net. *Proc. Natl. Acad. Sci. USA* **2013**, *110*, 12456–12461. [CrossRef] [PubMed]

12. Giamanco, K.A.; Morawski, M.; Matthews, R.T. Perineuronal net formation and structure in aggrecan knockout mice. *Neuroscience* **2010**, *170*, 1314–1327. [CrossRef] [PubMed]
13. Kwok, J.C.; Carulli, D.; Fawcett, J.W. In vitro modeling of perineuronal nets: Hyaluronan synthase and link protein are necessary for their formation and integrity. *J. Neurochem.* **2010**, *114*, 1447–1459. [CrossRef] [PubMed]
14. Kwok, J.C.; Dick, G.; Wang, D.; Fawcett, J.W. Extracellular matrix and perineuronal nets in CNS repair. *Dev. Neurobiol.* **2011**, *71*, 1073–1089. [CrossRef] [PubMed]
15. Yamaguchi, Y. Lecticans: Organizers of the brain extracellular matrix. *Cell. Mol. Life Sci.* **2000**, *57*, 276–289. [CrossRef] [PubMed]
16. Kitagawa, H. Using sugar remodeling to study chondroitin sulfate function. *Biol. Pharm. Bull.* **2014**, *37*, 1705–1712. [CrossRef] [PubMed]
17. Gama, C.I.; Tully, S.E.; Sotogaku, N.; Clark, P.M.; Rawat, M.; Vaidehi, N.; Goddard, W.A.; Nishi, A.; Hsieh-Wilson, L.C. Sulfation patterns of glycosaminoglycans encode molecular recognition and activity. *Nat. Chem. Biol.* **2006**, *2*, 467–473. [CrossRef] [PubMed]
18. Deepa, S.S.; Carulli, D.; Galtrey, C.; Rhodes, K.; Fukuda, J.; Mikami, T.; Sugahara, K.; Fawcett, J.W. Composition of perineuronal net extracellular matrix in rat brain: A different disaccharide composition for the net-associated proteoglycans. *J. Biol. Chem.* **2006**, *281*, 17789–17800. [CrossRef] [PubMed]
19. Carulli, D.; Rhodes, K.E.; Brown, D.J.; Bonnert, T.P.; Pollack, S.J.; Oliver, K.; Strata, P.; Fawcett, J.W. Composition of perineuronal nets in the adult rat cerebellum and the cellular origin of their components. *J. Comp. Neurol.* **2006**, *494*, 559–577. [CrossRef] [PubMed]
20. Fader, S.M.; Imaizumi, K.; Yanagawa, Y.; Lee, C.C. Wisteria Floribunda Agglutinin-Labeled Perineuronal Nets in the Mouse Inferior Colliculus, Thalamic Reticular Nucleus and Auditory Cortex. *Brain Sci.* **2016**, *6*, 13. [CrossRef] [PubMed]
21. Yamada, J.; Jinno, S. Molecular heterogeneity of aggrecan-based perineuronal nets around five subclasses of parvalbumin-expressing neurons in the mouse hippocampus. *J. Comp. Neurol.* **2017**, *525*, 1234–1249. [CrossRef] [PubMed]
22. Vitellaro-Zuccarello, L.; Bosisio, P.; Mazzetti, S.; Monti, C.; De Biasi, S. Differential expression of several molecules of the extracellular matrix in functionally and developmentally distinct regions of rat spinal cord. *Cell Tissue Res.* **2007**, *327*, 433–447. [CrossRef] [PubMed]
23. Brauer, K.; Härtig, W.; Bigl, V.; Brückner, G. Distribution of parvalbumin-containing neurons and lectin-binding perineuronal nets in the rat basal forebrain. *Brain Res.* **1993**, *631*, 167–170. [CrossRef]
24. Yamada, J.; Ohgomori, T.; Jinno, S. Perineuronal nets affect parvalbumin expression in GABAergic neurons of the mouse hippocampus. *Eur. J. Neurosci.* **2015**, *41*, 368–378. [CrossRef] [PubMed]
25. Galtrey, C.M.; Kwok, J.C.; Carulli, D.; Rhodes, K.E.; Fawcett, J.W. Distribution and synthesis of extracellular matrix proteoglycans, hyaluronan, link proteins and tenascin-R in the rat spinal cord. *Eur. J. Neurosci.* **2008**, *27*, 1373–1390. [CrossRef] [PubMed]
26. Bertolotto, A.; Manzardo, E.; Guglielmone, R. Immunohistochemical mapping of perineuronal nets containing chondroitin unsulfate proteoglycan in the rat central nervous system. *Cell Tissue Res.* **1996**, *283*, 283–295. [CrossRef] [PubMed]
27. Takahashi-Iwanaga, H.; Murakami, T.; Abe, K. Three-dimensional microanatomy of perineuronal proteoglycan nets enveloping motor neurons in the rat spinal cord. *J. Neurocytol.* **1998**, *27*, 817–827. [CrossRef] [PubMed]
28. Manuel, M.; Zytnicki, D. Alpha, beta and gamma motoneurons: Functional diversity in the motor system's final pathway. *J. Integr. Neurosci.* **2011**, *10*, 243–276. [CrossRef] [PubMed]
29. Zhao, R.-R.R.; Andrews, M.R.; Wang, D.; Warren, P.; Gullo, M.; Schnell, L.; Schwab, M.E.; Fawcett, J.W. Combination treatment with anti-Nogo-A and chondroitinase ABC is more effective than single treatments at enhancing functional recovery after spinal cord injury. *Eur. J. Neurosci.* **2013**, *38*, 2946–2961. [CrossRef] [PubMed]
30. Barritt, A.W.; Davies, M.; Marchand, F.; Hartley, R.; Grist, J.; Yip, P.; McMahon, S.B.; Bradbury, E.J. Chondroitinase ABC Promotes Sprouting of Intact and Injured Spinal Systems after Spinal Cord Injury. *J. Neurosci.* **2006**, *26*, 10856–10867. [CrossRef] [PubMed]

31. Smith, C.C.; Mauricio, R.; Nobre, L.; Marsh, B.; Wüst, R.C.; Rossiter, H.B.; Ichiyama, R.M. Differential regulation of perineuronal nets in the brain and spinal cord with exercise training. *Brain Res. Bull.* **2015**, *111*, 20–26. [CrossRef] [PubMed]
32. Wang, D.; Ichiyama, R.M.; Zhao, R.; Andrews, M.R.; Fawcett, J.W. Chondroitinase combined with rehabilitation promotes recovery of forelimb function in rats with chronic spinal cord injury. *J. Neurosci.* **2011**, *31*, 9332–9344. [CrossRef] [PubMed]
33. Barber, R.P.; Phelps, P.E.; Houser, C.R.; Crawford, G.D.; Salvaterra, P.M.; Vaughn, J.E. The morphology and distribution of neurons containing choline acetyltransferase in the adult rat spinal cord: An immunocytochemical study. *J. Comp. Neurol.* **1984**, *229*, 329–346. [CrossRef] [PubMed]
34. Koppe, G.; Bruckner, G.; Hartig, W.; Delpech, B.; Bigl, V. Characterization of proteoglycan-containing perineuronal nets by enzymatic treatments of rat brain sections. *Histochem. J.* **1997**, *29*, 11–20. [CrossRef] [PubMed]
35. Morawski, M.; Brückner, G.; Arendt, T.; Matthews, R.T. Aggrecan: Beyond cartilage and into the brain. *Int. J. Biochem. Cell Biol.* **2012**, *44*, 690–693. [CrossRef] [PubMed]
36. Lendvai, D.; Morawski, M.; Négyessy, L.; Gáti, G.; Jäger, C.; Baksa, G.; Glasz, T.; Attems, J.; Tanila, H.; Arendt, T.; et al. Neurochemical mapping of the human hippocampus reveals perisynaptic matrix around functional synapses in Alzheimer's disease. *Acta Neuropathol.* **2013**, *125*, 215–229. [CrossRef] [PubMed]
37. Favuzzi, E.; Marques-Smith, A.; Deogracias, R.; Winterflood, C.M.; Sánchez-Aguilera, A.; Mantoan, L.; Maeso, P.; Fernandes, C.; Ewers, H.; Rico, B. Activity-Dependent Gating of Parvalbumin Interneuron Function by the Perineuronal Net Protein Brevican. *Neuron* **2017**, *95*. [CrossRef] [PubMed]
38. Asher, R.A.; Morgenstern, D.A.; Fidler, P.S.; Adcock, K.H.; Oohira, A.; Braistead, J.E.; Levine, J.M.; Margolis, R.U.; Rogers, J.H.; Fawcett, J.W. Neurocan is upregulated in injured brain and in cytokine-treated astrocytes. *J. Neurosci.* **2000**, *20*, 2427–2438. [CrossRef] [PubMed]
39. Dours-Zimmermann, M.T.; Maurer, K.; Rauch, U.; Stoffel, W.; Fässler, R.; Zimmermann, D.R. Versican V2 Assembles the Extracellular Matrix Surrounding the Nodes of Ranvier in the CNS. *J. Neurosci.* **2009**, *29*, 7731–7742. [CrossRef] [PubMed]
40. Asher, R.A.; Morgenstern, D.A.; Shearer, M.C.; Adcock, K.H.; Pesheva, P.; Fawcett, J.W. Versican is upregulated in CNS injury and is a product of oligodendrocyte lineage cells. *J. Neurosci.* **2002**, *22*, 2225–2236. [PubMed]
41. Maurel, P.; Rauch, U.; Flad, M.; Margolis, R.K.; Margolis, R.U. Phosphacan, a chondroitin sulfate proteoglycan of brain that interacts with neurons and neural cell-adhesion molecules, is an extracellular variant of a receptor-type protein tyrosine phosphatase. *Proc. Natl. Acad. Sci. USA* **1994**, *91*, 2512–2516. [CrossRef] [PubMed]
42. Dwyer, C.A.; Katoh, T.; Tiemeyer, M.; Matthews, R.T. Neurons and Glia Modify Receptor Protein-tyrosine Phosphatase ζ (RPTPζ)/Phosphacan with Cell-specific O-Mannosyl Glycans in the Developing Brain. *J. Biol. Chem.* **2015**, *290*, 10256–10273. [CrossRef] [PubMed]
43. Haunsø, A.; Celio, M.R.; Margolis, R.K.; Menoud, P.-A. Phosphacan immunoreactivity is associated with perineuronal nets around parvalbumin-expressing neurones. *Brain Res.* **1999**, *834*, 219–222. [CrossRef]
44. Friese, A.; Kaltschmidt, J.A.; Ladle, D.R.; Sigrist, M.; Jessell, T.M.; Arber, S. Gamma and alpha motor neurons distinguished by expression of transcription factor Err3. *Proc. Natl. Acad. Sci. USA* **2009**, *106*, 13588–13593. [CrossRef] [PubMed]
45. Mueller, A.L.; Davis, A.; Sovich, S.; Carlson, S.S.; Robinson, F.R. Distribution of *N*-Acetylgalactosamine-Positive Perineuronal Nets in the Macaque Brain: Anatomy and Implications. *Neural Plast.* **2016**, *2016*. [CrossRef] [PubMed]
46. Jäger, C.; Lendvai, D.; Seeger, G.; Brückner, G.; Matthews, R.T.; Arendt, T.; Alpár, A.; Morawski, M. Perineuronal and perisynaptic extracellular matrix in the human spinal cord. *Neuroscience* **2013**, *238*, 168–184. [CrossRef] [PubMed]
47. Shneider, N.A.; Brown, M.N.; Smith, C.A.; Pickel, J.; Alvarez, F.J. Gamma motor neurons express distinct genetic markers at birth and require muscle spindle-derived GDNF for postnatal survival. *Neural Dev.* **2009**, *4*, 42. [CrossRef] [PubMed]
48. Eccles, J.C.; Eccles, R.M.; Iggo, A.; Lundberg, A. Electrophysiological studies on gamma motoneurones. *Acta Physiol. Scand.* **1960**, *50*, 32–40. [CrossRef] [PubMed]

49. Misawa, H.; Hara, M.; Tanabe, S.; Niikura, M.; Moriwaki, Y.; Okuda, T. Osteopontin is an alpha motor neuron marker in the mouse spinal cord. *J. Neurosci. Res.* **2012**, *90*, 732–742. [CrossRef] [PubMed]
50. Härtig, W.; Brauer, K.; Brückner, G. Wisteria floribunda agglutinin-labelled nets surround parvalbumin-containing neurons. *Neuroreport* **1992**, *3*, 869–872. [CrossRef] [PubMed]
51. Kalb, R.G.; Hockfield, S. Molecular evidence for early activity-dependent development of hamster motor neurons. *J. Neurosci.* **1988**, *8*, 2350–2360. [CrossRef] [PubMed]
52. Matthews, R.T.; Kelly, G.M.; Zerillo, C.A.; Gray, G.; Tiemeyer, M.; Hockfield, S. Aggrecan glycoforms contribute to the molecular heterogeneity of perineuronal nets. *J. Neurosci.* **2002**, *22*, 7536–7547. [PubMed]
53. Bignami, A.; Perides, G.; Rahemtulla, F. Versican, a hyaluronate-binding proteoglycan of embryonal precartilaginous mesenchyma, is mainly expressed postnatally in rat brain. *J. Neurosci. Res.* **1993**, *34*, 97–106. [CrossRef] [PubMed]
54. Ueno, H.; Suemitsu, S.; Okamoto, M.; Matsumoto, Y.; Ishihara, T. Sensory experience-dependent formation of perineuronal nets and expression of Cat-315 immunoreactive components in the mouse somatosensory cortex. *Neuroscience* **2017**, *355*, 161–174. [CrossRef] [PubMed]
55. Dauth, S.; Grevesse, T.; Pantazopoulos, H.; Campbell, P.H.; Maoz, B.M.; Berretta, S.; Parker, K.K. Extracellular matrix protein expression is brain region dependent. *J. Comp. Neurol.* **2016**, *524*, 1309–1336. [CrossRef] [PubMed]
56. Gage, G.J.; Kipke, D.R.; Shain, W. Whole animal perfusion fixation for rodents. *J. Vis. Exp.* **2012**. [CrossRef] [PubMed]
57. Phelps, P.E.; Barber, R.P.; Houser, C.R.; Crawford, G.D.; Salvaterra, P.M.; Vaughn, J.E. Postnatal development of neurons containing choline acetyltransferase in rat spinal cord: An immunocytochemical study. *J. Comp. Neurol.* **1984**, *229*, 347–361. [CrossRef] [PubMed]
58. Schindelin, J.; Arganda-Carreras, I.; Frise, E.; Kaynig, V.; Longair, M.; Pietzsch, T.; Preibisch, S.; Rueden, C.; Saalfeld, S.; Schmid, B.; et al. Fiji: An open-source platform for biological-image analysis. *Nat. Meth.* **2012**, *9*, 676–682. [CrossRef] [PubMed]
59. Mullen, R.J.; Buck, C.R.; Smith, A.M. NeuN, a neuronal specific nuclear protein in vertebrates. *Development* **1992**, *116*, 201–211. [PubMed]

10

A Single Dose of Atorvastatin Applied Acutely after Spinal Cord Injury Suppresses Inflammation, Apoptosis and Promotes Axon Outgrowth, Which Might be Essential for Favorable Functional Outcome

Katarina Bimbova [1], Maria Bacova [1], Alexandra Kisucka [1], Jaroslav Pavel [1], Jan Galik [1], Peter Zavacky [2], Martin Marsala [1,3], Andrea Stropkovska [1], Jana Fedorova [1], Stefania Papcunova [1], Jana Jachova [1] and Nadezda Lukacova [1,*]

1 Institute of Neurobiology of Biomedical Research Centre of Slovak Academy of Sciences, Soltesovej 4,6, 040 01 Kosice, Slovakia; bimbova@saske.sk (K.B.); bacova@saske.sk (M.B.); kisucka@saske.sk (A.K.); pavel@saske.sk (J.P.); galik@saske.sk (J.G.); mmarsala@ucsd.edu (M.M.); stropkovska@saske.sk (A.S.); jfedorova@saske.sk (J.F.); gedrova@saske.sk (S.P.); jachova@saske.sk (J.J.)

2 1st Department of Surgery, Louis Pasteur University Hospital, Faculty of Medicine University of Pavol Jozef Safarik, Trieda SNP 1, 041 66 Kosice, Slovakia; peterzavacky963@gmail.com

3 Neuroregeneration Laboratory, Department of Anesthesiology, University of California, 9500 Gilman Drive, San Diego, CA 92092-0100, USA

* Correspondence: lukacova@saske.sk

Abstract: The aim of our study was to limit the inflammatory response after a spinal cord injury (SCI) using Atorvastatin (ATR), a potent inhibitor of cholesterol biosynthesis. Adult Wistar rats were divided into five experimental groups: one control group, two Th9 compression (40 g/15 min) groups, and two Th9 compression + ATR (5 mg/kg, i.p.) groups. The animals survived one day and six weeks. ATR applied in a single dose immediately post-SCI strongly reduced IL-1β release at 4 and 24 h and considerably reduced the activation of resident cells at one day post-injury. Acute ATR treatment effectively prevented the excessive infiltration of destructive M1 macrophages cranially, at the lesion site, and caudally (by 66%, 62%, and 52%, respectively) one day post-injury, whereas the infiltration of beneficial M2 macrophages was less affected (by 27%, 41%, and 16%). In addition, at the same time point, ATR visibly decreased caspase-3 cleavage in neurons, astrocytes, and oligodendrocytes. Six weeks post-SCI, ATR increased the expression of neurofilaments in the dorsolateral columns and Gap43-positive fibers in the lateral columns around the epicenter, and from day 30 to 42, significantly improved the motor activity of the hindlimbs. We suggest that early modulation of the inflammatory response via effects on the M1/M2 macrophages and the inhibition of caspase-3 expression could be crucial for the functional outcome.

Keywords: spinal cord compression; inflammatory response; Atorvastatin; caspase-3; macrophages; Gap43; neurofilaments; gene expression

1. Introduction

Spinal cord injury (SCI) is one of the most devastating and complex clinical conditions, often leading to irreversible neurological deficits. The complex pathophysiology of a SCI, consisting of primary and secondary mechanisms, may explain the difficulty of finding a suitable therapy [1]. SCI is caused by two distinct events, which follow a somewhat overlapping temporal sequence: the acute (seconds to minutes after the injury) phase, the secondary (minutes to weeks after the injury) phase, and the chronic (months to years after the injury) phase [2,3]. In the acute phase, due to the direct mechanical insult, the spinal tissue undergoes a cascade of events followed by secondary damage affecting intact, neighboring tissue [4]. Inflammatory response is one of the key mechanisms of secondary injury (sub-acute phase). It includes the activation of resident cells (microglia, astrocytes), the recruitment of immune cells (macrophages and neutrophils) from the bloodstream to the site of the injury, and evident up-regulation of the NADPH oxidase (NOX) enzyme. The resident and immune cells release proinflammatory cytokines, including interleukins (IL-1β, IL-6) and tumor necrosis factor-α (TNF-α), all of which increase the extent of the inflammatory response. These events play an important role in secondary tissue damage and cell death [2,3,5,6]. During this period, the astrocytes begin to migrate out of the epicenter, producing molecules, such as proteoglycans and laminin, in the extracellular space. In the chronic phase of injury, there is continued necrosis, and demyelination in the white matter due to apoptotic oligodendrocytic death. Reactive astrocytes continue to invade the region surrounding the lesion center, leading to the formation of a cystic cavity surrounded by glial scar, which has been hypothesized to be a physical and biochemical barrier to axonal regeneration [7,8].

Research over the last few years has revealed numerous therapeutic approaches contributing to the modulation of the inflammation response and the reduction of the negative symptoms of a SCI [9–12]. Statins, the 3-hydroxyl-3-methylglutaryl-coenzyme A reductase inhibitors, are currently used for treatment of high cholesterol, coronary artherosclerosis, and atherosclerosis [13–15]. Atorvastatin (ATR), a drug with anti-inflammatory and immunomodulatory effects, has been widely studied in various ischemia-reperfusion and traumatic SCI models. When applied for several days before/after a SCI, it has been found to be neuroprotective [16–19]. It significantly reduced the release of pro-inflammatory cytokines and inhibited macrophage infiltration and microglial activation. In addition, this drug inhibited apoptosis and demyelination after traumatic injury and promoted the recovery of neurological functions [16,17].

Although pre- or post-long-lasting treatments with ATR have been shown to be effective in limiting pathology due to a traumatic SCI [17,18], the present study focused on treating animals in the very critical first moments after injury and on finding out whether an acute single dose of this clinically relevant drug would effectively minimize the negative impact of an acute, traumatic SCI. We found that ATR (5 mg/kg, i.p.) applied immediately after a Th9 compression favorably reduced the course of acute inflammation by decreasing the release of interleukin 1β 4 h and 1 d after a SCI. This statin significantly reduced macrophage infiltration, resident cell activation, and caspase-3 expression one day post-SCI and promoted axon outgrowth in the whole cranio-caudal extent after six weeks of survival. The mitigation of the strong inflammatory response soon after a SCI promoted regeneration at the lesion site and cranially and caudally from the epicenter and significantly improved the neurological outcome from day 30 to 42. These results strongly support the use of ATR as one of the first-line therapeutic drugs to treat an acute, traumatic SCI.

2. Results

2.1. Short-Term Survival (24 h)

2.1.1. Releasing of Pro-Inflammatory Cytokine IL-1β after Spinal Cord Trauma and the Atorvastatin Treatment

The activation of the inflammatory response after a spinal cord injury leads to the release of pro- and anti-inflammatory cytokines into the bloodstream [20]. We examined the effect of a single dose of ATR (5 mg/kg; i.p.) on the level of pro-inflammatory cytokine IL-1β in the blood serum at 4 and 24 h after a SCI. Figure 1 shows strong, up to 12-fold increase in the level of IL-1β (490.3 $\pm$ 82 pg/mL) at the acute (4 h) time point and rapid decrease in the cytokine level (84.8 $\pm$ 11.6 pg/mL) 24 h after the SCI. The concentration of IL-1β remained 2.9-fold higher after the SCI than the in naive spinal cord (29.3 $\pm$ 1.2 pg/mL). A single dose of Atorvastatin injected immediately after a Th9 compression decreased the release of IL-1β to 42.8 $\pm$ 7.3 pg/mL after 4 h. A similar level of IL-1β was maintained 24 h after the SCI and the ATR treatment (46.3 $\pm$ 4.6 pg/mL).

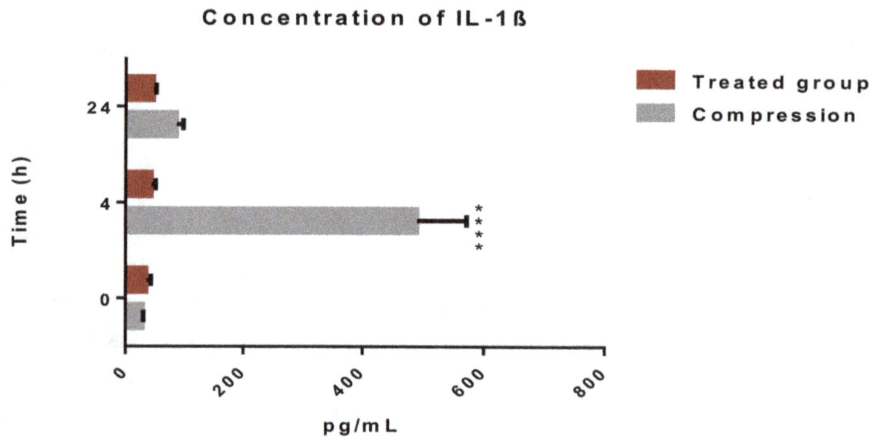

Figure 1. Concentration of pro-inflammatory cytokine IL-1β in the blood serum after a traumatic SCI and the ATR treatment. A significant elevation of IL-1β was noted 4 h after the SCI. ATR applied in a single dose (5 mg/kg; i.p.) immediately after the SCI reduced the release of IL-1β after 4 and 24 h. Data are the mean values of eight experiments ±SD. The results were statistically evaluated using two-way analysis of variance (ANOVA) and post hoc Tukey's HSD test; **** $p < 0.0001$. ATR—Atorvastatin; IL-1β—interleukin 1β; SCI—spinal cord injury.

2.1.2. Macrophage Response after a Spinal Cord Compression and the ATR Treatment

The ED-1 antibody, recognizing an intracellular antigen in activated macrophages, was used for identification of macrophages (ED-1) in immunostained cross-sections at the lesion site (Figure 2). No infiltrated ED-1 positive cells were detected in the intact spinal cord tissue; however, one day after the SCI, the macrophage infiltration was obvious (Figure 2B). Quantitative analysis revealed a higher number of ED-1 positive cells in the white matter (293 ± 22.9) than in the grey matter (257 ± 20.4). ATR significantly reduced the number of infiltrated macrophages in both the white (145 ± 40) and grey (109 ± 33) matter (Figure 2C,D).

Macrophages exhibit functional adaptability and can change phenotypes in response to stimuli [21]. One day after the SCI, both CD86 mRNA (M1 phenotype) and CD163 mRNA (M2 phenotype) were expressed at the lesion site and 1 cm cranially and caudally (Figure 2E,F). ATR significantly inhibited both the M1 and M2 phenotypes, but the decrease was more pronounced in the M1 phenotype, known to initiate a cascade of neurotoxic responses. Quantitative RT-PCR showed a significant decrease in CD86 mRNA expression at the lesion site ($p < 0.05$) and cranially from the site of the injury ($p < 0.01$) and significantly suppressed the expression of CD163 mRNA (anti-inflammatory M2 phenotype) cranially ($p < 0.05$) and at the injury site ($p < 0.01$) (Figure 2F).

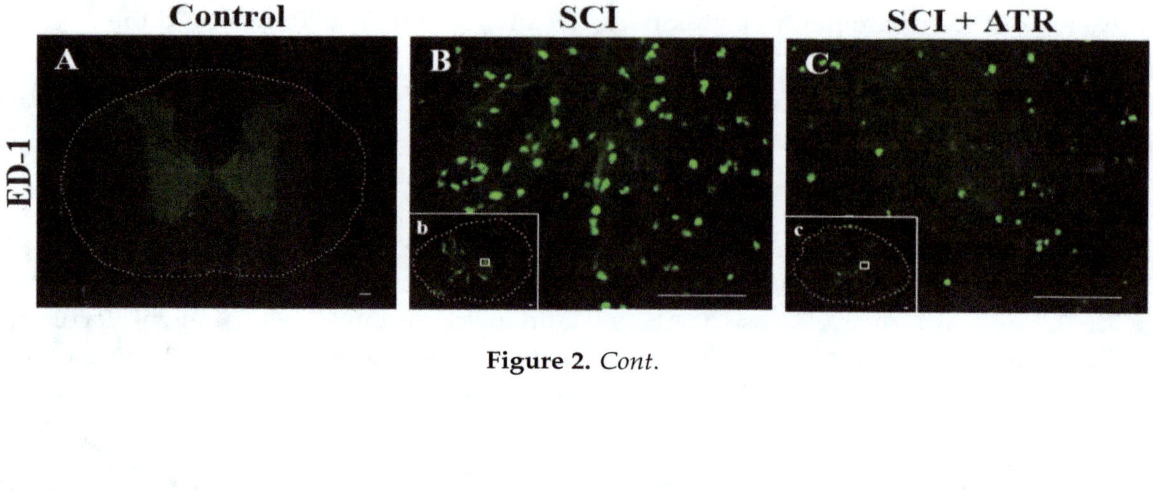

Figure 2. *Cont.*

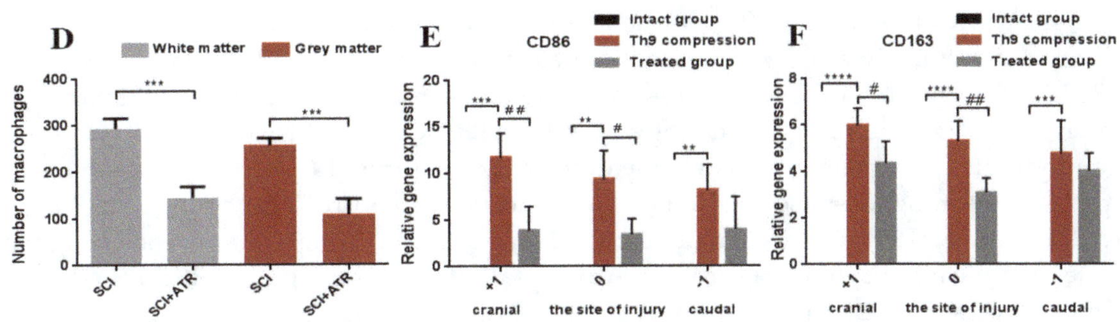

Figure 2. Infiltration of the macrophages in the spinal cord 24 h after a traumatic injury and the treatment with ATR (5 mg/kg; i.p.). Figures from immunohistochemical analysis show no appearance of the macrophages in the intact spinal tissue (**A**), marked macrophage infiltration at the lesion site (**B**) and a strong decrease in macrophage influx after the ATR treatment (**C**). ATR significantly reduced the number of infiltrated macrophages in the grey and white matter (**D**). CD86 mRNA (M1 macrophages) and CD163 mRNA (M2 macrophages) were confirmed by RT-PCR in the whole cranio-caudal extent of the spinal cord (**E**,**F**). Scale bars: (**A**,**b**,**c**—1000 µm; **B**,**C**—100 µm). Data are the mean values of nine experiments (4 IHC, 5 RT-PCR) ± SD. The results from the cell counting were statistically evaluated using a parametric *T*-Test and the results from the RT-PCR were evaluated with one-way ANOVA; # $p < 0.05$; ** $p < 0.01$; ## $p < 0.01$; *** $p < 0.001$; **** $p < 0.0001$. Atorvastatin—ATR; ED-1—macrophages; IHC—immunohistochemistry; SCI—spinal cord injury.

2.1.3. Changes in Glial Activation and Caspase-3 Activity

The GFAP antibody revealed a small stellate perikaryon of astrocytes, which had a few thin branched processes. Such morphology of GFAP-immunoreactive astrocytes was seen in the naive spinal cord (Figure 3A) and the in spinal tissue one day after the SCI. However, the activity of the astrocytes was more profound in the damaged regions within the impact area (Figure 3B). At the same time, the Iba-1 production, a marker for microglia, was strongly elevated (Figure 3E) at the site of the injury. The microglial cells were hypertrophied and massively distributed in the dorsal horn. Treatment with ATR (5 mg/kg; i.p.) decreased the extensive microglial activation (Figure 3F) and moderated the formation of reactive astrocytes at the lesion site (Figure 3C).

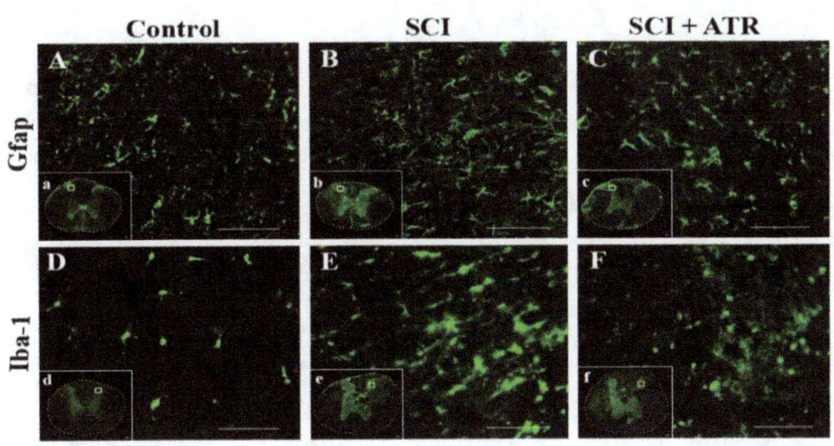

Figure 3. Representative images showing the activation of astrocytes and the microglia in the spinal cord after the Th9 compression and the atorvastatin treatment. Immunostaining of the astrocytes and microglial cells at the Th9 level of intact animals (**A**,**D**). Increased expression of the astrocytes (**B**) and the microglia (**E**) 24 h after the injury at the lesion site. The administration of ATR (5 mg/kg; i.p., immediately after the SCI) reduced the density of the activated astrocytes (**C**) and decreased the massive activation of the microglial cells (**F**). Scale bars: (**A**–**F**—100 µm; **a**–**f**—1000 µm). Atorvastatin—ATR; GFAP—astrocytes; Iba-1—microglia; SCI—spinal cord injury.

Figure 4A shows the course of astrogliosis in a 3 cm cranio-caudal extent 24 h after the SCI. The GFAP gene expression was overexpressed in the cranial ($p < 0.001$) and caudal ($p < 0.01$) segments after the SCI, but at the site of the injury this astrocyte marker was not significantly increased. GFAP mRNA expression was not markedly changed by the ATR treatment. However, compared with the controls, a moderate improvement was visible in the caudal segment (−1).

Caspases, including caspase-3, directly and indirectly control the changes in cells during apoptosis [22]. Strong mRNA expression of caspase-3 was confirmed one day after the Th9 compression in the whole cranio-caudal extent (Figure 4B). Atorvastatin (5 mg/kg; i.p.) significantly decreased the expression of caspase-3 mRNA in the cranial ($p < 0.0001$) and caudal ($p < 0.01$) segments. The results from the double immunostaining showed strong cleavage of caspase-3 in the oligodendrocytes, astrocytes, and neurons all around the lesion site 24 h after the Th9 compression (Figure 5). A marked reduction in apoptotic activity was noted after the ATR treatment in the oligodendrocytes and astrocytes in the dorsal and dorsolateral funiculi. Immunolabeled NeuN positive cells demonstrated a massive decrease in caspase-3 activity especially in the dorsal horns but also around the central canal. However, no cleavage of caspase-3 was observed in the microglial cells either after the SCI or after the ATR treatment at this time point.

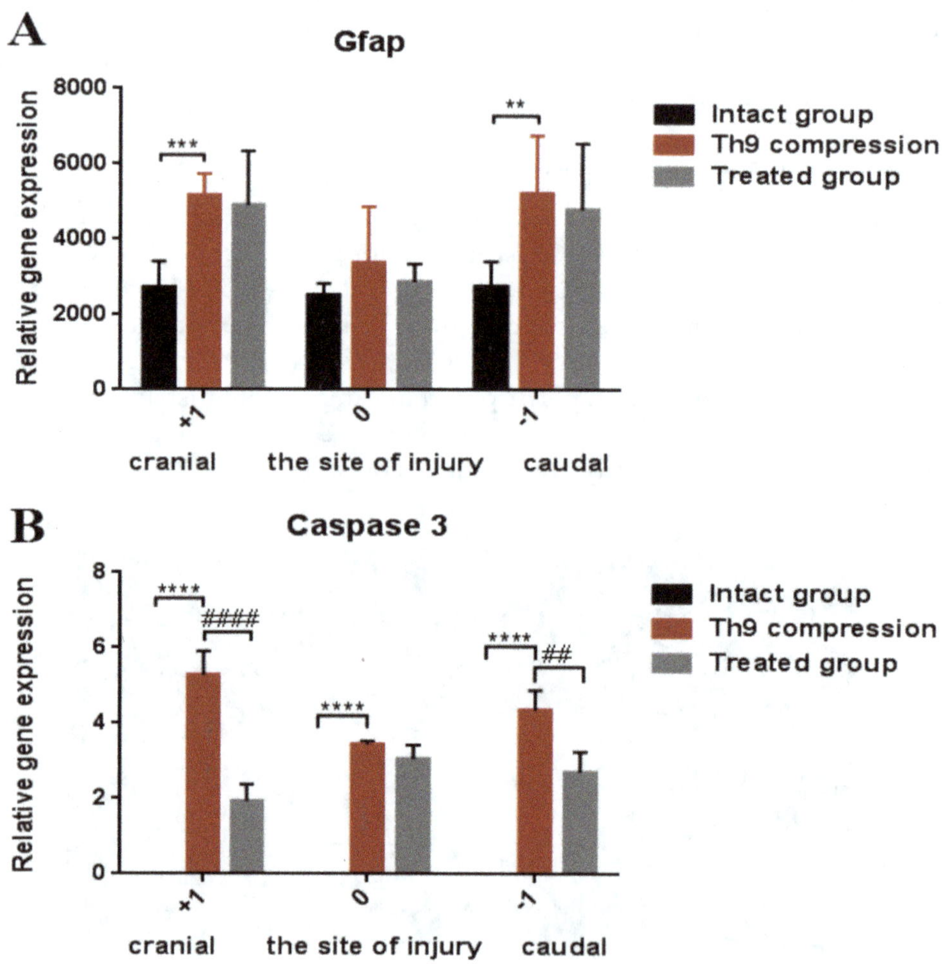

Figure 4. Gene expression showing astrogliosis (GFAP) and apoptosis (caspase-3) in the spinal cord 24 h after the Th9 compression and the atorvastatin (5 mg/kg; i.p.) treatment. The graphs show the relative quantities of GFAP (**A**) and caspase-3 (**B**) in rostro-caudal manner in the controls and 24 h after the SCI and SCI + ATR treatment. Data are the mean values of five experiments ±SD. The results were statistically evaluated using one-way ANOVA; ** $p < 0.01$; ## $p < 0.01$; *** $p < 0.001$; **** $p < 0.0001$; #### $p < 0.0001$. Atorvastatin—ATR; GFAP—astrocytes; SCI—spinal cord injury.

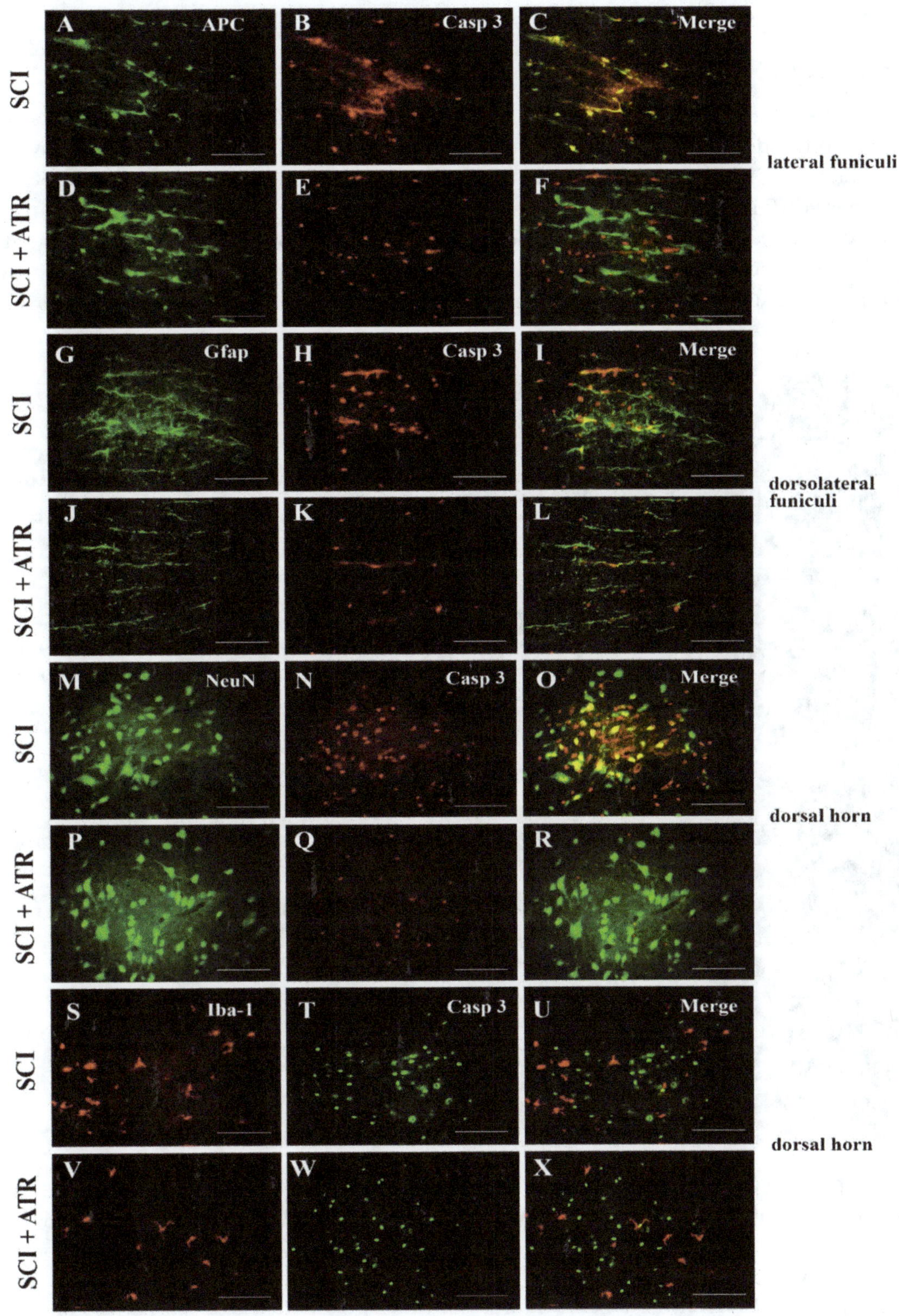

Figure 5. Set of microphotographs showing the immunofluorescent staining and co-localization of caspase-3 (red in B,E,H,K,N,Q; green in T,W) with APC (green), GFAP (green), NeuN (green), and Iba-1 (red) one day after the SCI and the ATR treatment. Double immunostaining demonstrates the cleavage of caspase-3 in the oligodendrocytes (**A**–**F**); astrocytes (**G**–**L**); neurons (**M**–**R**); and microglial cells (**S**–**X**) 0.5 cm caudally from the lesion site in the SCI and SCI + ATR groups. Scale bars: (**A**–**X**—100 μm). APC—adenomatous polyposis coli positive mature oligodendrocytes; ATR—Atorvastatin; Casp 3—caspase-3; GFAP—astrocytes, Iba-1—microglia; NeuN—neurons; SCI—spinal cord injury.

2.2. Long-Term Survival (Six Weeks)

2.2.1. Regenerative Capacity of the Spinal Cord

Six weeks after the SCI, numerous Iba-1 positive cells with rounded morphology were identified predominantly in the dorsal part of the spinal cord (Figure 6B). No obvious difference was observed visually between the SCI and ATR-treated SCI rats at six weeks in the dorsal horn (Figure 6C). As shown in Figure 6F, the GFAP immunoreactivity was markedly reduced in the ATR-treated group. Although ATR effectively reduced astrogliosis in the most affected dorsal horn of the caudal segment, the gene expression of GFAP showed no significant difference between the SCI and SCI + ATR groups in the cranial, injured, and caudal segments, each taken as a whole (Figure 7A).

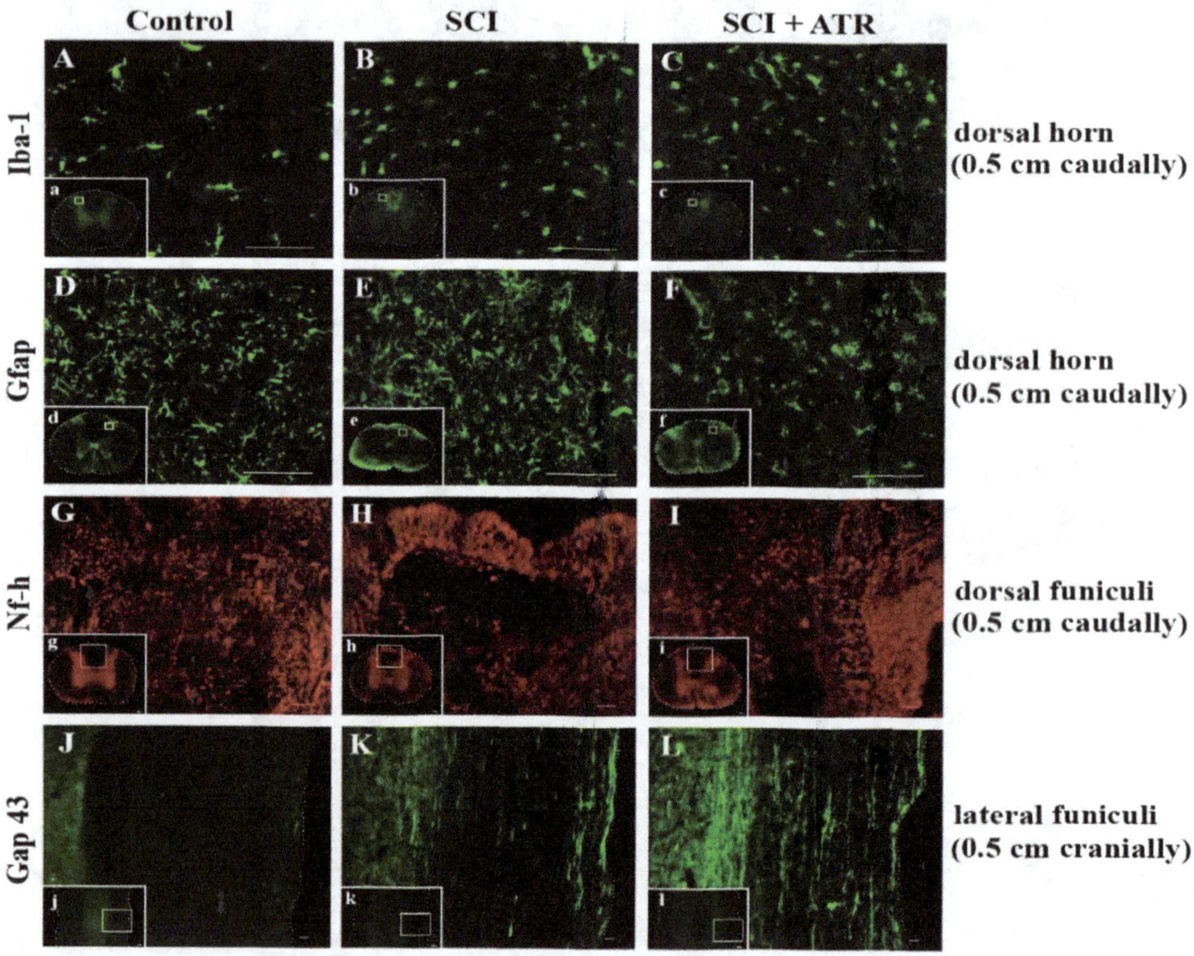

Figure 6. Effect of Atorvastatin on the glial cell activation and the regenerative capacity in the spinal cord six weeks after the SCI and the ATR treatment (5 mg/kg; i.p.). The microphotographs show visible changes in the activation of the microglia (green) (**A–C**) and astrocytes (green) (**D–F**) in the dorsal horn (0.5 cm caudally from the site of the injury) after the SCI and SCI + ATR. The regenerative capacity of Nf-h (red) is clearly visible in the dorsal funiculi caudally from the lesion site (**G–I**). Longitudinal spinal cord sections taken from the cranial segments show spontaneous axonal outgrowing (Gap43; green) after the SCI (**K**). More pronounced Gap43 immunoreactivity was visible in the ATR-treated group (**L**). Scale bars: (**A–F**—100 μm; **G–I**—200 μm; **J–L**—500 μm; **a–l**—1000 μm). ATR—Atorvastatin; Gap 43—outgrowing axons; GFAP—astrocytes; Iba-1—microglia; Nf-h—neurofilaments (heavy); SCI—spinal cord injury.

Nf-h immunoreactive axons were regularly distributed throughout the control spinal cord (Figure 6G). At six weeks, the Th9 compression resulted in massive damage to the white matter in the dorsal and lateral columns, with their partial obliteration by a cavity (Figure 6H). The ATR treatment increased the expression of neurofilaments in the dorsolateral part of the spinal cord (Figure 6I). However, compared with the SCI group, the Nf-h mRNA measured in the segments (cranial, injured, and caudal) in toto was not increased in the ATR-treated group (Figure 7C). Similar results were observed in the gene expression of Olig2 (Figure 7D).

Axonal sprouting and outgrowing in the damaged spinal cord is one of the key factors for tissue regeneration and motor function restoration. As shown in Figure 6K, spontaneous axonal overgrowing was very low six weeks post-SCI. Immufluorescence analysis of the longitudinal spinal cord sections revealed that the single dose of ATR (5 mg/kg, i.p.) strongly promoted the axons' outgrowth (Figure 6L). This effect was visible in the whole cranio-caudal extent. The results from the RT-PCR are shown in Figure 7B. The relative gene expression of Gap43 correlated with Gap 43 immunoreactivity. The ATR-treated group confirmed a significant improvement at the site of the injury ($p < 0.01$) and in the cranial segment ($p < 0.05$).

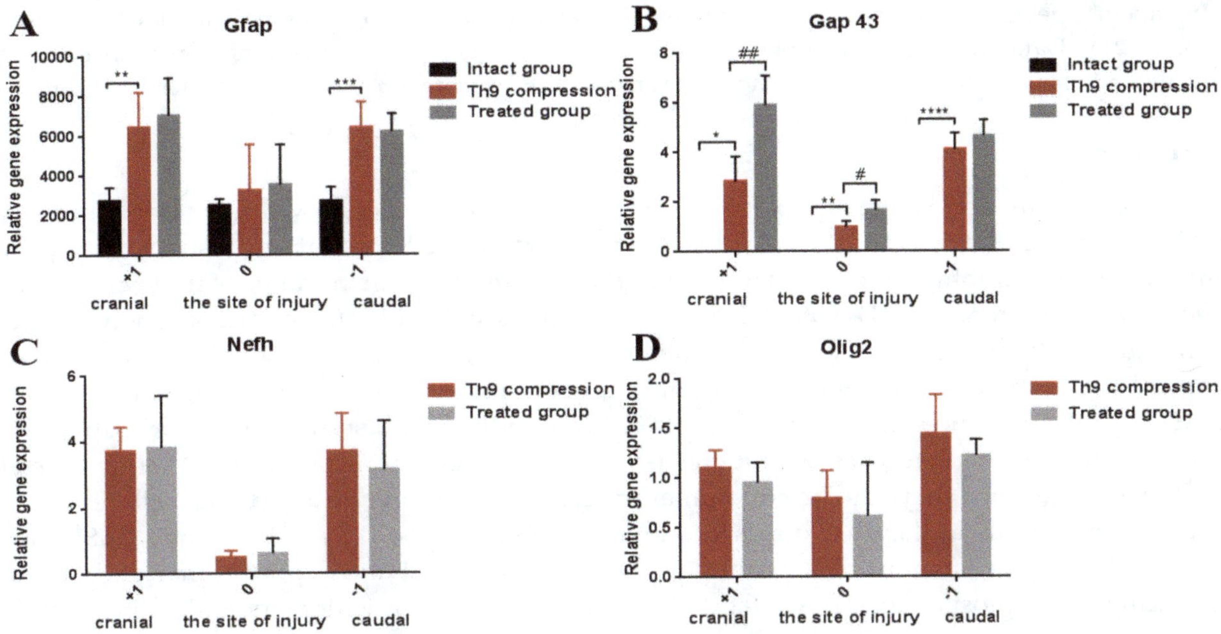

Figure 7. Graphs demonstrating the relative gene expression of GFAP, Gap 43, Nf-h, and Olig 2 in the spinal cord (site of the injury, cranially, and caudally) six weeks after the traumatic spinal cord injury and the ATR treatment. The lowest gene expression was observed at the lesion site. GFAP activation shows the changes in astrogliosis after the SCI and SCI + ATR (**A**). Markers of regenerative capacity (Gap 43, Nf-h, and Olig2) show a significant improvement in axonal outgrowing at the lesion site and in the cranial (+1) segment (**B**–**D**). The data are the mean values of five experiments ±SD. The results were statistically evaluated using a parametric *T*-test and one-way ANOVA; * $p < 0.05$; # $p < 0.05$; ** $p < 0.01$; ## $p < 0.01$; *** $p < 0.001$; **** $p < 0.0001$. Atorvastatin—ATR; Gap 43—outgrowing axons; GFAP—astrocytes; Nf-h—neurofilaments (heavy); Olig2—oligodendrocytes; SCI—spinal cord injury.

2.2.2. Neurological Outcome

Functional outcome was evaluated using the Basso–Beattie–Bresnahan (BBB) locomotor rating score representing the recovery stages for rat hindlimb motor function. One day post-injury, all the animals suffered from complete paraplegia (0.25 ± 0.39) and their motor function improved spontaneously up to day 42 (six weeks) with a mean neurological score of 9.7 ± 0.93 (Figure 8). Up until day 24, the development of the neurological score did not differ between the SCI and ATR-treated groups. However, the outcome was significantly different from day 30 to 42. At the end of survival, the mean score for motor outcome reached 11.06 ± 0.91 in the ATR-treated group.

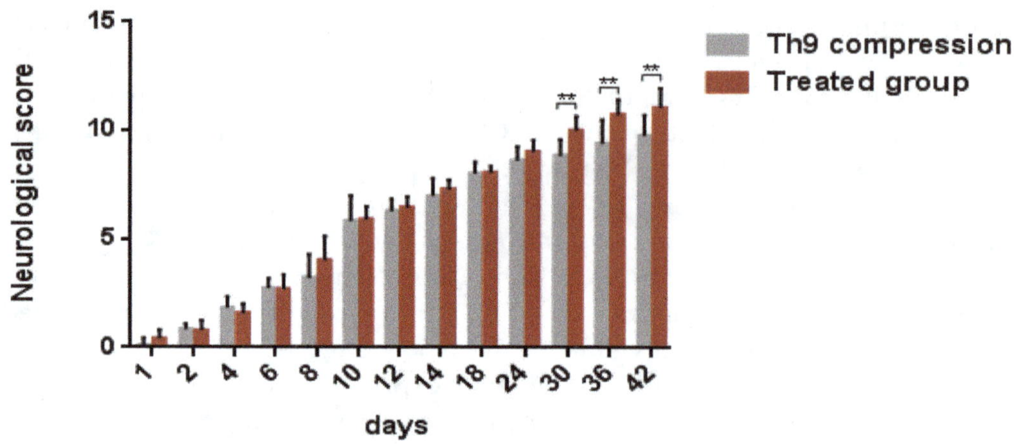

Figure 8. BBB scores showing the locomotor function of rats after the Th9 compression and the ATR treatment. The scoring points range from complete paraplegia (point zero) to normal hindlimb function (point 21). Data are the mean values of eighteen experiments ±SD. The results were statistically evaluated using a parametric *T*-test. Atorvastatin—ATR; BBB score—Basso-Beattie-Bresnahan score.

3. Discussion

Neuroinflammation is a complex immune response, which occurs within a short time period after SCI. It includes the activation and infiltration of numerous cell populations (astrocytes, microglia, T lymphocytes, neutrophils, and monocytes) and the release of a large number of non-cell mediators (interleukins, interferons, and TNFα) [23]. The first factors involved in the inflammatory response are pro- and anti- inflammatory cytokines and chemokines produced by endothelial cells and activated microglia [24]. In the CNS, the main pro-inflammatory cytokine is IL-1β, which is released just 2 h post-SCI [23,25]. In the present study, the levels of IL-1β in the blood serum were markedly (12-fold) elevated 4 h after the Th9 compression, but one day post-injury its concentration significantly decreased. Allan et al. [26] reported that this pro-inflammatory cytokine can directly affect glial cells, endothelial cells, and even neurons, as they all express interleukin 1 receptor type 1 (IL-1R1). In their rat SCI model, Nesic et al. [27] used infusions of IL1 antagonists 72 h after a SCI and reported markedly reduced injury-induced apoptosis, indicating that early expression of IL-1β is detrimental. It has also been shown that IL-1β promotes astrogliosis and triggers the astrocytic release of glutamate, nitric oxide, potassium, prostaglandins, cytokines, and chemokines [28], all of which were shown to be toxic to neurons at high concentrations [29–31]. The anti-inflammatory drug ATR applied in a single dose acutely after a Th9 compression significantly reduced the release of IL-1β.

Several studies have highlighted the therapeutic benefit of pre- and/or post-SCI application of ATR (long-lasting vs single and per-oral vs intraperitoneal). The present study produces new data showing the neuroprotective effect of a single dose of ATR applied immediately after a Th9 compression. First, ATR reduced the activation of the microglia within the most injured dorsolateral spinal cord and significantly reduced the infiltration of macrophages into the white and grey matter one day post-SCI. Papa et al. [9] showed that early microglial activation after spinal trauma is a key factor in the formation of a pathological environment, which supports injury progression. These authors demonstrated that early microglial inhibition induced a long-lasting recovery post-SCI (up to 63 days). As reported previously, microglia acquire pro-inflammatory phenotypes immediately after a SCI, which promote local inflammation and can lead to destructive (M1 phenotype) and beneficial (M2 phenotype) macrophage recruitment [9]. Based on their phenotype and activation status, macrophages may initiate the mechanisms of secondary injury or promote neuroregeneration of the spinal cord tissue [32]. One day after the SCI, we observed a significant increase in the expression of both the M1 and M2 phenotypes in each spinal cord region, but the presence of both macrophage phenotypes was not equal. The gene expression of the pro-inflammatory M1 macrophage marker was substantially higher compared with the M2 marker. ATR applied soon after the Th9 compression reduced the expression of both the M1 and M2 associated genes in all the evaluated areas, but a significant decrease was noted only in the cranial segments and at the lesion site. These segments are known to host a neuroprotective and neurotrophic environment [33]. Here, we also show that in the acute phase, ATR modulated the M1 macrophage phenotype more markedly than the M2 antigenic marker. Although the neuroprotective effect of ATR on macrophage infiltration has been shown in various SCI models, the precise time point of microglia/macrophage polarization and the factors controlling their shifts are still unclear. Khayrullina et al. [34] reported that acute inhibition of NOX2 (the enzyme that is a primary source of reactive oxygen species) with the specific inhibitor, gp91ds-tat, shifted microglial/macrophage polarization toward the M2 marker at seven days post-SCI. Although single acute gp91ds-tat treatment did not induce inflammatory effects beyond seven days, functional improvement continued through at least 28 days, indicating the importance of this single acute intervention. Bermudez et al. [35] also studied the correlation between NOX expression and microglial/macrophage polarization in a mouse SCI model. These authors confirmed that the expression of two NOX isoforms (NOX2 and NOX4) was temporally and polarization related, with an M1 preference for NOX2 acutely and NOX4 chronically; the M2 polarization marker was identified at acute time points only. While both the M1 and M2 microglia/macrophages express NOX isoforms, there is an influence of NOX on polarization. These data confirmed that NOX enzyme inhibition can alter the polarization status, which plays a significant role in the functional outcome. The regulation of the polarization of the M1/M2 macrophages after a SCI may also be related to neurotrophin-3 (NT-3) [36]. Electroacupuncture at GV acupuncture points, which can be used as an adjuvant therapy for a SCI, inhibited the proportion of M1 macrophages and proinflammatory cytokines, but at the other site it upregulated the M2 marker and NT-3 expression. Although we did not study the antioxidant effect of ATR, it seems that early ATR treatment, preferentially decreasing the M1 expression in segments with neuroprotective/neurotrophic environment could be involved in the oxidative response, thus reflecting the redox state of the lesion microenvironment. Pre-ischemic administration of ATR in a spinal cord ischemia-reperfusion model of a rabbit inhibited the depletion of antioxidative enzymes, reduced lipid peroxidation, and improved the extent of locomotor recovery [37]. In addition, increased levels of myeloperoxidase (MPO) were detected in the spinal cord following ischemia/reperfusion, suggesting leukocyte infiltration into the spinal cord. The authors have shown that ATR pre-treatment prevented MPO elevation. Secondly, astrocytes play a role in the mechanical and metabolic support of neurons. After spinal cord trauma, a select population of astrocytes, known as reactive astrocytes, upregulates the expression of intermediate filament proteins, proteoglycans, and other molecules and contributes to the inhibition of axonal outgrowth and glial scar formation [38–40]. One day after Th9 compression, we detected significant upregulation of GFAP mRNA in the areas surrounding the lesion site. Over time, the GFAP mRNA was only moderately reactivated at six weeks of survival. This finding might be associated with the regulation of the ion concentration in the extracellular space, the modulation of synaptic transmission, and the repair of the spinal parenchyma through the formation of a glial scar in the later post-SCI period [41]. Pannu et al. [16,17] injected ATR (5 mg/kg) through the whole period of survival, and they demonstrated a significant reduction of astrocyte activation. A single dose of ATR (5 mg/kg; i.p.) injected immediately after the SCI modulated the acute immune response, but we did not see its significant short- or long-lasting effect. It is also evident that although inflammation plays a very important role in the development of a glial scar, paradoxically, astrocyte activation by IL-1β can exert neuroprotective effects by stimulating the repair of the blood–brain barrier and decreasing its permeability [25]. Recently published data show that specific parts of the astrocytic scar have a supportive function for axon regeneration following a SCI [42] and might be induced by activated microglia [43]. Thirdly, early application of ATR could be crucial for limiting the secondary injury cascade after a SCI. One day after the Th9 compression, we noticed a sharp caspase-3 mRNA expression throughout the whole injured area. Moreover, the double immunostaining of caspase-3 with NeuN, APC, or GFAP showed marked apoptotic activity of these cells around the lesion site. Treatment with ATR, applied immediately after the Th9 compression, significantly reduced the expression of apoptotic markers. Immunohistochemical analysis showed the strong effect of the treatment on the reduction of caspase-3 cleavage in the oligodendrocytes, neurons, and astrocytes both cranially and caudally from the epicenter. Several recent studies have demonstrated the beneficial effect of ATR on the functional outcome through apoptosis inhibition. Gao et al. [18] showed that two doses of ATR (5 mg/kg; i.p.) injected one and two days after a weight-drop spinal cord injury significantly reduced caspase-3 and caspase-9 expression and activated autophagy, which was conducive to the recovery of neurological functions at seven days post-injury. Intraperitoneal injection of this drug was also effective in preventing early apoptosis at the lesion site within 2 h post-SCI administration [19]. ATR-treated rats showed a significant decrease in caspase-3 activity and a decrease in the number of TUNEL-positive cells at the injury site 4 h post-SCI, followed by an improvement in locomotion at four weeks post-SCI. While the treatment with ATR prevented excessive caspase-3 activation, it also inhibited the massive extension of the inflammatory response. Our results indicate that early inhibition of caspase-3 activity in the oligodendrocytes, neurons, and astrocytes may have a role in mitigating neurodegeneration, as well as in the remarkable functional outcome seen from day 30 to 42 after the Th9 compression. Gao et al. [44] also pointed out the positive effect of the early inhibition of programmed cell death. After Simvastatin injection (two doses, 10 mg/kg; i.p.), they observed a significant improvement in locomotor functional recovery seven weeks after a weight-drop SCI. It has been suggested that oligodendrocyte apoptosis contributes to chronic demyelination of spared axons and exacerbates the extent of the injury, eventually leading to permanent functional deficits [45]. Lee et al. [45] demonstrated that preventing oligodendrocyte cell death improved the neurological score for 35 days after a SCI in mice.

We suggest that the neuroprotective effect of ATR registered soon after a SCI could be crucial for improving tissue regeneration and the functional outcome. Markers of axonal outgrowing (Gap 43) quantified by means of the RT-PCR showed improvement in each evaluated segment. Gap-43 immunoreactive axons were distinctly visible throughout the whole cranio-caudal extent, but the most extensive Gap-43 immunoreactive axons were seen in the lateral funiculi. Similarly, a very strong regenerative response was detected in the expression of the neurofilaments. Neurofilaments are particularly abundant in large myelinated axons and are essential for axon radial growth and caliber maintenance during development [46,47]. We detected a loss of neurofilament-positive axons six weeks after the Th9 compression in areas infiltrated with Iba-1 positive cells. Massive regeneration of neurofilament immunoreactive axons was detected in the injured dorsolateral funiculi after the ATR treatment, although neurofilament mRNA measured in toto did not show a significant improvement. Wang et al. [48] have reported that neurofilament gene transcriptional regulation is crucial for neurofilament expression predominantly in axonal regeneration. We have also recently pointed out the role of neurofilaments in modulating spinal microcircuits leading to a better functional outcome [49]. Although the Olig2 transcription factor, an essential regulator of oligodendrocyte development, has been seen to improve locomotor recovery and enhance myelination in a rat contusive spinal cord injury model [50], we did not see any neuroprotective effect of the ATR treatment in Olig2 mRNA.

This study underscores the protective effect of ATR applied immediately post-SCI. The results suggest that ATR, even in a single dose, has important neuroprotective potential. However, a set of research problems dealing with practical ATR application in a traumatic SCI injury currently remains unexplored.

4. Materials and Methods

4.1. Experimental Animals and Surgical Procedure

A total of 48 adult female Wistar rats (weighing 250–300 g) were used in the experiment. The rats were housed 5 per cage on a 12-h dark/light cycle in a temperature- and humidity-controlled environment. Female rats were used in order to relieve serious urinary tract complications after

SCI, such as hematuria (hemorrhagic cystitis). Ferrero. S.L. et al. [51] showed that after contusion injury, hematuria duration was significantly longer in males compared with females, despite similar bladder reflex onset times. All procedures were carried out in accordance with the protocols approved by the State Veterinary and Food Administration in Bratislava (decision No. 4434/16-221/3), as well as by the Animal Use Committee at the Institute of Neurobiology, Slovak Academy of Sciences, and in accordance with the EC Council Directive (2010/63/EU) regarding the use of animals in research. All efforts were made to minimize the number of rats and their suffering.

The animals were divided into five experimental groups as follows: (1) control animals ($n = 6$); (2–3) rats subjected to the Th9 compression surviving for 24 h ($n = 12$) and six weeks ($n = 9$); and (4–5) rats after the SCI treated with post-surgical Atorvastatin administration (5 mg/kg, i.p.; Fluka by Sigma Aldrich, St. Louis, MO, USA) surviving for 24 h ($n = 12$) and six weeks ($n = 9$).

The surgical procedure was performed under isoflurane anesthesia (2–4%; AbbVie, BA, Slovak Republic; in 1.5–2.0 L/min oxygen), delivered by mask. After laminectomy at the Th9 segment, SCI was induced using a compression device with a weight of 40 g/15 min. The body temperature was maintained at 37 °C during the whole surgical procedure. After the Th9 compression, the rats received the antibiotic drug Amoksiklav (Sandoz Pharmaceuticals, Ljubljana, Slovenia; 30 mg/kg, i.m.) and the analgesic drug Novasul (Richterpharma, Wels, Austria; 2 mL/kg, i.m.) for three days. The Atorvastatin group of animals was treated with a single dose of Atorvastatin (5 mg/kg, i.p.), applied immediately after the SCI. The animals were housed in separated cages to recover with access to food and water ad libitum. The bladder expression of the rats after the SCI was required twice a day until the bladder reflex was restored (14–18 days).

4.2. Enzyme-Linked Immunosorbent Assay (ELISA)

Blood from the rats' tail vein (250–300 µL) was taken before the SCI, 4 and 24 h after trauma (4 animals/group). Each sample was centrifuged 10 min at 10,000 rpm to obtain the blood serum. The supernatants were kept at −70 °C until the ELISA procedure was performed. The level of IL-1β was measured using a Rat IL-1β ELISA Kit (Thermo Fisher Scientific, Waltham, MA, USA) according to the manufacturer's instructions.

4.3. Immunohistochemistry

At the end of the experiments, the rats ($n = 16$) were deeply anesthetized with thiopental (Valeant Czech Pharma s.r.o., Prague, Czech Republic; 50 mg/kg, i.p.) and perfused transcardially with 300 mL saline followed by 300 mL 4% paraformaldehyde in 0.1 M phosphate-buffered saline (PBS; pH 7.4, Sigma-Aldrich, St. Louis, MO, USA). Spinal cord blocks (0.5 cm cranially and caudally from the epicenter of the injury and the site of the injury) were post-fixed in the same fixative overnight and subsequently cryopreserved in a solution of 30% sucrose in PBS at 4 °C for 2 days. Afterwards, each tissue block was cut into transverse serial and longitudinal sections (25 µm thick) on a cryostat (Leica CM1850, Wetzlar, Germany). The sections were washed (3 × 10 min) in PBS with 0.3% Triton X-100 (Sigma-Aldrich, St. Louis, MO, USA) and blocked for 30 min at room temperature in a PBS solution containing 5% normal goat, rabbit, or donkey serum and 0.3% Triton X-100. For the processing of macrophages, microglia, astrocytes, neurofilaments, and outgrowing axons, the sections were incubated overnight at 4 °C with the following primary antibodies: ED-1 (mouse, 1:400 Biorad, Hercules, CA, USA), IBA-1 (goat, 1:1000 abcam, Cambridge, UK), GFAP (mouse, 1:600 Burlington, MA, USA), Nf-h (mouse, 1:1000 Danvers, MA, USA), and Gap43 (mouse, 1:500 abcam, Cambridge, UK). For the identification of caspase-3-expressing cells, double immunostaining was used. Anti-caspase-3 antibody (rabbit, 1:500 abcam, Cambridge, UK) was incubated overnight at 4 °C in combination with neuronal specific NeuN (mouse, 1:1000 abcam, Cambridge, UK), APC (mouse, 1:200 Millipore, Darmstadt, Germany), IBA-1, and GFAP antibodies. After washing (3 × 10 min) in PBS with 0.3% Triton X-100, the sections were incubated in the following secondary antibodies: FITC goat anti-mouse IgG (1:200); FITC rabbit anti-goat IgG (1:125); RRX goat anti-mouse IgG (1:600) (Jackson Immunoresearch,

West Grove, PA, USA); AF donkey anti-rabbit IgG (1:500); AF donkey anti-goat IgG (1:500) (Thermo Fisher Scientific, Waltham, MA, USA) for 2 h at room temperature. Immunolabeled spinal cord sections were mounted with Prolong (Invitrogen by Thermo Fisher Scientific, Carlsbad, CA, USA). Images were captured using an Olympus BX51 (Tokyo, Japan) fluorescent microscope.

4.4. Cell Counting

The ED-1 positive cells were counted using ImageJ 1.47 software (Wayne Rasband, National Institutes of Health, Bethesda, MD, USA). The number of immunostained macrophages (ED-1) was quantified at the lesion site from 25 μm thick transverse sections. The ED-1 positive cells were counted in the grey and white matter from 20 immunofluorescently labeled sections.

4.5. Tissue Processing for RT-PCR

Total RNA from the Th7-Th10 spinal cord ($n = 20$) was obtained using a Trizol Reagent (Thermo Fisher Scientific, Waltham, MA, USA) according to the manufacturer's instructions. The concentration of RNA in each sample was measured using NanoDrop 2000 c (Thermo Fisher Scientific, Waltham, MA, USA). The isolated RNA (2000 ng/μL) was reverse transcribed into cDNA in duplicates using a High-capacity cDNA Reverse Transcription Kit (AB applied biosystems by Thermo Fisher Scientific, Waltham, MA, USA) and a T1000™ Thermal Cycler (Bio-Rad, Hercules, CA, USA). cDNA samples (20 μL) were stored at −20 °C until real-time PCR was performed.

Immediately before the RT-PCR reaction, the cDNA samples were diluted with 80 μL nuclease-free water (Thermo Fisher Scientific, Waltham, MA, USA). The amplification of cDNA was performed using the CFX96™ Real-Time System (Bio-Rad, Hercules, CA, USA). The reaction mixture (20 μL) was composed of 10 μL TaqMan® Gene Expression MasterMix (AB applied biosystems by Thermo Fisher Scientific, Waltham, MA, USA), 1 μL TaqMan® Gene Expression Assays (AB applied biosystems by Thermo Fisher Scientific, Waltham, MA, USA)—βactin (Rn00667869); Gap43 (Rn01474579); Cd163 (Rn1492519); Cd86 (Rn00571654); GFAP (Rn00566603); Olig2 (Rn01767116); Casp3 (Rn00563902); Nf-h (Rn00709325), 4 μL nuclease-free water and 5 μL of cDNA sample. The amplifications were run under the following conditions: 10 min at 95 °C followed by 50 cycles of 15 s/95 °C and 1 min/60 °C. Gene expression was normalized with β-actin (reference gene). As a calibration product, samples from previous reactions were used. The relative quantity of gene expression was assigned using Bio-Rad CFX Manager. For statistical analyses, GraphPad Prism version 6.01 (La Jolla, CA, USA) was used.

4.6. Behavioral Assessment

The neurological outcome of animals was tested using the Basso–Beattie–Bresnahan (BBB) locomotor rating scale ranging from 0 (complete paralysis) to 21 points (normal movement with trunk stability) [52]. Each rat was scored in an open field for a period of 5 min by two examiners. The locomotor assessment was carried out one day after the SCI, every other day for the first two weeks, and then once a week until six weeks post-injury.

4.7. Statistical Analysis

The data from the BBB locomotor test was analyzed using Student's parametric *T*-Test. One-way analysis of variance (ANOVA) was used to determine the statistical significance ($p < 0.05$) of the differences between the compression group, ATR-treated group, and control group. All these data were analyzed using GraphPad Prism version 6.01 (La Jolla, CA, USA) and were expressed as mean values with standard deviation (SD). The data from the ELISA were analyzed using two-way ANOVA, in which the time after the spinal cord injury was the first independent variable and with or without ATR was the second independent variable. These data were analyzed using StatSoft, Inc. (2013), version 12.

5. Conclusions

Atorvastatin (5 mg/kg, i.p.) injected in a single dose immediately after spinal cord trauma, significantly reduced the early inflammatory response and sharply decreased the expression of caspase-3 in neurons, astrocytes, and oligodendrocytes 24 h post-SCI. Acute ATR treatment effectively prevented the excessive infiltration of destructive M1 macrophages around the lesion site, while the infiltration of beneficial M2 macrophages was less affected. This statin significantly improved the regeneration capacity of the injured tissue at six weeks, leading to the promotion of axonal outgrowth and increasing neurofilament expression. We can conclude that the early modulation of the inflammatory response via effects on the M1/M2 macrophages and the inhibition of caspase-3 expression strongly promote tissue regeneration in later periods.

Acknowledgments: This research was supported by APVV grant No. 15/0766, VEGA grants 2/0168/17, 2/0160/16, and the project: Formation and development of a diagnostic procedure in the treatment of trauma—injured spinal cord (ITMS 26220220202), supported by the Research & Development Operational Programme funded by the ERDF. We are grateful to Zuzana Barkacs for her technical assistance.

Author Contributions: Study concept and design of experiments: Nadezda Lukacova, Katarina Bimbova. Spinal cord compression at Th9 segment: Katarina Bimbova and Peter Zavacky. Post-surgical animal care and behavioral assessment: Katarina Bimbova, Maria Bacova, Jana Fedorova and Andrea Stropkovska. Transcardial perfusion, immunohistochemical, and molecular analyses: Katarina Bimbova, Alexandra Kisucka and Jana Jachova. Data analyses: Katarina Bimbova, Maria Bacova and Stefania Papcunova. Writing of the paper: Katarina Bimbova, Jan Galik, Martin Marsala, Jaroslav Pavel and Nadezda Lukacova.

References

1. Blesch, A.; Tuszynski, M.H. Spinal cord injury: Plasticity, regeneration and the challenge of translational drug development. *Trends Neurosci.* **2009**, *32*, 41–47. [CrossRef] [PubMed]
2. Fehlings, M.G.; Nguyen, D.H. Immunoglobulin G: A Potential Treatment to Attenuate Neuroinflammation Following Spinal Cord Injury. *J. Clin. Immunol.* **2010**, *30*, S109–S112. [CrossRef] [PubMed]
3. Oyinbo, C.A. Secondary injury mechanisms in traumatic spinal cord injury: A nugget of this multiply cascade. *Acta Neurobiol. Exp.* **2011**, *71*, 281–299.
4. Tator, C.H. Update on the pathophysiology and pathology of acute spinal cord injury. *Brain Pathol.* **1995**, *5*, 407–413. [CrossRef] [PubMed]
5. Donnelly, D.J.; Popovich, P.G. Inflammation and its role in neuroprotection, axonal regeneration and functional recovery after spinal cord injury. *Exp. Neurol.* **2008**, *209*, 378–388. [CrossRef] [PubMed]
6. Silva, A.N.; Sousa, N.; Reis, R.L.; Salgado, A.J. From basics to clinical: A comprehensive review on spinal cord injury. *Prog. Neurobiol.* **2014**, *114*, 25–57. [CrossRef] [PubMed]
7. Silver, J.; Miller, J.H. Regeneration beyond the glial scar. *Nat. Rev. Neurosci.* **2004**, *5*, 146–156. [CrossRef] [PubMed]
8. Saxena, T.; Deng, B.; Stelzner, D.; Hasenwinkel, J.; Chaiken, J. Raman spectroscopic investigation of spinal cord injury in a rat model. *J. Biomed. Opt.* **2011**, *16*, 027003. [CrossRef] [PubMed]
9. Papa, S.; Caron, I.; Erba, E.; Panini, N.; De Paola, M.; Mariani, A.; Colombo, C.; Ferrari, R.; Pozzer, D.; Zanier, E.R.; et al. Early modulation of pro-inflammatory microglia by minocycline loaded nanoparticles confers long lasting protection after spinal cord injury. *Biomaterials* **2016**, *75*, 13–24. [CrossRef] [PubMed]
10. Wang, Z.; Nong, J.; Shultz, R.B.; Zhang, Z.; Kim, T.; Tom, V.J.; Ponnappan, R.K.; Zhong, Y. Local delivery of minocycline from metal ion-assisted self-assembled complexes promotes neuroprotection and functional recovery after spinal cord injury. *Biomaterials* **2017**, *112*, 62–71. [CrossRef] [PubMed]
11. Machova, U.L.; Karova, K.; Ruzicka, J.; Kloudova, A.; Shannon, C.; Dubisova, J.; Murali, R.; Kubinova, S.; Sykova, E.; Jhanwar-Uniyal, M.; et al. The Anti-inflammatory compound curcumin enhances locomotor and sensory recovery after spinal cord injury in rats by immunomodulation. *Int. J. Mol. Sci.* **2016**, *17*, 49. [CrossRef] [PubMed]
12. Wang, Y.; Zu, J.N.; Li, J.; Chen, C.; Xi, C.; Yan, J. Curcumin promotes the spinal cord repair via inhibition of glial scar formation and inflammation. *Neurosci. Lett.* **2014**, *560*, 51–56. [CrossRef] [PubMed]

13. Blauw, G.J.; Lagaay, A.M.; Smelt, A.H.; Westendorp, R.G. Stroke, statins, and cholesterol. A meta-analysis of randomized, placebo-controlled, double-blind trials with HMG-CoA reductase inhibitors. *Stroke* **1997**, *28*, 946–950. [CrossRef] [PubMed]
14. Komukai, K.; Kubo, T.; Kitabata, H.; Matsuo, Y.; Ozaki, Y.; Takarada, S.; Okumoto, Y.; Shiono, Y.; Orii, M.; Shimamura, K.; et al. Effect of atorvastatin therapy on fibrous cap thickness in coronary atherosclerotic plaque as assessed by optical coherence tomography: The EASY-FIT study. *J. Am. Coll. Cardiol.* **2014**, *64*, 2207–2217. [CrossRef] [PubMed]
15. Pordal, A.H.; Hajmiresmail, S.J.; Assadpoor-Piranfar, M.; Hedayati, M.; Ajami, M. Plasma oxysterol level in patients with coronary artery stenosis and its changes in response to the treatment with atorvastatin. *Med. J. Islam. Repub. Iran* **2015**, *29*, 192. [PubMed]
16. Pannu, R.; Barbosa, E.; Singh, A.K.; Singh, I. Attenuation of acute inflammatory response by atorvastatin after spinal cord injury in rats. *J. Neurosci. Res.* **2005**, *79*, 340–350. [CrossRef] [PubMed]
17. Pannu, R.; Christie, D.K.; Barbosa, E.; Singh, I.; Singh, A.K. Post-trauma Lipitor treatment prevents endothelial dysfunction, facilitates neuroprotection, and promotes locomotor recovery following spinal cord injury. *J. Neurochem.* **2007**, *101*, 182–200. [CrossRef] [PubMed]
18. Gao, S.; Zhang, Z.; Shen, Z.; Gao, K.; Chang, L.; Guo, Y.; Li, Z.; Wang, W.; Wang, A. Atorvastatin activates autophagy and promotes neurological function recovery after spinal cord injury. *Neural Regen. Res.* **2016**, *11*, 977–982. [CrossRef] [PubMed]
19. Déry, M.A.; Rousseau, G.; Benderdour, M.; Beaumont, E. Atorvastatin prevents early apoptosis after thoracic spinal cord contusion injury and promotes locomotion recovery. *Neurosci. Lett.* **2009**, *453*, 73–76. [CrossRef] [PubMed]
20. Alves, E.S.; Lemos, V.A.; Silva, F.R.; Lira, F.S.; Santos, R.V.T.; Rosa, J.P.P.; Caperuto, E.; Tufik, S.; Mello, M.T. Low-Grade Inflammation and Spinal Cord Injury: Exercise as Therapy? *Mediat. Inflamm.* **2013**, *2013*, 971841. [CrossRef]
21. Gensel, J.C.; Zhang, B. Macrophage activation and its role in repair and pathology after spinal cord injury. *Brain Res.* **2015**, *1619*, 1–11. [CrossRef] [PubMed]
22. Aydemir, S.; Dogan, D.; Kocak, A.; Dilsiz, N. The effect of melatonin on spinal cord after ischemia in rats. *Spinal Cord* **2016**, *54*, 360–363. [CrossRef] [PubMed]
23. Rowland, J.W.; Hawryluk, G.W.; Kwon, B.; Fehlings, M.G. Current status of acute spinal cord injury pathophysiology and emerging therapies: Promise on the horizon. *Neurosurg. Focus* **2008**, *25*, 1–17. [CrossRef] [PubMed]
24. Carlson, S.L.; Parrish, M.E.; Springer, J.E.; Doty, K.; Dosset, L. Acute Inflammatory Response in Spinal Cord Following Impact Injury. *Exp. Neurol.* **1998**, *151*, 77–88. [CrossRef] [PubMed]
25. Rust, R.; Kaiser, J. Insights into the Dual Role of Inflammation after Spinal Cord Injury. *J. Neurosci.* **2017**, *37*, 4658–4660. [CrossRef] [PubMed]
26. Allan, S.M.; Tyrrel, P.J.; Rothwell, N.J. Interleukin-1 and neuronal injury. *Nat. Rev. Immunol.* **2005**, *5*, 629–640. [CrossRef] [PubMed]
27. Nesic, O.; Xu, G.Y.; McAdoo, D.; High, K.W.; Hulsebosch, C.; Perez-Polo, R. IL-1 Receptor Antagonist Prevents Apoptosis and Caspase-3 Activation after Spinal Cord Injury. *J. Neurotrauma* **2004**, *18*, 947–956. [CrossRef] [PubMed]
28. Basu, A.; Krady, J.K.; Levison, S.W. Interleukin-1: A master regulator of neuroinflammation. *J. Neurosci. Res.* **2004**, *78*, 151–156. [CrossRef] [PubMed]
29. David, S.; Lacroix, S. Role of the immune response in tissue damage and repair in the injured spinal cord. In *Clinical Neuroimmunology*, 3rd ed.; Antel, J., Birnbaum, G., Hartung, H.P., Vincent, A., Eds.; Oxford University Press: New York, NY, USA, 2005; pp. 53–63, ISBN 0-19-851068-3.
30. Lukacova, N.; Kolesárová, M.; Kuchárová, K.; Pavel, J.; Kolesár, D.; Radonák, J.; Marsala, M.; Chalimoniuk, M.; Langfort, J.; Marsala, J. The effect of a spinal cord hemisection on changes in nitric oxide synthase pools in the site of injury and in regions located far away from the injured site. *Cell. Mol. Neurobiol.* **2006**, *26*, 1367–1385. [CrossRef] [PubMed]
31. Lourenço, C.F.; Ferreira, N.R.; Santos, R.M.; Lukacova, N.; Barbosa, R.M.; Laranjinha, J. The pattern of glutamate-induced nitric oxide dynamics in vivo and its correlation with nNOS expression in rat hippocampus, cerebral cortex and striatum. *Brain Res.* **2014**, *1554*, 1–11. [CrossRef] [PubMed]

32. Kong, X.; Gao, J. Macrophage polarization: A key event in the secondary phase of acute spinal cord injury. *J. Cell. Mol. Med.* **2017**, *21*, 941–954. [CrossRef] [PubMed]
33. Devaux, S.; Cizkova, D.; Quanico, J.; Franck, J.; Nataf, S.; Pays, L.; Hauberg-Lotte, L.; Maass, P.; Kobarg, J.H.; Kobeissy, F.; et al. Proteomic Analysis of the Spatio-temporal Based Molecular Kinetics of Acute Spinal Cord Injury Identifies a Time- and Segment-specific Window for Effective Tissue Repair. *Mol. Cell. Proteom.* **2016**, *15*, 2641–2670. [CrossRef] [PubMed]
34. Khayrullina, G.; Bermudez, S.; Byrnes, K.R. Inhibition of NOX2 reduces locomotor impairment, inflammation, and oxidative stress after spinal cord injury. *J. Neuroinflamm.* **2015**, *12*, 172. [CrossRef] [PubMed]
35. Bermudez, S.; Khayrullina, G.; Zhao, Y.; Byrnes, K.R. NADPH oxidase isoform expression is temporally regulated and may contribute to microglial/macrophage polarization after spinal cord injury. *Mol. Cell. Neurosci.* **2016**, *77*, 53–64. [CrossRef] [PubMed]
36. Zhao, J.; Wang, L.; Li, Y. Electroacupuncture alleviates the inflammatory response via effects on M1 and M2 macrophages after spinal cord injury. *Acupunct. Med.* **2017**, *35*, 224–230. [CrossRef] [PubMed]
37. Nazli, Y.; Colak, N.; Alpay, M.F.; Uysal, S.; Uzunlar, A.K.; Cakir, O. Neuroprotective effect of atorvastatin in spinal cord ischemia-reperfusion injury. *Clinics* **2015**, *70*, 52–60. [CrossRef]
38. Raisman, G. Formation of synapses in the adult rat after injury: Similarities and differences between a peripheral and a central nervous site. *Philos. Trans. R. Soc. Lond. B Biol. Sci.* **1977**, *278*, 349–359. [CrossRef] [PubMed]
39. Codeluppi, S.; Svensson, C.I.; Hefferan, M.P.; Valencia, F.; Silldorff, M.D.; Oshiro, M.; Marsala, M.; Pasquale, E.B. The Rheb-mTOR pathway is upregulated in reactive astrocytes of the injured spinal cord. *J. Neurosci.* **2009**, *29*, 1093–1104. [CrossRef] [PubMed]
40. Lukovic, D.; Stojkovic, M.; Moreno-Manzano, V.; Jendelova, P.; Sykova, E.; Bhattacharya, S.S.; Erceg, S. Concise review: Reactive astrocytes and stem cells in spinal cord injury: Good guys or bad guys? *Stem Cells* **2015**, *33*, 1036–1041. [CrossRef] [PubMed]
41. Kucharikova, A.; Schreiberova, A.; Zavodska, M.; Gedrova, S.; Hricova, L.; Pavel, J.; Galik, J.; Marsala, M.; Lukáčová, N. Repeated Baclofen treatment ameliorates motor dysfunction, suppresses reflex activity and decreases the expression of signaling proteins in reticular nuclei and lumbar motoneurons after spinal trauma in rats. *Acta Histochem.* **2014**, *116*, 344–353. [CrossRef] [PubMed]
42. Anderson, M.A.; Burda, J.E.; Ren, Y.; Ao, Y.; O'Shea, T.M.; Kawaguchi, R.; Coppola, G.; Khakh, B.S.; Deming, T.J.; Sofroniew, M.V. Astrocyte scar formation aids central nervous system axon regeneration. *Nature* **2016**, *532*, 195–200. [CrossRef] [PubMed]
43. Liddelow, S.A.; Guttenplan, K.A.; Clarke, L.E.; Bennett, F.C.; Bohlen, C.J.; Schirmer, L.; Bennett, M.L.; Münch, A.E.; Chung, W.S.; Peterson, T.C.; et al. Neurotoxic reactive astrocytes are induced by activated microglia. *Nature* **2017**, *541*, 481–487. [CrossRef] [PubMed]
44. Gao, K.; Shen, Z.; Yuan, Y.; Han, D.; Song, C.; Guo, Y.; Mei, X. Simvastatin inhibits neural cell apoptosis and promotes locomotor recovery via activation of Wnt/β-catenin signaling pathway after spinal cord injury. *J. Neurochem.* **2016**, *138*, 139–149. [CrossRef] [PubMed]
45. Lee, J.Y.; Kang, S.R.; Yune, T.Y. Fluoxetine prevents oligodendrocyte cell death by inhibiting microglia activation after spinal cord injury. *J. Neurotrauma* **2015**, *32*, 633–644. [CrossRef] [PubMed]
46. Nishida, F.; Sisti, M.S.; Zanuzzi, C.N.; Barbeito, C.G.; Portiansky, E.L. Neurons of the rat cervical spinal cord express vimentin and neurofilament after intraparenchymal injection of kainic acid. *Neurosci. Lett.* **2017**, *643*, 103–110. [CrossRef] [PubMed]
47. Lépinoux-Chambaud, C.; Eyer, J. Review on intermediate filaments of the nervous system and their pathological alterations. *Histochem. Cell Biol.* **2013**, *140*, 13–22. [CrossRef] [PubMed]
48. Wang, H.; Wu, M.; Zhan, C.; Ma, E.; Yang, M.; Yang, X.; Li, Y. Neurofilament proteins in axonal regeneration and neurodegenerative diseases. *Neural Regen. Res.* **2012**, *7*, 620–626. [PubMed]
49. Gedrova, S.; Galik, J.; Marsala, M.; Zavodska, M.; Pavel, J.; Sulla, I.; Gajdos, M.; Lukac, I.; Kafka, J.; Ledecky, V.; et al. Neuroprotective effect of local hypothermia in a computer-controlled compression model in minipig: Correlation of tissue sparing along the rostro-caudal axis with neurological outcome. *Exp. Ther. Med.* **2017**, *15*, 254–270. [CrossRef] [PubMed]

50. Hwang, D.H.; Kim, B.G.; Kim, E.J.; Lee, S.I.; Joo, I.S.; Suh-Kim, H.; Sohn, S.; Kim, S.U. Transplantation of human neural stem cells transduced with Olig2 transcription factor improves locomotor recovery and enhances myelination in the white matter of rat spinal cord following contusive injury. *BMC Neurosci.* **2009**, *10*, 117. [CrossRef] [PubMed]
51. Ferrero, S.L.; Brady, T.D.; Dugan, V.P.; Armstrong, J.E.; Hubscher, C.H.; Johnson, R.D. Effects of Lateral Funiculus Sparing, Spinal Lesion Level, and Gender on Recovery of Bladder Voiding Reflexes and Hematuria in Rats. *J. Neurotrauma* **2015**, *32*, 200–208. [CrossRef] [PubMed]
52. Basso, D.M.; Beattie, M.S.; Bresnahan, J.C. A sensitive and reliable locomotor rating scale for open field testing in rats. *J. Neurotrauma* **1995**, *12*, 1–21. [CrossRef] [PubMed]

11

The Effect of Human Mesenchymal Stem Cells Derived from Wharton's Jelly in Spinal Cord Injury Treatment is Dose-Dependent and can be Facilitated by Repeated Application

Petr Krupa [1,2], Irena Vackova [2], Jiri Ruzicka [2], Kristyna Zaviskova [2,3], Jana Dubisova [2,3], Zuzana Koci [2,3], Karolina Turnovcova [2], Lucia Machova Urdzikova [2], Sarka Kubinova [2], Svatopluk Rehak [1] and Pavla Jendelova [2,3,*]

1 Department of Neurosurgery, Charles University, Medical Faculty and University Hospital Hradec Králové, Sokolska 581, 50005 Hradec Kralove, Czech Republic; petr.krupa@fnhk.cz (P.K.); rehak@lfhk.cuni.cz (S.R.)

2 Institute of Experimental Medicine, Czech Academy of Sciences, Vídeňská 1083, 14220 Prague 4, Czech Republic; irena.vackova@biomed.cas.cz (I.V.); j.ruzicka@biomed.cas.cz (J.R.); kristyna.zaviskova@biomed.cas.cz (K.Z.); jana.dubisova@biomed.cas.cz (J.D.); zuzana.koci@biomed.cas.cz (Z.K.); karolina.turnovcova@biomed.cas.cz (K.T.); urdzikl@biomed.cas.cz (L.M.U.); sarka.k@biomed.cas.cz (S.K.)

3 Department of Neuroscience, Charles University, Second Faculty of Medicine, 15006 Prague 5, Czech Republic

* Correspondence: jendel@biomed.cas.cz

Abstract: Human mesenchymal stem cells derived from Wharton's jelly (WJ-MSCs) were used for the treatment of the ischemic-compression model of spinal cord injury in rats. To assess the effectivity of the treatment, different dosages (0.5 or 1.5 million cells) and repeated applications were compared. Cells or saline were applied intrathecally by lumbar puncture for one week only, or in three consecutive weeks after injury. Rats were assessed for locomotor skills (BBB, rotarod, flat beam) for 9 weeks. Spinal cord tissue was morphometrically analyzed for axonal sprouting, sparing of gray and white matter and astrogliosis. Endogenous gene expression (*Gfap*, *Casp3*, *Irf5*, *Cd86*, *Mrc1*, *Cd163*) was studied with quantitative Real-time polymerase chain reaction (qRT PCR). Significant recovery of functional outcome was observed in all of the treated groups except for the single application of the lowest number of cells. Histochemical analyses revealed a gradually increasing effect of grafted cells, resulting in a significant increase in the number of GAP43+ fibers, a higher amount of spared gray matter and reduced astrogliosis. mRNA expression of macrophage markers and apoptosis was downregulated after the repeated application of 1.5 million cells. We conclude that the effect of hWJ-MSCs on spinal cord regeneration is dose-dependent and potentiated by repeated application.

Keywords: spinal cord injury; human mesenchymal stem cells; Wharton's jelly; inflammatory response; neuroregeneration; astrogliosis; axonal growth

---

1. Introduction

Spinal cord injury (SCI) is a serious mutilating injury, resulting in loss of motor, sensory, and autonomic functions, and remains a challenging medical and social problem even in the 21st century. The final neurological deficit is determined by two mechanisms—primary and secondary injury. Primary injury represents the mechanism and strength of the direct trauma. Secondary injury is characterized by the local immune reaction followed by apoptosis of the injured and vulnerable neurons, tissue atrophy with cavitation, and glial scar formation [1]. Since there is no specific treatment for primary injury, and the endogenous potential to regenerate the spinal cord neurons is very limited [2], several treatments are focused on neuroprotection and/or reducing the impact of secondary pathological processes. Promising results in alleviation of the pathological chain of secondary damage were found in the last decade by application of mesenchymal stem cells (MSCs).

MSCs are multipotent cells with multi-differentiation and self-renewal capacity. Many types of adult and embryogenic tissue have been proven as a source of MSCs—adipose tissue, peripheral blood, lung, heart, corneal stroma, dental pulp, placenta, endometrium, amniotic membrane, and umbilical cord blood and tissue (Wharton's jelly). Under special conditions in vitro, they are capable of differentiating into various tissue cells such as osteocytes or osteoblasts, adipocytes, and chondrocytes [3–5]. However, the regenerative potential of MSCs as a therapeutic tool can be provided mainly by the paracrine effect, interacting with the environment around the injured tissue. In nervous tissue repair and regeneration, MSCs support revascularization, modulate inflammatory response [6], produce different growth factors and cytokines [7], and protect vulnerable cells from oxidative stress, causing stress-induced apoptosis [8]. Therefore, it was recently suggested by Caplan [9] that they should be renamed to medicinal signaling cells (MSCs).

In the current study, we used MSCs isolated from human Wharton's jelly (WJ-MSCs). Wharton's jelly is the primitive gelatinous connective tissue of the umbilical cord, first described by Thomas Wharton in 1656. Compared to other sources of MSCs (bone marrow, adipose tissue), WJ-MSCs are more primitive with higher proliferating potential [10], have lower immunogenicity because of a lower major histocompatibility complex class I (MHC-I) and the absence of major histocompatibility complex class II (MHC-II) expression [11], and are proven to be non-tumorigenic [12]. Furthermore, WJ-MSCs can be easily and non-invasively obtained from discarded umbilical tissue, and represent neither potential danger for the donor, nor ethical concerns [13]. They are highly proliferative and can be easily expanded.

The delivery route of stem cells is a frequently discussed issue, as the mode of delivery is an important factor in translation to clinical practice. Therefore, several studies have compared the intraspinal, intrathecal (or intracisternal), intraarterial and intravenous application of MSCs. Regardless of the delivery route, MSC treatment has improved functional recovery after SCI. Whilst the engraftment of the transplanted cells was higher in animals with intraspinal delivery [14,15], injections into the parenchyma of the spinal cord may further damage the spinal cord tissue; therefore, less invasive methods, such as intrathecal or intravenous delivery, are preferable. Indeed, the cells grafted via lumbar puncture, or intracisternally have shown the best functional recovery, even though they often remained in the intrathecal space [16,17] or accumulated around the anterior spinal artery [18]. Rats intrathecally grafted with human bone marrow MSCs (hBM-MSCs) had reduced inflammatory reactions and apoptosis, improved functional recovery, and the glial scar formation had been rearranged after SCI, though no cells were detected in the spinal cord parenchyma two months after transplantation [19,20]. Because of the relatively short survival time of MSCs in the host tissue the repetitive delivery of MSCs may prolong the beneficial effects induced by MSC application by potentiating their regenerative potential [18].

The main goal of this study was to assess the dose of the applied WJ-MSCs, and the difference between single and repetitive application on functional recovery and tissue repair after SCI in rats. WJ-MSCs were applied intrathecally by a lumbar puncture into rats with balloon-induced spinal cord compression lesion. This model simulates the compression of the human spinal cord by an unreduced dislocation or a fracture dislocation of the spine. It is assumed that both mechanical and vascular factors are involved in the pathogenesis of spinal cord injury in this model. Moreover, it is simple and reproducible and requires minimal surgical preparation of the animal (no laminectomy) [21]. The functional outcome was assessed using a set of behavioral tests (BBB, flat beam test, and rotarod). Furthermore, histological and immunohistochemical analyses were performed to evaluate the sparing of gray and white matter, axonal sprouting, and formation of glial scar. Finally, quantitative PCR analyses of selected endogenous genes were performed.

2. Results

2.1. Cell Culture

hWJ-MSCs phenotype, their multipotent differentiation potential, and high proliferation capacity was evaluated prior to transplantation (see Supplement 1, Figures S1–S3).

2.2. Behavioral Analysis

2.2.1. BBB Test

Recovery of the hind limb locomotor function was evaluated every week starting the first week after SCI. The BBB score was calculated as a mean value from the scores of both legs (Figure 1A). One week after SCI, all tested animals had severe paraparesis or paraplegia. The average score was 1.28 ± 0.15. No differences between the groups were observed. The second week after SCI animals in all groups showed new motions in one or two joints. Among the groups, a significant difference was found between the control group (2.1 ± 0.43) and the group treated with a single dose of 1.5 M hWJ-MSCs (5.28 ± 0.59) ($p < 0.05$). In the third week after SCI, a rapid improvement of the locomotor functions was observed in the groups treated with a single dose of 1.5 M, and the groups with repeated treatment of 0.5 and 1.5 M, respectively. All three groups recovered significantly better than the control group ($p < 0.05$, $p < 0.001$). Animals treated with only 0.5 M showed little improvement over the control group, which was not statistically significant. In the following weeks, improvement of movement and strength of the hind limbs continued but not so rapidly as was seen during the first three weeks. From the fourth week onward, until the end of the experiment, rats treated with 1.5 M and 3 × 0.5 M and 3 × 1.5 M had comparable results, which were significantly better than the control group and animals treated by 0.5 M ($p < 0.01$, $p < 0.001$). No significant difference between the control group and the 0.5 M group was found. The final results at the end of the ninth week were 4.29 ± 0.57 for the control group, 5.19 ± 0.36 for 0.5 M, 9.81 ± 0.88 for 3 × 0.5 M, 8.67 ± 0.88 for 1.5 M and 9.21 ± 0.45 for 3 × 1.5 M. Animals in the groups with repetitive treatment were mostly able to achieve effective weight support of their body when standing, or even walking. The gap between scores 8 (and lower) and 9 (and higher) is substantial when comparing the strength of the muscles of the hindlimbs.

(Two-way RM ANOVA, Treatment; $F = 8.481$, $p < 0.001$; for p values of post hoc pair-to-pair test, see Supplement 2).

2.2.2. Rotarod Test

Coordination of the limb movements was tested by a rotarod test (Figure 1B). All animals were trained in this task before surgery at a fixed speed of 10 rpm. Testing was then performed every two weeks—2nd, 4th, 6th, and 8th week after SCI. Due to the severity of the lesion and limited recovery, no significant differences were observed between the groups.

(Two-way RM ANOVA, Treatment; $F = 0.490$, $p = 0.743$; for p values of post hoc pair-to-pair test, see Supplement 2).

2.2.3. Beam Walk Test

Advanced locomotor skills and coordination of the hind limbs was measured by walking on the flat beam. Results were evaluated using a 0–7 scale modified from Metz and Whishaw. All animals were firstly trained in this task before surgery and then tested every week starting the second week after SCI (Figure 1C). Due to the severity of the lesion, most of the rats showed minimal ability to cross the beam and often just stayed and balanced at the starting point of the beam. The best scores (7th week after SCI 3.1 ± 0.33) were obtained in animals treated by 3 × 1.5 M, which were significantly better, when compared to all of the other groups. For the first three weeks, animals treated with 0.5 M achieved significantly better results than the control group, but in subsequent weeks they gradually worsened and the significant difference was lost. This was most probably due to the gaining of weight, lack of motivation, and fear of falling off the beam.

(Two-way RM ANOVA, Treatment; $F = 20.656$, $p < 0.001$; for p values of post hoc pair-to-pair test, see Supplement 2).

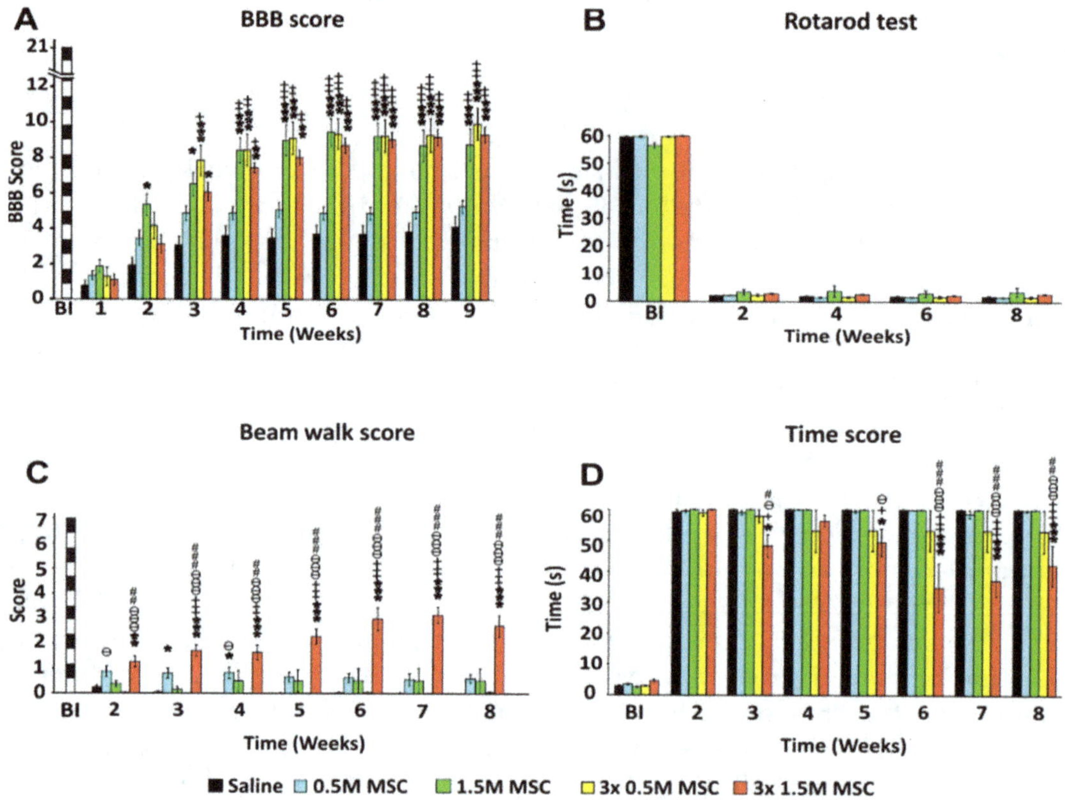

Figure 1. Recovery of locomotor functions following hWJ-MSCs transplantation after SCI. Treatments by a different number of administrated cells. The locomotor skills of saline- or stem cell-treated rats were measured using the BBB (**A**), rotarod (**B**), beam walk score (**C**), and time score (**D**). Animals treated with a higher single dose and by repetitive dose of hWJ-MSCs achieved significantly higher scores in the open-field BBB test when compared to saline controls and animals treated by 0.5 M hWJ-MSCs (**A**). Strength and limb coordination was measured by rotarod test (**B**), where no significant differences were found. The flat beam test (**C**), which is focused on advanced locomotor skills, demonstrated significantly higher scores in the group treated by 3 × 1.5 M hWJ-MSCs. Time score (**D**) reflects the time the rat needs to cross the beam and shows the overall stability of the rat. Animals treated by 3 × 1.5 M achieved significantly better times than the rest of the rats. * $p < 0.05$ versus saline; ** $p < 0.01$ versus saline; *** $p < 0.001$ versus saline; + $p < 0.05$ versus 0.5 M MSCs; ++ $p < 0.01$ versus 0.5 M MSCs; +++ $p < 0.001$ versus 0.5 M MSCs; # $p < 0.05$ versus 3 × 0.5 M MSCs; ## $p < 0.01$ versus 3 × 0.5 M MSCs; ### $p < 0.001$ versus 3 × 0.5 M MSCs; ɵ $p < 0.05$ versus 1.5 M MSCs; ɵɵ $p < 0.01$ versus 1.5 M MSCs; ɵɵɵ $p < 0.001$ versus 1.5 M MSCs. BBB = Basso, Beattie, and Bresnahan test; BI = before injury; MSC = human Wharton Jelly mesenchymal stem cell; SCI = spinal cord injury.

In addition to the beam score, we measured the time needed to cross the beam (maximally for 60 s). During the pre-training, healthy rats were able to cross the beam in approximately 3.0 s (Figure 1D). The measurement was performed weekly starting the second week after SCI. Two weeks after SCI not all the rats were able to cross the beam and did not move from the starting line. In the following weeks, a significant improvement was observed between the rats treated by 3 × 1.5 M and the other groups. The best score was achieved in the sixth week in the group 3 × 1.5 M, when rats traversed the beam at an average time of 34.9 ± 7 s.

(Two-way RM ANOVA, Treatment; $F = 5.001$, $p = 0.002$; for p values of post hoc pair-to-pair test, see Supplement 2).

2.3. *Histology and Immunohistochemistry*

2.3.1. Gray and White Matter Sparing

The total area of spared gray/white matter was measured on the 15 cross sections of the spinal cord 9 weeks after the SCI (7 sections cranially and caudally to the center of the lesion, which was determined as the section with the smallest area of the residual spinal cord tissue). Values were averaged and compared to the control, which was set as 100%. Concerning the gray matter preservation (Figure 2A), a significant difference was found between the group 3 × 1.5 M and the control ($p < 0.05$), and a strong trend was observed when compared to the group of 0.5 M ($p = 0.051$). Comparison of the white matter sparing showed no significant difference between the groups as a whole (Figure 2B). Similarly to the gray matter, in the center of the lesion and in the surrounding tissue, we observed significantly more spared white matter in animals treated with 3 × 1.5 M and 1.5 M when compared to the control group and rats treated with 0.5 M.

(Two-way RM ANOVA, Treatment; gray matter − $F = 3.341$, $p = 0.03$, white matter − $F = 1.290$, $p = 0.307$; for p values of post hoc pair-to-pair test, see Supplement 3).

2.3.2. Astrogliosis and Distribution of Protoplasmic Astrocytes

The total area of the glial scar formed around the central cavity was measured on 15 GFAP-CY3 stained cross sections of the spinal cord 9 weeks after the SCI (7 sections cranially and caudally to the center of the lesion, which was determined as the section with the smallest area of the residual spinal cord tissue). Values were averaged and are presented as a ratio of scar tissue to the whole section in percentages (Figure 2C). Groups treated with 3 × 1.5 M as well as 3 × 0.5 M and 1.5 M had a significantly smaller GFAP positive area around the main cavity compared to the control group ($p < 0.05$). The group treated by 0.5 M showed no significant difference compared to saline-treated rats.

(Two-way RM ANOVA, Treatment; $F = 4.026$, $p = 0.015$; for p values of post hoc pair-to-pair test, see Supplement 3).

On the same slices, the number of protoplasmic astrocytes was counted (Figure 2D). Rats treated by 3 × 0.5 M and 1.5 M as well as 3 × 1.5 M had a significantly lower number of protoplasmic astrocytes compared to the control group.

(Two-way RM ANOVA, Treatment; $F = 3.997$, $p = 0.015$; for p values of post hoc pair-to-pair test, see Supplement 3).

2.3.3. Axonal Sprouting

Axonal sprouting was determined as the number of $GAP43^+$ fibers, which were manually counted on the 15 cross sections of the spinal cord 9 weeks after the SCI (7 sections cranially and caudally to the center of the lesion, which was determined as the section with the smallest area of the residual spinal cord tissue). Values were averaged and compared to the control, which was set as 100%. The significant effect of the cell treatment was not only dose-dependent, but further improved after repeated application (Figure 2E). Treatment with the lowest dose—0.5 M, had no or minimal effect on axonal sprouting (102 ± 4%). In the other cell-treated groups, the number of positive fibers was gradually increasing with the higher number of grafted cells (1.5 M 140 ± 4%), and repeated application had a significantly stronger effect than a single dose (3 × 0.5 M 168 ± 10%) and (3 × 1.5 M 212 ± 18%) ($p < 0.05$).

(One-way ANOVA, Treatment; $H_4 = 21.844$, $p < 0.001$).

2.4. *qRT-PCR*

Expression of Intrinsic Genes after Stem Cell Transplantation, after SCI

Samples from the spinal cord for qPCR analysis were taken 4 (Figure 3A) and 9 weeks (Figure 3B) after the cell transplantation. A comparison was made against the saline-treated rats, which were set as 0. The expression of genes, which are related to the M1 (*Irf5*, *Cd86*) and M2 (*Mrc1*, *Cd163*) macrophage phenotypes, astrogliosis (*Gfap*), and apoptosis (*Casp3*), was analyzed. Pro-inflammatory genes *Irf5* and *CD86* were, 4 weeks after the transplantation of the cells, insignificantly upregulated in the groups treated by 1.5 M and 3 × 0.5 M but, 9 weeks after the transplantation, were downregulated in all groups except the 3 × 0.5 M. Statistical significance against the saline group was found only in the group 3 × 1.5 M ($p < 0.05$).

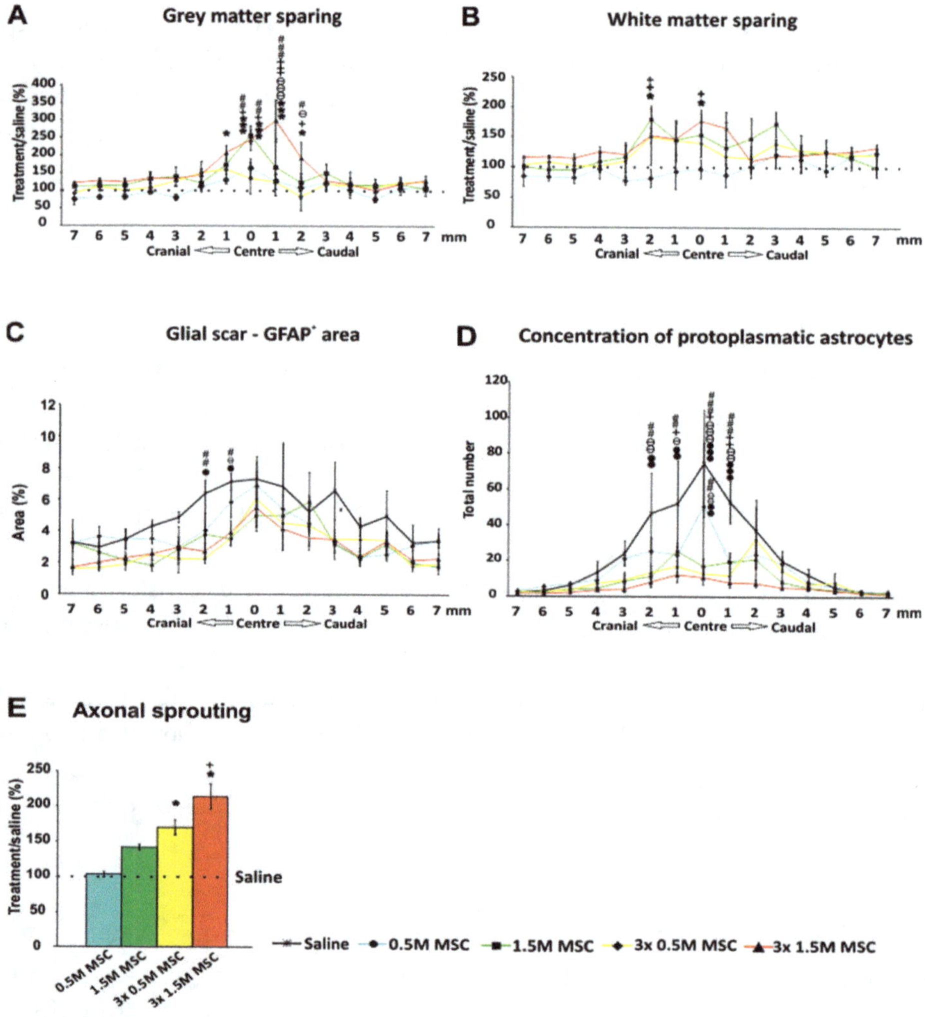

Figure 2. Immunohistochemical and histological analysis 9 weeks after SCI. The total area of spared gray matter was significantly higher in the group treated by 3 × 1.5 M hWJ-MSCs, mainly in the slices near the center of the lesion (**A**). Analysis of the white matter sparing showed similar results to the gray matter, resulting in mild yet still significant preservation in the group treated by 3 × 1.5 M hWJ-MSCs (**B**). The GFAP-CY3 positive area showing the glial scar formation around the central cavity was slightly smaller in all treated groups compared to the control, with a significant difference near the center of the lesion against the groups treated by repetitive doses (**C**). The average number of protoplasmic astrocytes near the center of the lesion was significantly higher in the control group than in the cell-treated groups (**D**). The average number (15 slices per rat; 5 rats) of GAP43+ fibers presented as relative when compared to the control, which is set as 100%. A gradually significant increase with the total number of applied MSCs is shown (**E**).

The dotted line represents the value of saline-treated rats (100%). * $p < 0.05$ versus saline; *** $p < 0.001$ versus saline; + $p < 0.05$ versus 0.5 M MSCs; ++ $p < 0.01$ versus 0.5 M MSCs; +++ $p < 0.001$ versus 0.5 M MSCs; # $p < 0.05$ versus 3 × 0.5 M MSCs; ## $p < 0.01$ versus 3 × 0.5 M MSCs; ### $p < 0.001$ versus 3 × 0.5 M MSCs; ɵ $p < 0.05$ versus 1.5 M MSCs; ɵɵ $p < 0.01$ versus 1.5 M MSCs; ɵɵɵ $p < 0.001$ versus 1.5 M MSCs; • $p < 0.05$ versus 3 × 1.5 M MSCs; •• $p < 0.01$ versus 3 × 1.5 M MSCs; ••• $p < 0.001$ versus 3 × 1.5 M MSCs. MSCs = human Wharton Jelly mesenchymal stem cells; SCI = spinal cord injury; GFAP-CY3 = glial fibrillary acidic protein cyanine 3; GAP43 = growth-associated protein 43.

The anti-inflammatory related genes *Mrc1* and *Cd163* were, 9 weeks after the transplantation, downregulated in all subjected groups with a significant difference in groups 1 × 0.5 M ($p < 0.05$) and 3 × 1.5 M ($p < 0.001$). However, groups treated by a total number of 1.5 M cells (1.5 M and 3 × 0.5 M) were, 4 weeks after transplantation, insignificantly upregulated; thus, their dynamics changed throughout the experiment.

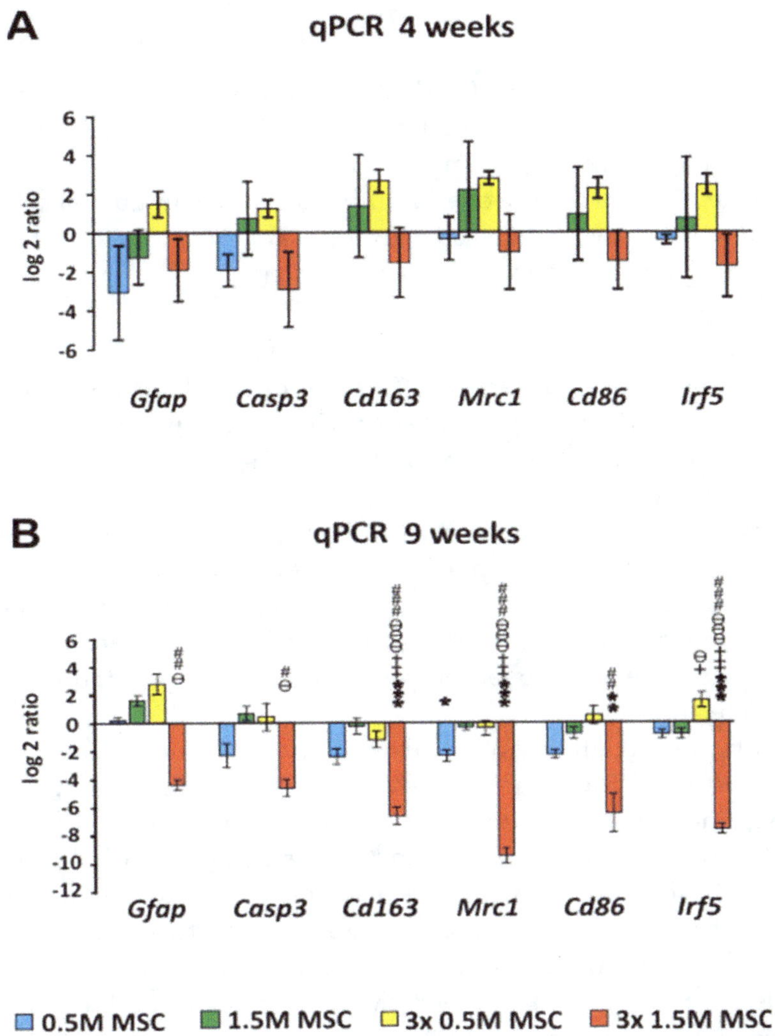

Figure 3. mRNA expression of selected genes 4 and 9 weeks after WJ-MSCs transplantation into the SCI. The graphs show the log2-fold changes of the ΔΔCt values of the indicated genes in comparison to the animals treated with the saline, which were set to 0 and are represented as x axis in the graphs. The expression of genes, which are related to the M1 (*Irf5*, *Cd86*) and M2 (*Mrc1*, *Cd163*) macrophage phenotypes, astrogliosis (*Gfap*), and apoptosis (*Casp3*) are shown 4 weeks after the SCI (**A**) and 9 weeks after the SCI (**B**). All of them were significantly downregulated in the group treated by 3 × 1.5 M and remained stable throughout the whole experiment.

Data are expressed as mean ± SEM. * $p < 0.05$ versus saline; ** $p < 0.01$ versus saline; *** $p < 0.001$ versus saline; + $p < 0.05$ versus 0.5 M MSCs; ++ $p < 0.01$ versus 0.5 M MSCs; +++ $p < 0.001$ versus 0.5 M MSCs; # $p < 0.05$ versus 3 × 0.5 M MSCs; ## $p < 0.01$ versus 3 × 0.5 M MSCs; ### $p < 0.001$ versus 3 × 0.5 M MSCs; ө $p < 0.05$ versus 1.5 M MSCs; өө $p < 0.01$ versus 1.5 M MSCs; өөө $p < 0.001$ versus 1.5 M MSCs. MSC: human Wharton Jelly mesenchymal stem cell; SCI: spinal cord injury; *Mrc1*: mannose receptor C type 1; *Casp3*: Caspase-3; *Gfap*: glial fibrillary acidic protein.

Four weeks after the cell implantation, *Gfap*, except in the 3 × 0.5 M group, was downregulated in all groups; 9 weeks after the cell implantation, it remained downregulated only in the 3 × 1.5 M group, with a significant difference that corresponds with the immunohistochemical analysis of the astrogliosis that was lowest in this group. The expression of *Casp3* insignificantly decreased in the 0.5 M and 3 × 1.5 M groups and remained stable throughout the entire experiment.

(One-way ANOVA, Treatment; *Gfap* − $H_4 = 18.454$, $p = 0.001$, *Casp3* − $H_4 = 15.153$, $p = 0.004$, *Cd163* − $F = 20.243$, $p < 0.001$, *Mrc1* − $F = 59.317$, $p < 0.001$, *Cd86* − $H_4 = 19.170$, $p < 0.001$, *Irf5* − $F = 47.495$, $p < 0.001$; for p values of post hoc pair-to-pair test, see Supplement 4).

2.5. Cell Survival

Survival of the transplanted cells (0.5 M and 1.5 M) was evaluated by staining with the antibody against HuNu, two weeks after the transplantation. Surviving cells were detected as green clusters. Most of the cells remained at the site of the implantation—caught between the folds of arachnoidea mater in the cauda equinae. There was, however, a difference in the number of cells present. While after 0.5 M application only a few cells were detected, the application of 1.5 M resulted in a greater number of trapped cells. No homing into the lesion site was observed.

3. Discussion

The present study aimed to determine the effect and optimal dosage of transplanted stem cells derived from Wharton's jelly into injured spinal cord. Cultured human WJ-MSCs were intrathecally implanted into spinal cord compression lesions of Wistar rats, and the impact on the recovery of the spinal cord tissue was described.

We compared single and triple repeated intrathecal delivery of hWJ-MSCs with a different number of cells (0.5 M and 1.5 M) in each application. Since cell survival in the vertebral canal is rather low [20,22,23], we hypothesized that, by repeated application, the trophic and immunomodulatory effect of the cells can be substantially increased. The route of MSC delivery varies in previous studies, and local or systemic approaches have been proposed and investigated, but the optimal method of delivery has yet to be determined.

We have chosen intrathecal delivery in our experiments. It eliminates the risk of direct surgical implantation without the need for deep analgesia and anaesthesia for the animal, and yet still guarantees a wide dissemination of cells through the subarachnoid space and around the lesion site [24]. The procedure can be done either by lumbar puncture or by suboccipital puncture of the cisterna magna. In our study, we chose lumbar puncture because it is more relevant to clinical medicine, where, especially in adult neurosurgery, it is an everyday occurrence. Additionally, repeated application via lumbar puncture is a lesser burden for animals than a suboccipital puncture of the cisterna magna. Since cell survival in the vertebral canal is rather low (approximately 14 days), repeated application substantially increased the trophic and immunomodulatory effect of the cells and could even be feasible in human patients.

Despite reports showing that intralesional transplantation provides better accumulation of the effector cells in the injury site [25], meta-analyses did not prove any statistical significant differences in locomotor improvement after delivery of MSCs using intravenous, intraparenchymal, and intrathecal administration [15,26]. Moreover, Pal et al. compared hBM-MSC injection into the spinal cord parenchyma and application via lumbar puncture. They reported that, while both i.t. and intraspinal transplantation showed improvement in histological evaluation, only the i.t.-transplanted group performed better in all behavioral tests [27]. Recently intranasal delivery of BM-MSCs with their successful migration into the spinal cord canal was reported, but compared to direct intrathecal delivery, there was significantly lower number of cells detected and the locomotor recovery was insignificant [28].

Besides the determination of transplantation route, optimal timing of transplantation is one of the most important factors to be considered. The subacute phase, defined as the time period between 3 and 14 days post-SCI in rodents and 2 months in humans showed better cell survival as a result of the reduced aggressive host environment due to the inflammation response, and when compared to the acute phase and unlike the chronic phase, the glial scar formation has not yet been formed [18,29,30]. Therefore, we had cell application start 7 days after lesion induction. Another disputable question remains regarding the appropriate dosage of transplanted cells. The vast majority of studies proving the effect of MSCs on SCI have focused only on single transplantation of 0.2–1 M of cells [31–35]. Alternatively, repetition and higher dosage is considered to be superior to single delivery. Li et al. compared single, triple, and quintuple transplantations of 1 M BM-MSCs and concluded that triple delivery is the best [36]. Similar results were found by Cizkova et al. with the conclusion that high doses and/or repetition of the transplantation may lead to higher efficacy of cell survival, more engraftment into the host tissue, and an improvement in functional outcome.

No such experimental study with hWJ-MSCs has been conducted, so evidence of the effect of single vs. multiple deliveries, together with various amounts of cells, is in high demand.

Analysis of behavioral tests revealed that functional recovery of hind limb motion in treated rats was partially dependent on the number of applied cells, which is in agreement with findings by Himes et al., who used a similar number of hBM-MSCs [32]. Whereas the single dose of 0.5 M hWJ-MSCs showed no significant difference in BBB testing, other groups achieved similar significantly higher scores, regardless of repeated application. However, in the advanced motor function testing, such as crossing the beam, the effect was visible in animals with repeated injections. The dose-dependent effect of hBM-MSCs in more advanced motor tests (grid walk and inclined plane test) was also observed by Pal et al. who compared doses of 2 M and 5 M cells/kg body weight [27]. No effect was detected in the rotarod test, which requires a higher level of motor coordination and stepping. Our experimental setting was comparable to our previous study with the hBM-MSCs [20]. However, application of 0.5 M hBM-MSCs resulted in functional improvement similar to the one observed with single application of 1.5 M hWJ-MSCs. It is generally accepted that, due to the low ability of MSCs to survive in the donor tissue, as confirmed in our study, and their limited in vivo differentiation, the main therapeutic effect of MSCs lies in their ability to secrete trophic factors promoting local neovascularization, inhibiting cell death, and suppressing the immune response [37]. We did not perform any in vitro analysis of growth factors and bioactive molecules, which would compare the paracrine effect of hWJ-MSCs and hBM-MSCs. Though various studies include the analysis of secretory factors, results are not unified in terms of the strength of secretion of regeneration-associated neurotrophic factors. Balasubramanian et al. found that WJ-derived cells secreted higher levels of neurotrophic factors bFGF, NGF, NT3, NT4, and GDNF compared to BM and adipose tissue (AT)-derived cells [38]. Hsieh and colleagues compared MSCs derived from Wharton's jelly and bone marrow regarding their ability to regenerate infarcted myocardia; they described secretome differences that make Wharton's jelly-derived MSCs a more angiogenic, neuroprotective, and neurogenic option [39]. On the other hand, Amable et al. reported that WJ-MSCs secreted very low concentrations of VEGF-4.070 and 4.614 times lower than BM- and adipose tissue MSCs (AT-MSCs), respectively [10]. Most studies agree that hWJ-MSCs have a more effective immunosuppressive function compared to hBM-MSCs [40,41]. However, all those studies were performed in vitro, where the proliferation rate of the WJ-MSCs (cell doubling time 40 h) is much higher than the hBM-MSC doubling time of 70 h [42], resulting in more paracrine effective cells in the medium and thus higher overall secretome. Our results confirmed relatively short population doubling time of hWJ-MSCs, which was approximately 34 h compared to 84 h of hBM-MSCs (see Supplement 1, Figure S1). Another possible explanation of the lesser effect of the same number of transplanted cells in our study is the smaller size of WJ-MSCs when compared with BM-MSCs, which can result in higher dilution in the host environment, or even leakage through the canal after the lumbar puncture. On the other hand, due to a smaller size, more cells can fit into small volumes and these cells can more easily spread through the CSF in the canal. Therefore, the dose-dependent effect can be more visible in the case of hWJ-MSCs than in hBM-MSCs.

Immunohistochemical analyses showed that transplantation of hWJ-MSCs facilitates axonal sprouting and plays a role in decreasing glial scar formation. Astrogliosis, which is closely bound up with reactive astrocytes was significantly less present in cell-treated rats. Axonal sprouting was increasingly enhanced as the total number of transplanted cells increased. This is in agreement with the findings of Li et al., who described the effect of WJ-MSCs in SCI as mainly due to the decreased expression of interleukin-1β (IL-1β) and the increased expression of nerve growth factor (NGF), which plays an important role in axonal growth [43]. The same trend was present in the measuring of the white and gray matter preservation, which revealed a strong neuroprotective effect in gray matter, mainly in the center of the lesion and only in groups with the highest number of treated cells. A significant effect on tissue sparing was observed only in animals treated by single or triple implantation of 1.5 M hWJ-MSCs. All these finding are in contrast with behavioral analysis, where no differences between higher dosage cell-treated animal groups were found in the BBB test. It is evident that, for the simple locomotor test, such as the BBB test, a threshold of a minimum number of cells is required to trigger functional improvement. However, closer analyses of tissue microstructure have shown that an increased number of cells applied repeatedly further improve the neuroprotective and neuroregenerative properties of the hWJ-MSCs.

Overall, our results proved a substantial benefit from treatment of SCI with MSCs and are in many ways comparable to other studies that used human BM-MSCs, AT-MSCs, or UC-MSCs in rats [27,32,35,44–49] or dogs [50,51]. Meta-analysis from 2014 by Oliveri confirmed the beneficial effect of MSCs in traumatic spinal cord injury but could not detect any clear association between locomotor recovery and MSCs isolated from specific tissues [15]. Still, because of the relative easy harvesting of hWJ-MSCs from otherwise discarded tissue, we believe that hWJ-MSCs are the most suitable for potential wide use in clinics.

Most of the clinical studies with mesenchymal stromal stem cells were performed on chronic lesions with total paraplegia (Frankel A, AIS A), lasting months after the primary injury [52]. Despite some reports that note some neurological improvement after transplantation [53], the effect of WJ-MSCs in the chronic model of SCI must be elucidated. However, we suggest that this treatment should be proposed for patients with spinal trauma that causes "only" compression of the spinal cord, which is visible in the magnetic resonance imaging (MRI) of T2 and STIR sequences as a hyper intense area of the spinal cord—myelopathia. These patients usually have preserved residual motor and sensory functions (Frankel B and above) and have a good prognosis of recovery when the best medical therapy is applied. hWJ-MSCs, since they are allogenic, can be easily up-scaled, prepared in advance, cryopreserved, and made ready for use in a relatively short time. Therefore, repeated application of hWJ-MSCs could add another piece to the yet unsolvable puzzle of how to treat SCI.

4. Materials and Methods

4.1. Cell Culture

The collection and isolation of WJ-MSCs were performed by explant culture according to the methodology described by Koci et al. [54]. In brief, human WJ-MSCs were obtained from discarded human umbilical cords from healthy full-term neonates after spontaneous delivery, with the informed consent of the donors using the guidelines approved by the Institutional Committee at University Hospital (Pilsen, Czech Republic). About 10–15 cm per umbilical cord were aseptically transported into sterile phosphate buffered saline (PBS; IKEM, Prague, Czech Republic) with antibiotic-antimycotic solution (Sigma, St. Louis, MO, USA) at 4 °C. After the removal of blood vessels, the remaining tissue was cut into small pieces (cca 1 mm^3) and put into Nunc culture dishes (Schoeller, Thermo Fisher Scientific, Waltham, MA, USA) containing the alpha-Minimum Essential Medium (αMEM; East Port, Prague, Czech Republic), supplemented with 5% platelet lysate (IKEM, Prague, Czech Republic) and gentamicin 10 mg/mL (Sandoz, Holzkirchen, Germany), and cultivated at 37 °C in a humidified atmosphere containing 5% CO_2. After 10 days, the explants were removed from the culture dishes, and the remaining adherent cells were cultured for 3 weeks or until 90% confluence and passaged using 0.05% Trypsin/EDTA (Life Technologies, Carlsbad, CA, USA). After passaging, the cells were seeded into culture flasks (Nunc; Schoeller, Thermo Fisher Scientific, Waltham, MA, USA) at a density of 5×10^3 cells/cm^2. The medium was changed twice a week. Cells of the 3rd passage were characterized by flow cytometry and their growth properties and differentiation potential was assessed (see Supplementary Material 1). For the transplantation, cells in the 3rd passage were used.

4.2. Animals

As an experimental model, adult Wistar male rats were used. Animals were obtained from the breeding facility of the Academy of Sciences of the Czech Republic. All experiments were performed in accordance with the European Communities Council Directive of 22nd of September 2010 (2010/63/EU) regarding the use of animals in research and were approved 8 September 2014 by the Professional Committee for Laboratory Animal Welfare of the Institute of Experimental Medicine, Academy of Sciences of the Czech Republic in Prague as the experimental project number 53/2014. All animals were approximately 10 weeks old, with weight varying between 275–305 g (n = 90). The first group of animals (n = 47), surviving 9 weeks, was used for behavioral testing, histological, immunohistochemical, and qPCR analysis (9W). The second group of animals (n = 39) was used for qPCR evaluation 4 weeks (4W) after SCI and was not included in behavioral testing. An additional four animals in the two groups (n = 4) were used for evaluation of surviving cells two weeks after transplantation of 0.5 and 1.5 M hWJ-MSCs.

4.3. Spinal Cord Injury Model

The surgical procedure was performed in an operating theatre under standard conditions. As a model of SCI, a balloon-induced ischemic-compression lesion was used [21,55]. At the beginning of the surgery, the animals were anesthetized with Isoflurane (Forane; Abbott Laboratories, Queenborough, UK), analgesia was induced by intramuscular injection of carprofen (Rimadyl, Cymedica, Horovice, Czech Republic, 4 mg/kg), and surgical prophylaxis was maintained by intramuscular injection gentamicin sulfate (Sandoz, Holzkirchen, Germany 5 mg/kg). After the skin incision, the paravertebral muscles were separated at the level of thoracic vertebra T7–T12 and laminectomy of T 10 was performed. A sterile 2-french Fogarty catheter was carefully inserted into the epidural space until the center of the balloon rested on the level of thoracic vertebra 8 (T8). The balloon was rapidly inflated with 15 μL saline and kept for 5 min. During this procedure, 3% isoflurane in air was administered at a flow rate of 0.3 L/min, and the animal's body temperature was kept at 37 °C with a heating pad. After 5 min, the catheter was rapidly deflated and removed, and separated muscles and incised skin were sutured by single non-absorbable stitches. The lesioned animals were assisted in feeding and urination until they had recovered sufficiently to perform these functions on their own. The animals received gentamicin sulfate (5 mg/kg) for 7 days to prevent postoperative infections and were allowed to feed and drink ad libitum.

4.4. Transplantation

Transplantation of hWJ-MSCs was performed on the 7th, 14th, and 21st day after the SCI. Treatment was given intrathecally by a lumbar puncture between L3 and L4 or L4 and L5 through a 25 G needle under the short-time general anaesthesia described above. Firstly, a small volume of CSF was taped as a proof of the subarachnoid space. During the injection of the saline with hWJ-MSCs there was a movement of the rats tail as a response to irritation of the nerve roots of cauda equina. After injection the needle was rested in situ for 30 s to prevent backflow of the content. Animals were divided into 5 groups with variable treatment. The first group (**0.5 M**) received a single transplantation of 0.5 M hWJ-MSCs in 50 μL saline on the 7th day after SCI (n = 12). The second group (**1.5 M**) received a single transplantation of 1.5 M hWJ-MSCs in 50 μL saline on the 7th day after SCI (n = 9). The third group (**3 × 0.5 M**) received a triple transplantation of 0.5 M hWJ-MSCs in 50 μL saline on the 7th, 14th, and 21st day after SCI (n = 8). The fourth group (**3 × 1.5 M**) received a triple transplantation of 1.5 M hWJ-MSCs in 50 μL saline on the 7th, 14th, and 21st day after SCI (n = 7). The control group (**saline**) received a single or triple injection of 50 μL saline on the 7th (14th and 21st) day after SCI (n = 11). No differences between simple and repetitive transplantation of the saline were found, so the results were pooled together as a single control when compared with other types of treatment. The day before the transplantation, all animals received cyclosporine A by an intraperitoneal injection (10 mg/kg), which continued daily until the end of the experiment.

4.5. Behavioral Analysis

4.5.1. BBB Test

The BBB open field test, originally described by Basso, Beattie, and Bresnaham [56] was used to assess the joint movement, weight support, forelimb-hindlimb coordination, paw placement and stability of the body. The rats were placed on the floor surrounded by boundaries making a rectangular shape. Results were evaluated in the range of 0–21 points: 0 indicated complete lack of motor capability and 21 indicated the best possible score (healthy rat). Measurements were performed every week for 8 weeks starting the first week after SCI.

4.5.2. Rotarod Test

A rotarod unit machine (Ugo Basile, Comerio, Italy) was used to test the advanced degree of motor coordination of the limbs according to the method first described by Dunham and Miya [57]. Ability to balance on a rotating rod was recorded. Each animal was taught this task one week before surgery. Animals were placed on a rotating rod at a fixed speed of 10 rpm before surgery and 5 rpm after surgery and were left to walk for 60 s. There were four trials per day within five consecutive days. Between trials there was always a 5 min break. The latency to fall off the rod onto the floor was measured.

4.5.3. Beam Walk Test

In the flat beam test, we tested the ability to cross a 1 m long narrow beam with a flat surface. Rats were placed on one side of the beam, and on the other side an escape box was placed. The latency and the trajectory to traverse the beam were recorded by a video tracking system (TSE-Systems Inc., Bad Homburg, Germany) for a maximum of 60 s. Performance of locomotor coordination was evaluated using a 0–7 point scale modified from Metz and Whishaw [58].

4.6. Histological and Immunohistochemical Analyses

At the end of the experiment (9 weeks after the SCI), all animals were anesthetized with ketamine (100 mg/kg) and xylazine (20 mg/kg) and transcardially perfused with a phosphate buffer solution (250 mL), followed by a 4% paraformaldehyde solution in a phosphate buffer (250 mL). The spinal cord was dissected and removed from the spinal column and embedded in paraffin wax. Serial cross sections (5 μm thick) were obtained by microtome within a 2-cm-long segment around the center of the lesion. Samples of five animals from each group were analyzed for the total volume of spared white and gray matter, axonal sprouting, and the extent of glial scar. Sections were stained with Luxol fast blue and Cresyl violet to distinguish the white and gray matter, with anti-GAP43 antibody to evaluate axonal sprouting or by anti-GFAP primary antibody to visualize the glial scar and reactive astrocytes.

4.6.1. Cresyl Violet-Luxol Staining

For visualizing white and gray matter of the spinal cord, Cresyl violet and Luxol fast blue staining were used. Samples from five animals from each group were obtained. Each sample of the spinal cord was cut at 1 mm intervals. A total number of 15 cross sections, including the center of the lesion, were observed with an Axioskop 2 plus microscope (Zeiss, Oberkochen, Germany). Acquired images were analyzed for the total area of spared gray and white matter by ImageJ software (NIH, Bethesda, MD, USA) (Figure 4A).

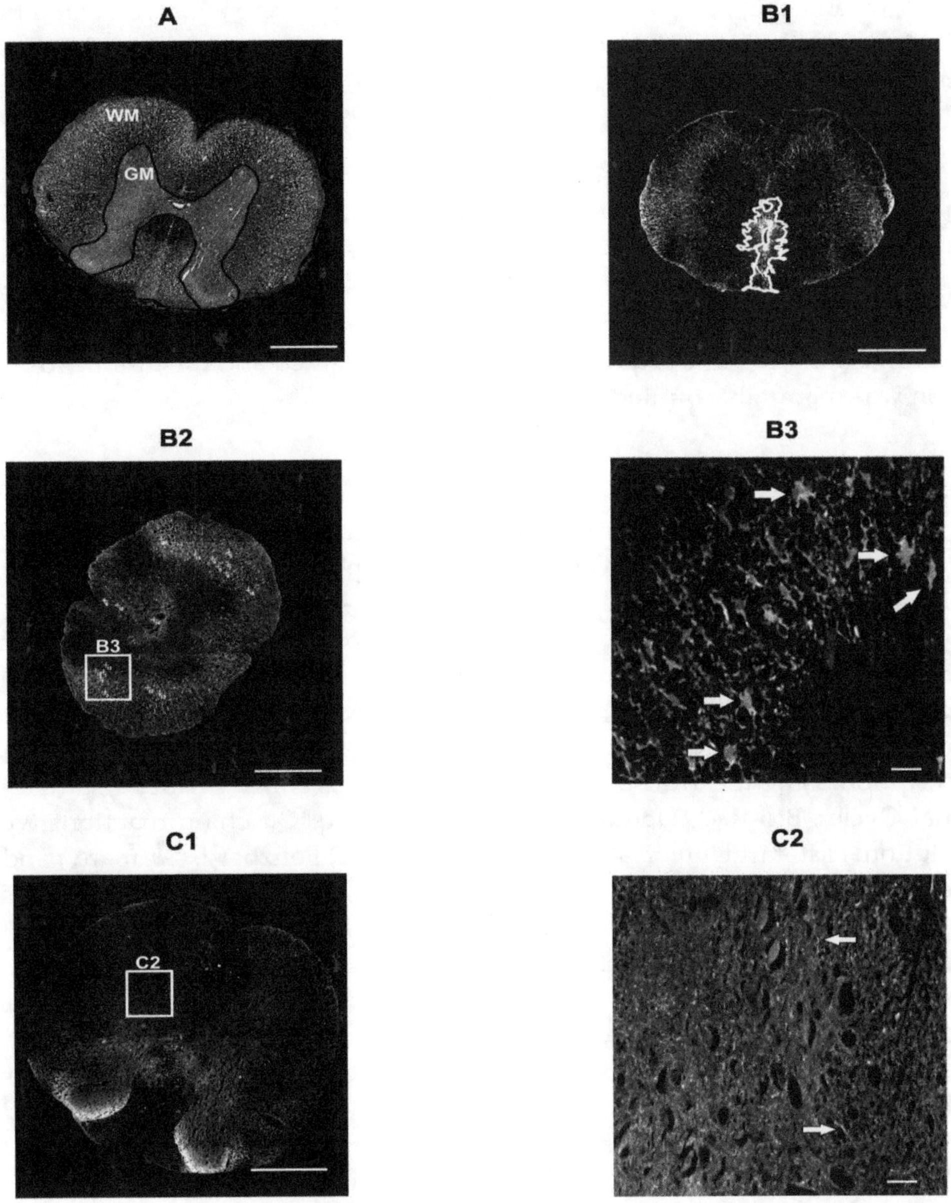

Figure 4. Illustrative images of morphometric and immunohistochemical analyses 9 weeks after SCI. Microscopic image of a section stained with Cresyl violet and Luxol fast blue to distinguish the white (WM) and gray (GM) matter (**A**). Scale bar: 500 μm. The marked glial scar around the main cavity (**B1**) and the total number of protoplasmatic astrocytes (**B2**) with a detailed inset (**B3**) from slices stained with GFAP-CY3. Scale bars: 500 μm (**B1**,**B2**), 10 μm (**B3**). Illustrative image of a section labeled with a GAP43^{+} antibody (**C1**) with a detailed inset (**C2**).

Arrows point at GAP43^{+} fibers, which were manually counted as described in the Methods section. Scale bars: 500 μm (**C1**), 20 μm (**C2**). SCI: spinal cord injury; GM: gray matter; WM: white matter; GFAP-CY3: glial fibrillary acidic protein cyanine 3; GAP43: growth-associated protein 43.

4.6.2. GFAP Staining

To determine the extent of the glial scar, immunohistochemical analysis of a CY3-conjugated primary antibody against GFAP (Sigma, St. Louis, MO, USA) was used. Samples from five animals from each group were obtained. Each sample of the spinal cord was cut at 1 mm intervals. A total number of 15 cross sections, including the center of the lesion, was observed with an Axioskop 2 plus microscope (Zeiss, Oberkochen, Germany). The acquired images were analyzed using ImageJ software (NIH, Bethesda, MD, USA). The GFAP positive area around the central cavity (Figure 4(B1)) together with the number of protoplasmic astrocytes (Figure 4(B2,B3)) was measured on each section.

4.6.3. GAP43 Staining

The newly sprouted axons were visualized immunohistochemically using a primary antibody against GAP43 (Millipore, Billerica, MA, USA). Samples from five animals from each group were obtained. Each sample of the spinal cord was cut at 1 mm intervals. A total number of 15 cross sections, including the center of the lesion, were observed with an Axioskop 2 plus microscope (Zeiss, Oberkochen, Germany). The acquired images were analyzed and the number of GAP43-positive fibers per section was manually counted (Figure 4(C1,C2)).

4.7. *qRT-PCR*

To evaluate the up- or downregulation of expression rat target genes (*Gfap*, *Mrc1*, *Irf5*, *Cd163*, *Cd86*, *Casp3*) the quantitative real-time reverse transcription polymerase chain reaction (qRT-PCR) was used. Expression was evaluated at 4 and 9 weeks after hWJ-MSC administration (five animals from each group). Studied RNA was isolated from the paraffin cross sections of injured spinal cord around the center of the lesion using the High Pure RNA Paraffin Kit (Roche, Penzberg, Germany) following the manufacturer's recommendations. The amount of RNA was measured by a spectrophotometer (NanoPhotometerTM P-Class, Munchen, Germany). cDNA was obtained from the isolated RNA by a reverse transcription using the Transcriptor Universal cDNA Master (Roche), and a thermal cycler (T100™ Thermal Cycler, Bio-Rad, Hercules, CA, USA). The qPCR chain reactions were performed using cDNA solution, FastStart Universal Probe Master (Roche, Penzberg, Germany) and the following TagMan® Gene Expression Assays (Life Technologies): Casp3/Rn00563902_m1, Gfap/Rn00566603_m1, Cd86/Rn00571654_m1, Irf5/Rn01500522_m1, Mrc1/Rn01487342_m1, and Cd163/Rn01492519_m1.

The final solution of 25 ng extracted RNA diluted in 10 μL of solution was amplified on a StepOnePlus™ real-time PCR cycler (StepOnePlus™, Life Technologies, Carlsbad, CA, USA). The process of amplification was repeatedly performed under the same standard conditions: 120 s at 50 °C, 300 s at 95 °C, followed by 40 cycles of 15 s at 95 °C and 60 s at 60 °C. Each array included also a negative control (water). As a reference gene, Gapdh was used. The ΔΔCt method was used for relative quantification of gene expression. All results were analyzed with StepOnePlus® software (StepOnePlus™, Life Technologies, Carlsbad, CA, USA). Differences between the transplanted and control (saline) groups were analyzed for statistical significance with ΔCt values level, using a one-way ANOVA test with a post hoc pair-to-pair test. Differences were considered statistically significant if $p < 0.05$. Data are expressed as the mean ± the standard error of mean. The values of saline-treated animals were set as zero.

4.8. Statistical Analyses

Presented graphs with obtained data are shown as the mean ± SEM. The statistical significance between the groups treated by WJ-MSCs and the saline (control) group was assessed using either one-way ANOVA, or two-way ANOVA in the case of a second factor (time). Differences between the groups in behavioral tests and in areal measuring of the gray/white matter sparing and GFAP positive area of glial scar were assessed by two-way repeated measurement (RM) ANOVA. The Student–Newman–Keuls (SNK) post hoc pair-to-pair test was used to specify for which groups and at which time points the changes were significant. Statistical evaluation of the expression of the rat target genes was performed with one-way ANOVA test with a post hoc pair-to-pair test. In case of non-parametric values Kruskal–Wallis one-way ANOVA on ranks test was used. (All in Sigmastat 3.1, Sistat Software Inc., San Jose, CA, USA). Differences were considered statistically significant if $p < 0.05$.

5. Conclusions

Implantation of human MSCs derived from Wharton's jelly improves functional outcome, by modulating the inflammatory response, inducing axonal sprouting and remodeling the glial scar. The effect is dose-dependent, with the best result achieved by repeated delivery.

Author Contributions: P.K.: study conception and design, experimentation, collection and/or assembly of data, data analysis and interpretation, manuscript writing, and final approval of the manuscript; I.V.: study conception and design, and provision of study material; J.R.: study conception and design; L.M.U.: study conception and design; K.Z.: collection and/or assembly of data; J.D.: collection and/or assembly of data; Z.K.: collection and/or assembly of data, data analysis and interpretation, and manuscript writing; K.T.: collection and/or assembly of data; S.K.: qRT PCR data analysis and interpretation, manuscript writing; S.R.: study conception and design, and financial support; P.J.: study conception and design, data analysis and interpretation, manuscript writing, financial support, and final approval of the manuscript.

Acknowledgments: This study was supported by the Czech Science Foundation GACR P304/12/G069; GACR 17-03765S, Operational Programme Research, Development and Education in the framework of the project "Center of Reconstructive Neuroscience", registration number CZ.02.1.01/0.0./0.0/15_003/0000419 and from EATRIS-CZ (LM2015064). K.Z.. S.K., I.V., L.M.U. and P.J. were members of the BIOCEV (CZ.1.05/1.1.00/02.0109) and their work was supported by the Ministry of Education, Youth and Sports of CR within the LQ1604 National Sustainability Program II (Project BIOCEV-FAR).

References

1. Fawcett, J.W.; Asher, R.A. The glial scar and central nervous system repair. *Brain Res. Bull.* **1999**, *49*, 377–391. [CrossRef]
2. Zai, L.J.; Wrathall, J.R. Cell proliferation and replacement following contusive spinal cord injury. *Glia* **2005**, *50*, 247–257. [CrossRef] [PubMed]
3. Mbalaviele, G.; Jaiswal, N.; Meng, A.; Cheng, L.; Van Den Bos, C.; Thiede, M. Human mesenchymal stem cells promote human osteoclast differentiation from CD34+ bone marrow hematopoietic progenitors. *Endocrinology* **1999**, *140*, 3736–3743. [CrossRef] [PubMed]
4. Woodbury, D.; Schwarz, E.J.; Prockop, D.J.; Black, I.B. Adult rat and human bone marrow stromal cells differentiate into neurons. *J. Neurosci. Res.* **2000**, *61*, 364–370. [CrossRef]
5. Toma, C.; Pittenger, M.F.; Cahill, K.S.; Byrne, B.J.; Kessler, P.D. Human mesenchymal stem cells differentiate to a cardiomyocyte phenotype in the adult murine heart. *Circulation* **2002**, *105*, 93–98. [CrossRef] [PubMed]
6. Bai, L.; Lennon, D.P.; Eaton, V.; Maier, K.; Caplan, A.I.; Miller, S.D.; Miller, R.H. Human bone marrow-derived mesenchymal stem cells induce th2-polarized immune response and promote endogenous repair in animal models of multiple sclerosis. *Glia* **2009**, *57*, 1192–1203. [CrossRef] [PubMed]
7. Park, C.W.; Kim, K.S.; Bae, S.; Son, H.K.; Myung, P.K.; Hong, H.J.; Kim, H. Cytokine secretion profiling of human mesenchymal stem cells by antibody array. *Int. J. Stem Cells* **2009**, *2*, 59–68. [CrossRef] [PubMed]
8. Torres-Espin, A.; Corona-Quintanilla, D.L.; Fores, J.; Allodi, I.; Gonzalez, F.; Udina, E.; Navarro, X. Neuroprotection and axonal regeneration after lumbar ventral root avulsion by re-implantation and mesenchymal stem cells transplant combined therapy. *Neurotherapeutics* **2013**, *10*, 354–368. [CrossRef] [PubMed]

9. Caplan, A.I. Mesenchymal stem cells: Time to change the name! *Stem Cells Transl. Med.* **2017**, *6*, 1445–1451. [CrossRef] [PubMed]
10. Amable, P.R.; Teixeira, M.V.; Carias, R.B.; Granjeiro, J.M.; Borojevic, R. Protein synthesis and secretion in human mesenchymal cells derived from bone marrow, adipose tissue and wharton's jelly. *Stem Cell Res. Ther.* **2014**, *5*, 53. [CrossRef] [PubMed]
11. Zhou, C.; Yang, B.; Tian, Y.; Jiao, H.; Zheng, W.; Wang, J.; Guan, F. Immunomodulatory effect of human umbilical cord wharton's jelly-derived mesenchymal stem cells on lymphocytes. *Cell. Immunol.* **2011**, *272*, 33–38. [CrossRef] [PubMed]
12. Kim, D.W.; Staples, M.; Shinozuka, K.; Pantcheva, P.; Kang, S.D.; Borlongan, C.V. Wharton's jelly-derived mesenchymal stem cells: Phenotypic characterization and optimizing their therapeutic potential for clinical applications. *Int. J. Mol. Sci.* **2013**, *14*, 11692–11712. [CrossRef] [PubMed]
13. Zhang, J.; Li, Y.; Chen, J.; Yang, M.; Katakowski, M.; Lu, M.; Chopp, M. Expression of insulin-like growth factor 1 and receptor in ischemic rats treated with human marrow stromal cells. *Brain Res.* **2004**, *1030*, 19–27. [CrossRef] [PubMed]
14. Bao, X.; Wei, J.; Feng, M.; Lu, S.; Li, G.; Dou, W.; Ma, W.; Ma, S.; An, Y.; Qin, C.; et al. Transplantation of human bone marrow-derived mesenchymal stem cells promotes behavioral recovery and endogenous neurogenesis after cerebral ischemia in rats. *Brain Res.* **2011**, *1367*, 103–113. [CrossRef] [PubMed]
15. Oliveri, R.S.; Bello, S.; Biering-Sorensen, F. Mesenchymal stem cells improve locomotor recovery in traumatic spinal cord injury: Systematic review with meta-analyses of rat models. *Neurobiol. Dis.* **2014**, *62*, 338–353. [CrossRef] [PubMed]
16. Saito, F.; Nakatani, T.; Iwase, M.; Maeda, Y.; Murao, Y.; Suzuki, Y.; Fukushima, M.; Ide, C. Administration of cultured autologous bone marrow stromal cells into cerebrospinal fluid in spinal injury patients: A pilot study. *Restor. Neurol. Neurosci.* **2012**, *30*, 127–136. [PubMed]
17. Forostyak, S.; Jendelova, P.; Sykova, E. The role of mesenchymal stromal cells in spinal cord injury, regenerative medicine and possible clinical applications. *Biochimie* **2013**, *95*, 2257–2270. [CrossRef] [PubMed]
18. Cizkova, D.; Novotna, I.; Slovinska, L.; Vanicky, I.; Jergova, S.; Rosocha, J.; Radonak, J. Repetitive intrathecal catheter delivery of bone marrow mesenchymal stromal cells improves functional recovery in a rat model of contusive spinal cord injury. *J. Neurotrauma* **2011**, *28*, 1951–1961. [CrossRef] [PubMed]
19. Cheng, I.; Mayle, R.E.; Cox, C.A.; Park, D.Y.; Smith, R.L.; Corcoran-Schwartz, I.; Ponnusamy, K.E.; Oshtory, R.; Smuck, M.W.; Mitra, R.; et al. Functional assessment of the acute local and distal transplantation of human neural stem cells after spinal cord injury. *Spine J.* **2012**, *12*, 1040–1044. [CrossRef] [PubMed]
20. Urdzikova, L.M.; Ruzicka, J.; LaBagnara, M.; Karova, K.; Kubinova, S.; Jirakova, K.; Murali, R.; Sykova, E.; Jhanwar-Uniyal, M.; Jendelova, P. Human mesenchymal stem cells modulate inflammatory cytokines after spinal cord injury in rat. *Int. J. Mol. Sci.* **2014**, *15*, 11275–11293. [CrossRef] [PubMed]
21. Vanicky, I.; Urdzikova, L.; Saganova, K.; Cizkova, D.; Galik, J. A simple and reproducible model of spinal cord injury induced by epidural balloon inflation in the rat. *J. Neurotrauma* **2001**, *18*, 1399–1407. [CrossRef] [PubMed]
22. Antonic, A.; Sena, E.S.; Lees, J.S.; Wills, T.E.; Skeers, P.; Batchelor, P.E.; Macleod, M.R.; Howells, D.W. Stem cell transplantation in traumatic spinal cord injury: A systematic review and meta-analysis of animal studies. *PLoS Biol.* **2013**, *11*, e1001738. [CrossRef] [PubMed]
23. Ruzicka, J.; Machova-Urdzikova, L.; Gillick, J.; Amemori, T.; Romanyuk, N.; Karova, K.; Zaviskova, K.; Dubisova, J.; Kubinova, S.; Murali, R.; et al. A comparative study of three different types of stem cells for treatment of rat spinal cord injury. *Cell Transplant* **2017**, *26*, 585–603. [CrossRef] [PubMed]
24. Amemori, T.; Ruzicka, J.; Romanyuk, N.; Jhanwar-Uniyal, M.; Sykova, E.; Jendelova, P. Comparison of intraspinal and intrathecal implantation of induced pluripotent stem cell-derived neural precursors for the treatment of spinal cord injury in rats. *Stem Cell Res. Ther.* **2015**, *6*, 257. [CrossRef] [PubMed]
25. Paul, C.; Samdani, A.F.; Betz, R.R.; Fischer, I.; Neuhuber, B. Grafting of human bone marrow stromal cells into spinal cord injury: A comparison of delivery methods. *Spine* **2009**, *34*, 328–334. [CrossRef] [PubMed]
26. Sareen, D.; Gowing, G.; Sahabian, A.; Staggenborg, K.; Paradis, R.; Avalos, P.; Latter, J.; Ornelas, L.; Garcia, L.; Svendsen, C.N. Human induced pluripotent stem cells are a novel source of neural progenitor cells (iNPCs) that migrate and integrate in the rodent spinal cord. *J. Comp. Neurol.* **2014**, *522*, 2707–2728. [CrossRef] [PubMed]

27. Pal, R.; Gopinath, C.; Rao, N.M.; Banerjee, P.; Krishnamoorthy, V.; Venkataramana, N.K.; Totey, S. Functional recovery after transplantation of bone marrow-derived human mesenchymal stromal cells in a rat model of spinal cord injury. *Cytotherapy* **2010**, *12*, 792–806. [CrossRef] [PubMed]
28. Ninomiya, K.; Iwatsuki, K.; Ohnishi, Y.; Ohkawa, T.; Yoshimine, T. Intranasal delivery of bone marrow stromal cells to spinal cord lesions. *J. Neurosurg. Spine* **2015**, *23*, 111–119. [CrossRef] [PubMed]
29. Okada, S.; Ishii, K.; Yamane, J.; Iwanami, A.; Ikegami, T.; Katoh, H.; Iwamoto, Y.; Nakamura, M.; Miyoshi, H.; Okano, H.J.; et al. In vivo imaging of engrafted neural stem cells: Its application in evaluating the optimal timing of transplantation for spinal cord injury. *FASEB J.* **2005**, *19*, 1839–1841. [CrossRef] [PubMed]
30. Parr, A.M.; Kulbatski, I.; Tator, C.H. Transplantation of adult rat spinal cord stem/progenitor cells for spinal cord injury. *J. Neurotrauma* **2007**, *24*, 835–845. [CrossRef] [PubMed]
31. Chen, C.; Chen, F.; Yao, C.; Shu, S.; Feng, J.; Hu, X.; Hai, Q.; Yao, S.; Chen, X. Intrathecal injection of human umbilical cord-derived mesenchymal stem cells ameliorates neuropathic pain in rats. *Neurochem. Res.* **2016**, *41*, 3250–3260. [CrossRef] [PubMed]
32. Himes, B.T.; Neuhuber, B.; Coleman, C.; Kushner, R.; Swanger, S.A.; Kopen, G.C.; Wagner, J.; Shumsky, J.S.; Fischer, I. Recovery of function following grafting of human bone marrow-derived stromal cells into the injured spinal cord. *Neurorehabilit. Neural Repair* **2006**, *20*, 278–296. [CrossRef] [PubMed]
33. Amemori, T.; Jendelova, P.; Ruzickova, K.; Arboleda, D.; Sykova, E. Co-transplantation of olfactory ensheathing glia and mesenchymal stromal cells does not have synergistic effects after spinal cord injury in the rat. *Cytotherapy* **2010**, *12*, 212–225. [CrossRef] [PubMed]
34. Cho, S.R.; Kim, Y.R.; Kang, H.S.; Yim, S.H.; Park, C.I.; Min, Y.H.; Lee, B.H.; Shin, J.C.; Lim, J.B. Functional recovery after the transplantation of neurally differentiated mesenchymal stem cells derived from bone marrow in a rat model of spinal cord injury. *Cell Transplant.* **2009**, *18*, 1359–1368. [CrossRef] [PubMed]
35. Hu, S.L.; Luo, H.S.; Li, J.T.; Xia, Y.Z.; Li, L.; Zhang, L.J.; Meng, H.; Cui, G.Y.; Chen, Z.; Wu, N.; et al. Functional recovery in acute traumatic spinal cord injury after transplantation of human umbilical cord mesenchymal stem cells. *Crit. Care Med.* **2010**, *38*, 2181–2189. [CrossRef] [PubMed]
36. Li, H.; Wen, Y.; Luo, Y.; Lan, X.; Wang, D.; Sun, Z.; Hu, L. Transplantation of bone marrow mesenchymal stem cells into spinal cord injury: A comparison of delivery different times. *Zhongguo Xiu Fu Chong Jian Wai Ke Za Zhi* **2010**, *24*, 180–184. [PubMed]
37. Bollini, S.; Gentili, C.; Tasso, R.; Cancedda, R. The regenerative role of the fetal and adult stem cell secretome. *J. Clin. Med.* **2013**, *2*, 302–327. [CrossRef] [PubMed]
38. Balasubramanian, S.; Thej, C.; Venugopal, P.; Priya, N.; Zakaria, Z.; Sundarraj, S.; Majumdar, A.S. Higher propensity of wharton's jelly derived mesenchymal stromal cells towards neuronal lineage in comparison to those derived from adipose and bone marrow. *Cell Biol. Int.* **2013**, *37*, 507–515. [CrossRef] [PubMed]
39. Hsieh, J.Y.; Wang, H.W.; Chang, S.J.; Liao, K.H.; Lee, I.H.; Lin, W.S.; Wu, C.H.; Lin, W.Y.; Cheng, S.M. Mesenchymal stem cells from human umbilical cord express preferentially secreted factors related to neuroprotection, neurogenesis, and angiogenesis. *PLoS ONE* **2013**, *8*, e72604. [CrossRef] [PubMed]
40. Drela, K.; Lech, W.; Figiel-Dabrowska, A.; Zychowicz, M.; Mikula, M.; Sarnowska, A.; Domanska-Janik, K. Enhanced neuro-therapeutic potential of wharton's jelly-derived mesenchymal stem cells in comparison with bone marrow mesenchymal stem cells culture. *Cytotherapy* **2016**, *18*, 497–509. [CrossRef] [PubMed]
41. Shi, C. Recent progress toward understanding the physiological function of bone marrow mesenchymal stem cells. *Immunology* **2012**, *136*, 133–138. [CrossRef] [PubMed]
42. Li, X.; Bai, J.; Ji, X.; Li, R.; Xuan, Y.; Wang, Y. Comprehensive characterization of four different populations of human mesenchymal stem cells as regards their immune properties, proliferation and differentiation. *Int. J. Mol. Med.* **2014**, *34*, 695–704. [CrossRef] [PubMed]
43. Li, C.; Chen, X.; Qiao, S.; Liu, X.; Liu, C.; Zhu, D.; Su, J.; Wang, Z. Effects of wharton's jelly cells of the human umbilical cord on acute spinal cord injury in rats, and expression of interleukin-1beta and nerve growth factor in spinal cord tissues. *Artif. Cells Nanomed. Biotechnol.* **2016**, *44*, 1254–1258. [CrossRef] [PubMed]
44. Lee, K.H.; Suh-Kim, H.; Choi, J.S.; Jeun, S.S.; Kim, E.J.; Kim, S.S.; Yoon, D.H.; Lee, B.H. Human mesenchymal stem cell transplantation promotes functional recovery following acute spinal cord injury in rats. *Acta Neurobiol. Exp.* **2007**, *67*, 13–22.

45. Nakajima, H.; Uchida, K.; Guerrero, A.R.; Watanabe, S.; Sugita, D.; Takeura, N.; Yoshida, A.; Long, G.; Wright, K.T.; Johnson, W.E.; et al. Transplantation of mesenchymal stem cells promotes an alternative pathway of macrophage activation and functional recovery after spinal cord injury. *J. Neurotrauma* **2012**, *29*, 1614–1625. [CrossRef] [PubMed]
46. Oh, J.S.; Park, I.S.; Kim, K.N.; Yoon, D.H.; Kim, S.H.; Ha, Y. Transplantation of an adipose stem cell cluster in a spinal cord injury. *Neuroreport* **2012**, *23*, 277–282. [CrossRef] [PubMed]
47. Park, S.I.; Lim, J.Y.; Jeong, C.H.; Kim, S.M.; Jun, J.A.; Jeun, S.S.; Oh, W.I. Human umbilical cord blood-derived mesenchymal stem cell therapy promotes functional recovery of contused rat spinal cord through enhancement of endogenous cell proliferation and oligogenesis. *J. Biomed. Biotechnol.* **2012**, *2012*, 362473. [CrossRef] [PubMed]
48. Shang, A.J.; Hong, S.Q.; Xu, Q.; Wang, H.Y.; Yang, Y.; Wang, Z.F.; Xu, B.N.; Jiang, X.D.; Xu, R.X. Nt-3-secreting human umbilical cord mesenchymal stromal cell transplantation for the treatment of acute spinal cord injury in rats. *Brain Res.* **2011**, *1391*, 102–113. [CrossRef] [PubMed]
49. Matyas, J.J.; Stewart, A.N.; Goldsmith, A.; Nan, Z.; Skeel, R.L.; Rossignol, J.; Dunbar, G.L. Effects of bone-marrow-derived msc transplantation on functional recovery in a rat model of spinal cord injury: Comparisons of transplant locations and cell concentrations. *Cell Transplant.* **2017**, *26*, 1472–1482. [CrossRef] [PubMed]
50. Gabr, H.; El-Kheir, W.A.; Farghali, H.A.; Ismail, Z.M.; Zickri, M.B.; El Maadawi, Z.M.; Kishk, N.A.; Sabaawy, H.E. Intrathecal transplantation of autologous adherent bone marrow cells induces functional neurological recovery in a canine model of spinal cord injury. *Cell Transplant.* **2015**, *24*, 1813–1827. [CrossRef] [PubMed]
51. Ryu, H.H.; Kang, B.J.; Park, S.S.; Kim, Y.; Sung, G.J.; Woo, H.M.; Kim, W.H.; Kweon, O.K. Comparison of mesenchymal stem cells derived from fat, bone marrow, wharton's jelly, and umbilical cord blood for treating spinal cord injuries in dogs. *J. Vet. Med. Sci.* **2012**, *74*, 1617–1630. [CrossRef] [PubMed]
52. Satti, H.S.; Waheed, A.; Ahmed, P.; Ahmed, K.; Akram, Z.; Aziz, T.; Satti, T.M.; Shahbaz, N.; Khan, M.A.; Malik, S.A. Autologous mesenchymal stromal cell transplantation for spinal cord injury: A phase I pilot study. *Cytotherapy* **2016**, *18*, 518–522. [CrossRef] [PubMed]
53. Mendonca, M.V.; Larocca, T.F.; de Freitas Souza, B.S.; Villarreal, C.F.; Silva, L.F.; Matos, A.C.; Novaes, M.A.; Bahia, C.M.; de Oliveira Melo Martinez, A.C.; Kaneto, C.M.; et al. Safety and neurological assessments after autologous transplantation of bone marrow mesenchymal stem cells in subjects with chronic spinal cord injury. *Stem Cell Res. Ther.* **2014**, *5*, 126. [CrossRef] [PubMed]
54. Koci, Z.; Vyborny, K.; Dubisova, J.; Vackova, I.; Jager, A.; Lunov, O.; Jirakova, K.; Kubinova, S. Extracellular matrix hydrogel derived from human umbilical cord as a scaffold for neural tissue repair and its comparison with extracellular matrix from porcine tissues. *Tissue Eng. Part C Methods* **2017**, *23*, 333–345. [CrossRef] [PubMed]
55. Parr, A.M.; Kulbatski, I.; Zahir, T.; Wang, X.; Yue, C.; Keating, A.; Tator, C.H. Transplanted adult spinal cord-derived neural stem/progenitor cells promote early functional recovery after rat spinal cord injury. *Neuroscience* **2008**, *155*, 760–770. [CrossRef] [PubMed]
56. Yang, J.R.; Liao, C.H.; Pang, C.Y.; Huang, L.L.; Chen, Y.L.; Shiue, Y.L.; Chen, L.R. Transplantation of porcine embryonic stem cells and their derived neuronal progenitors in a spinal cord injury rat model. *Cytotherapy* **2013**, *15*, 201–208. [CrossRef] [PubMed]
57. Dunham, N.W.; Miya, T.S. A note on a simple apparatus for detecting neurological deficit in rats and mice. *J. Am. Pharm. Assoc.* **1957**, *46*, 208–209. [CrossRef]
58. Metz, G.A.; Whishaw, I.Q. The ladder rung walking task: A scoring system and its practical application. *J. Vis. Exp.* **2009**. [CrossRef] [PubMed]

12

Combined Transcriptomics, Proteomics and Bioinformatics Identify Drug Targets in Spinal Cord Injury

Jure Tica [1], Elizabeth J. Bradbury [2] and Athanasios Didangelos [3,*]

1 Imperial College London, Alexander Fleming Building, London SW7 2AZ, UK; j.tica16@imperial.ac.uk
2 King's College London, Wolfson CARD, Institute of Psychiatry, Psychology & Neuroscience, London SE1 1UL, UK; elizabeth.bradbury@kcl.ac.uk
3 Department of Infection, Immunity and Inflammation, University of Leicester, Leicester LE1 7RH, UK
* Correspondence: ad482@leicester.ac.uk

Abstract: Spinal cord injury (SCI) causes irreversible tissue damage and severe loss of neurological function. Currently, there are no approved treatments and very few therapeutic targets are under investigation. Here, we combined 4 high-throughput transcriptomics and proteomics datasets, 7 days and 8 weeks following clinically-relevant rat SCI to identify proteins with persistent differential expression post-injury. Out of thousands of differentially regulated entities our combined analysis identified 40 significantly upregulated versus 48 significantly downregulated molecules, which were persistently altered at the mRNA and protein level, 7 days and 8 weeks post-SCI. Bioinformatics analysis was then utilized to identify currently available drugs with activity against the filtered molecules and to isolate proteins with known or unknown function in SCI. Our findings revealed multiple overlooked therapeutic candidates with important bioactivity and established druggability but with unknown expression and function in SCI including the upregulated purine nucleoside phosphorylase (PNP), cathepsins A, H, Z (CTSA, CTSH, CTSZ) and proteasome protease PSMB10, as well as the downregulated ATP citrate lyase (ACLY), malic enzyme (ME1) and sodium-potassium ATPase (ATP1A3), amongst others. This work reveals previously unappreciated therapeutic candidates for SCI and available drugs, thus providing a valuable resource for further studies and potential repurposing of existing therapeutics for SCI.

Keywords: spinal cord injury; transcriptomics; proteomics; bioinformatics

---

1. Introduction

Severe injury to the mammalian spinal cord causes irreversible tissue damage and in most cases, results in permanent loss of sensorimotor function below the affected site. At the molecular level SCI is characterized by neuronal death and loss of axons, aggressive inflammation, maladaptive tissue remodelling, excessive accumulation of extracellular matrix and scarring [1,2]. These events cause permanent pathological changes at the injury site and prevent neuronal regeneration and axonal growth. With the exception of reducing acute inflammation using corticosteroids, a therapeutic approach which remains controversial [3], followed by chronic rehabilitation physiotherapy, there are no approved therapies for SCI and to date, no drugs can reverse tissue damage or facilitate regrowth of surviving axons through the lesion site. There are few experimental therapies currently under investigation, including antibodies against highly neurotoxic myelin debris proteins (i.e., anti-Nogo antibodies [4]), stabilization of axonal microtubules using paclitaxel/taxol and epothilone B to facilitate the regrowth of damaged axons [5,6] and chondroitinase ABC, an enzyme that digests the growth inhibitory glycosaminoglycan moieties in proteoglycans, which accumulate abundantly in the fibrotic scar that develops after severe SCI and prevent neuronal growth through the injury site [7–9]. The complexity of the spinal tissue and the very severe inflammatory, fibrotic and neurodegenerative pathology together with the fact that the SCI patient population is relatively small in comparison to other neurological disorders, make the process of drug discovery difficult.

One possible approach to facilitate the discovery of novel pathological mechanisms and therapeutic targets is to utilize high-throughput -omics such as transcriptomics and proteomics. Contemporary high-throughput methods allow the interrogation of thousands of differentially regulated transcripts or proteins in multiple biological replicates in single quantitative experiments [10]. When combined with rigorous computational analysis of the large data that they return, –omics experiments can provide systems-wide insight into the pathological changes taking place in disease and allow the screening of multi-molecular changes instead of limited focusing towards single genes or proteins.

In this article, we sought to identify previously unappreciated and potentially promising therapeutic candidates for SCI by combining high-throughput transcriptomics and proteomics to profile gene and protein expression changes following clinically-relevant models of rat SCI. To ensure careful filtering of potential therapeutic candidates, we only retrieved molecules that were significantly regulated at the mRNA and protein level in tandem and showed consistent differential expression at 7 days (subacute) and 8 weeks (chronic) post-injury. We subsequently isolated druggable proteins and mined their potential function in SCI. This work could provide the basis for future mechanistic and preclinical studies investigating bioactive molecules with disease-modifying potential in SCI. Importantly, all transcriptomics and proteomics data, as well as the source code for the computational analysis that we developed, are available and freely accessible online via the *Mendeley Data* repository (Elsevier; https://data.mendeley.com) and our analysis is based on highly-cited freely accessible bioinformatics tools.

2. Results

2.1. Transcriptomics and Proteomics Analysis 7 Days and 8 Weeks after Rat SCI

SCI is a complex disorder which involves multiple different cell types and tissue substrates (neurons and axons, microglia and infiltrating immune cells, astrocytes, vascular cells, meningeal cells and others). It is also affected by the immune privilege of the central nervous system and the vascular limitations of the blood-brain-barrier. Multiparametric high-throughput approaches that examine large-scale transcript and protein changes in tandem can offer a broad understanding of molecular changes in SCI. To this end, we combined high-throughput transcriptomics and proteomics and at two different time-points (7 days and 8 weeks) after SCI to capture consistent and persistent molecular changes post-SCI and to identify proteins with important bioactivity and drug-targeting potential.

First, we performed an intersection of differentially regulated genes identified in a publicly available rat SCI microarray performed recently by Chamankhah and colleagues [11], to identify molecules that were significantly up or downregulated at the mRNA level, both at 7 days and 8 weeks post-SCI. Injury was performed by clip-compression using a 35 g aneurysm clip for 60 s, producing moderate to severe SCI [11]. We chose to use this transcriptomics study because it was performed by an experienced group, it had identical time-points to our proteomics analysis (see below) and importantly, compression SCI shares pathological similarities to contusion injury. This transcriptomics analysis compared uninjured (control) T7 spinal cord segments (n = 4) versus injured spinal cord, either at 7 days (n = 4) or 8 weeks (n = 4) post-injury. All microarray data was made freely accessible online from the authors [11] via the gene expression omnibus (GEO-NCBI: https://www.ncbi.nlm.nih.gov/geo/query/acc.cgi?acc=GSE45006). Moreover, all differentially regulated transcripts from 7 days and 8 weeks post-SCI were downloaded from GEO-NCBI and have been publicly deposited as easily accessible excel files in Mendeley Data: control versus 7 days post-SCI microarray: https://goo.gl/XqbbgN; control versus 8 weeks post-SCI microarray: https://goo.gl/BXYEeT. Only genes that had adjusted p-value ≤ 0.05 were accepted in the analysis. 902 were significantly upregulated at both 7 days and 8 weeks versus 835 genes significantly downregulated at both time-points.

Second, to expand the transcriptomics findings to protein expression post-SCI, we used high-throughput proteomics datasets obtained from spinal tissue LC-MS/MS (liquid chromatography-tandem mass spectrometry) performed in our lab. High-throughput analysis at the protein level is biologically important given that transcripts tend to be short-lived in comparison to proteins and mRNA expression does not necessarily reflect protein expression or accumulation at tissue sites, especially given the substantial tissue remodelling that takes place in injured tissues.

To improve the relative enrichment of different protein species and the depth of protein identifications, we used a solubility-based tissue protein subfractionation method previously developed by us, which allows separate analysis of cellular and extracellular proteins by LC-MS/MS and is based on using 0.08% SDS to isolate cellular proteins followed by 4 M guanidine for extracellular matrix and insoluble proteins [10,12,13]. Control (uninjured) versus injured rat spinal cord proteomics comparisons were made again at 7 days and 8 weeks post-SCI, matching the transcriptomics data. Relative estimation of protein abundance in tissue samples by LC-MS/MS was performed using spectral counting [14]. This comparison returned 115 proteins that were significantly upregulated and 149 proteins that were significantly downregulated in tandem, at both 7 days and 8 weeks post-SCI. All protein identification datasets, differentially regulated proteins and statistically analysed spectral counts from 7 days and 8 weeks post-SCI are publicly deposited as easily accessible excel files in Mendeley Data: 7 days proteomics: https://goo.gl/k93LwN; 8 weeks proteomics: https://goo.gl/qYoTJz.

2.2. *Integration of Transcriptomics and Proteomics Datasets to Identify Persistently Differentially Regulated Molecules*

To filter entities with consistent and persistent differential regulation at the mRNA and protein level and at 7 days and 8 weeks post-SCI, we integrated the transcriptomics and proteomics datasets described above. To ensure stringent selection, we accepted only molecules that were significantly differentially regulated (control vs. injured; *t*-test $p \leq 0.05$) in all 4 high-throughput datasets (transcriptomics and proteomics, 7 days and 8 weeks post-SCI). This combined analysis returned a filtered signature of only 40 upregulated (Figure 1a–c) and 48 downregulated (Figure 1d–f) molecules, at the transcript and protein level and both at 7 days and 8 weeks post-SCI. These consistent signatures are summarised as heatmaps, which display differential expression from shotgun proteomics (upregulated; Figure 1a and downregulated; Figure 1d) as well as protein-protein interaction networks, which highlight the interconnectivity of the differentially regulated proteins (upregulated; Figure 1b and downregulated; Figure 1e). Figure 1c,f depict 10 upregulated and downregulated proteins respectively, with the highest network betweenness centrality, a measure of how associated and central a protein is in comparison to other network proteins and offers an unbiased assessment of its relative biological importance [15]. Conceivably, proteins with high betweenness centrality and therefore extensive biological association with other proteins, might be considered as good drug targets given that they likely have an important function in the system either in isolation or as part of a functional pathway.

2.2.1. 40 Persistently Upregulated Proteins

The network of the 40 upregulated entities (Figure 1a,b) contains multiple proteins involved in extracellular matrix metabolism, including minor glycoproteins galectin 3 (LGALS3), lumican (LUM) and decorin (DCN) together with annexin A2 (ANXA2) and both alpha chains of collagen-1 (COL1A1 and COL1A2). The upregulated network (Figure 1a,b) also contains cytoskeletal proteins such as LIMA1 (actin-binding), CALD1 (actin-binding caldesmon), AIF1 (microglia/macrophage cytoskeletal protein commonly known as IBA1), LCP1 (plastin-2, T cell actin-binding protein), filamin A (FLNA) and vimentin (VIM) an abundant non-epithelial cytoskeletal protein with key collagen-1 mRNA-stabilising function.

Consistently upregulated proteins also include 5 cathepsins (lysosomal proteases); A (CTSA), B (CTSB), D (CTSD), H (CTSH) and Z (CTSZ) (Figure 1a,b) covering a large spectrum of cellular and extracellular proteolytic substrates. Cathepsin upregulation, proteolytic activity and lysosomal involvement are often associated with inflammatory tissue remodelling and loss of normal tissue function as well as activation of cell death pathways. Cathepsins are typically associated with activated macrophages and other immune cells [16]. The multicatalytic proteasome proteinase PSMB10 and dipeptidase PEPD, the latter with an important function in collagen-1 metabolism, are also present (Figure 1a,b). VIM, CTSD and ANX A2 have high betweenness centrality (Figure 1c), followed by FLNA and COL1A1 (Figure 1c), indicating relative biological importance in the system. The persistent upregulation of these proteins highlights the dominance of inflammation and scarring after SCI, driving pathological matrix remodelling and extensive proteolysis.

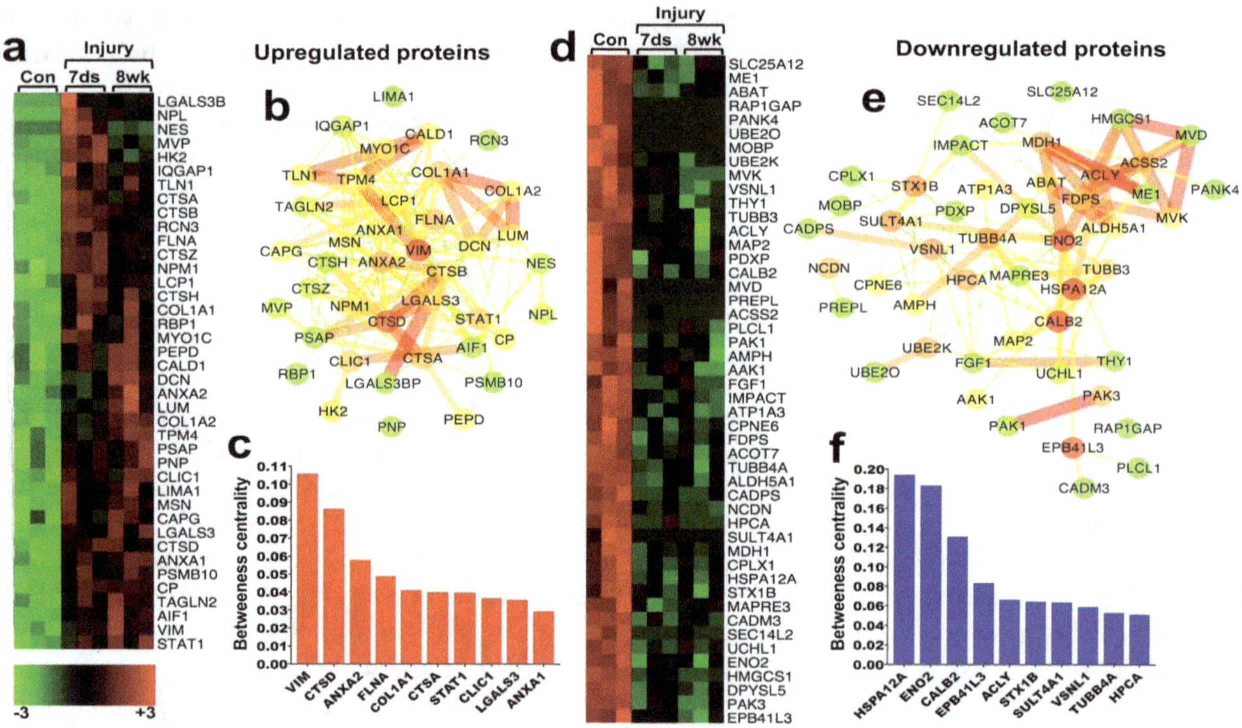

Figure 1. Persistently differentially regulated molecules at the mRNA and protein level 7 days and 8 weeks post-spinal cord injury (SCI): (**a**) 40 molecules that were consistently and significantly upregulated (t-test $p \leq 0.05$, Con vs. 7 ds and Con vs. 8 weeks) in all transcriptomics and proteomics datasets, at both 7 days and 8 weeks post-SCI. Heat-map displays differential protein expression quantified by spectral counting using shotgun proteomics. Heat-map values were normalised from −3 (green; low spectral counts) to +3 (red; high spectral counts). (**b**) The 40 persistently upregulated molecules were collected into a protein-protein interaction network using StringDB and Cytoscape. Node colours indicate protein betweenness centrality (how connected a protein is with others in the network); green nodes: low score; red nodes: high score. The width and colour of edges indicates protein-protein interaction score obtained from StringDB (green and slim: low interaction; red and broad: high interaction). Betweenness centrality and interaction scores were calculated and visualised in Cytoscape. (**c**) Ten upregulated proteins with the highest betweenness centrality score from network (**b**) are depicted. (**d**) 48 molecules that were consistently and significantly downregulated (t-test $p \leq 0.05$, Con vs. 7 ds and Con vs. 8 weeks) in all transcriptomics and proteomics datasets, at both 7 days and 8 weeks post-SCI. Heat-map displays differential protein expression quantified by spectral counting. (**e**) The 48 persistently downregulated molecules were collected into a protein-protein interaction network using StringDB and Cytoscape as above. (**f**) Ten downregulated proteins with the highest betweenness centrality from network (**e**) are depicted.

2.2.2. 48 Persistently Downregulated Proteins

Unsurprisingly, the network of the 48 persistently downregulated proteins (Figure 1d,e) contains multiple neuronal proteins with direct involvement in synaptic transmission including CPLX1 (complexin-1) and STX1B (syntaxin-1B) involved in synaptic vesicle function, ABAT (mitochondrial aminobutyrate aminotransferase) and ALDH5A1 (mitochondrial aldehyde dehydrogenase), both involved in the degradation of the neurotransmitter GABA, CPNE6 (copine-6; dendrite formation), HPCA (neuron-specific calcium-binding hippocalcin; regulates calcium channels), ME1 (malic enzyme) and AMPH (amphiphysin; involved in synaptic exocytosis). The persistent downregulation of synaptic-associated proteins is likely the result of neurodegeneration following SCI.

The downregulated network also contains 7 proteins involved in cholesterol and lipid synthesis and metabolism including MVD and MVK (mevalonate decarboxylase and kinase respectively), FDPS (farnesyl diphosphate/pyrophosphate kinase), HMGCS1 (catalyses synthesis of mevalonate from acetyl-CoA), ACSS2 (acetyl-CoA synthetase), ACLY (ATP citrate lyase) involved in acetyl-CoA metabolism) and SEC14L2 (supernatant protein factor). The central nervous system-specific heat-shock protein 70, 12A (HSPA12A) has the highest betweenness centrality (Figure 1f) reflecting the role of chaperone heat-shock proteins in multiple biological functions. Neuron-specific gamma-enolase (ENO2 or NSE) with a catalytic role in the synthesis of pyruvate and CALB2 (calretinin; a neuron- specific calcium-binding protein) follow HSPA12A in betweenness centrality (Figure 1f). The consistent downregulation of proteins involved in cholesterol metabolism is very interesting and such mechanisms in SCI are not well understood. One likely hypothesis is their involvement in myelin synthesis [17] and as such, their restoration might promote myelination after SCI. In contrast, downregulation of cholesterol synthesis has been associated with the highly effective regenerative capacity that is observed in peripheral nerves [18].

2.3. *Identification of Druggable Proteins in SCI*

To examine further the tight list of 40 upregulated and 48 downregulated molecules, we first looked for proteins that could be targeted using currently available, clinically-approved or experimental drugs/bioactive chemicals and second, we asked whether these druggable proteins have been cited in studies related to SCI. Druggable proteins were predicted using DGIdb v3 [19] and further validated with StitchDB v5 [20]. The relevance of druggable proteins to SCI was then examined using an automated PubMed text-mining tool that we developed for this study (source code deposited online: https://goo.gl/vRScJ3). Druggable proteins were searched in PubMed in conjunction to the terms "spinal cord injury" and "spinal injury" as well as with the words "trauma," "contusion" or "transection" replacing "injury" in the query.

DGIdb and StitchDB identified 15 upregulated druggable proteins, 10 of which returned at least one citation in SCI and 19 downregulated druggable proteins, 7 with at least one citation in SCI. These are summarised in Figure 2a. Druggable proteins are plotted against the number of drugs predicted to act against them (x axis) versus their betweenness centrality (y axis), to visualise druggability versus relative biological importance Figure 2a. Next, StitchDB-validated druggable proteins and their protein-protein as well as protein-drug interactions are illustrated in 4 networks. Figure 2b: 10 upregulated proteins with SCI citations plus 60 associated drugs; Figure 2c: 5 upregulated proteins with no SCI references plus 22 associated drugs; Figure 2d: 7 downregulated proteins with SCI citations plus 33 associated drugs; Figure 2e: 12 downregulated druggable proteins with no SCI citations plus 34 linked drugs. The predicted drugs from networks in Figure 2b–e were also text-mined in PubMed for potential reference to SCI (as described above) and the number of retrieved articles is shown in Figure 2f–i. All identified drugs from each network (Figure 2b–e) are listed here (https://goo.gl/zwbuq1) together with the number of citations retrieved from text-mining using SCI terms (as explained above) and compared to terms "brain," "spinal cord" and "central nervous system" for comparison. Links to the drug database PubChem is also provided for fast screening of essential drug information.

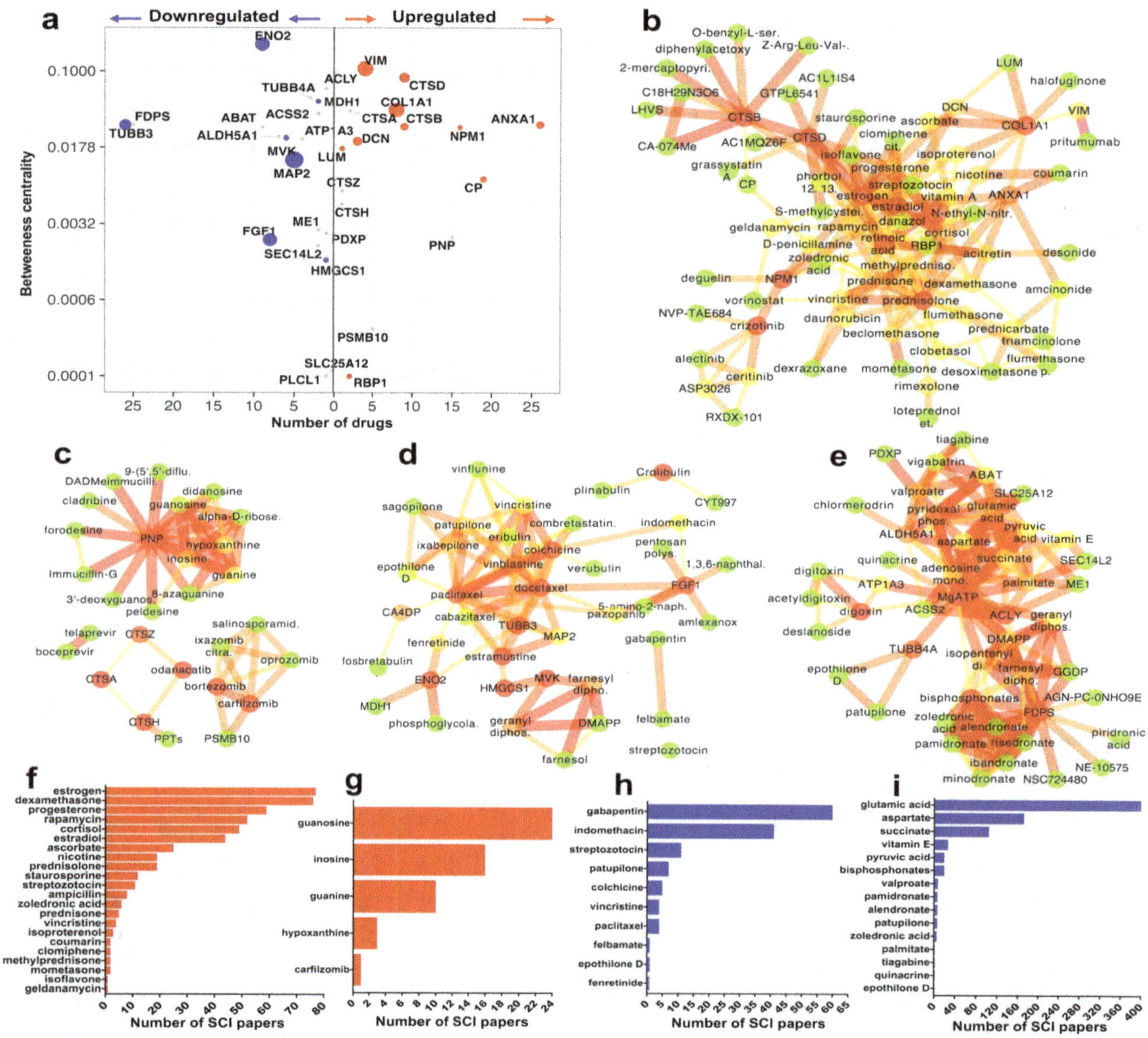

Figure 2. Mining druggable proteins using DGIdb and StitchDB: (**a**) DGIdb analysis followed by StitchDB identified 15 upregulated druggable proteins 10 of which returned at least one citation in SCI and 19 downregulated druggable proteins 7 of which with at least one citation in SCI. Proteins are summarised in 3 dimensions. Druggable proteins are plotted against the number of drugs predicted to act against them (x axis) versus their network betweenness centrality (y axis) to visualise druggability versus relative biological importance. The size of nodes (3rd dimension) indicates the number of PubMed articles citing these proteins in SCI. Grey nodes are proteins with no SCI citations in PubMed. (**b**) Protein-protein-drug interaction network of the 10 upregulated druggable proteins with at least one citation in SCI. The network was made using StitchDB and visualised in Cytoscape. Nodes and edges are colour-coded according to their betweenness centrality while the width and colour of edges indicates the strength of interaction between molecules (proteins and drugs) as predicted by StitchDB. (**c**) Protein-protein-drug interaction network of the 5 upregulated druggable proteins with no citations in SCI. (**d**) Protein-protein-drug interaction network of the 7 downregulated druggable proteins with at least one citation in SCI. (**e**) Protein-protein-drug interaction network of the 12 upregulated druggable proteins with no citations in SCI. (**f–i**) Predicted drugs from networks were text-mined in PubMed for potential reference to SCI and the number of articles is presented; (**f**) drugs interacting with proteins in network (**b**); (**g**) drugs interacting with proteins in network (**c**); (**h**) drugs interacting with proteins in network (**d**); (**i**) drugs interacting with proteins in network (**e**).

2.3.1. Upregulated Druggable Proteins with SCI Citations (Figure 2b,f)

In the group of upregulated proteins with SCI citations (Figure 2b), the association of annexin A1 (ANXA1) with classic corticosteroids (cortisone, dexamathasone, prednisone, amcinonide and associated steroids and hormones, i.e. estradiol and progesterone) dominates the network (Figure 2b). The potent anti-inflammatory effect of corticosteroids in tissues is thought to be exerted, at least in part, by regulating the synthesis and function of ANXA1 [21]. Interestingly, while ANXA1 has received limited attention in SCI, corticosteroids have been extensively used to reduce acute SCI inflammation (Figure 2f) but their efficacy in alleviating long-term pathology is debatable and their use is controversial [22,23]. Steroid hormones estradiol and progesterone are also well studied (Figure 2f) and are considered neuroprotective in SCI [24].

Another notable cluster in Figure 2b includes the well-studied cathepsins B and D (CTSB, CTSD) and the numerous mostly experimental inhibitors that block their proteolytic activity. Both CTSB and CTSD are likely involved in the degradation of axonal components after SCI [25] but notably anti-cathepsin drugs have not been used in SCI thus far in either preclinical or clinical studies. NPM1 (nucleophosmin; Figure 2b) is associated with anti-neoplastic drugs crizotinib and deguelin (plus associated compounds). While inhibition of NPM1 was recently noted to block neuronal apoptosis after SCI in one study [26], neither deguelin nor crizotinib have been tested in SCI (Figure 2f).

Although vimentin (VIM; Figure 2b) has been cited extensively in SCI, mainly as a non-specific marker of proliferating (astrocytes, ependymal cells, fibroblasts) or invading (macrophages, endothelial cells, progenitors) mesenchymal cells in the injury site, it has not been tested as a putative drug target thus far. The cytoskeletal protein, which has very high betweenness centrality (Figure 2a), is recently gaining attention as a potential target in glioma and other cancers using antibodies against its ectodomain (pritumumab [27]). In SCI, anti-vimentin antibodies could be conceivably used for the removal of vimentin-positive cells but the selectivity of such an approach against a protein that is highly abundant in multiple cell types, some with potentially neuroprotective roles [28], is questionable.

The archetypal matrix and fibrosis protein collagen-1 (chain COL1A1; Figure 2b) is persistently upregulated after SCI, it has high betweenness centrality (Figure 2f) and is associated with the anti-fibrosis collagen expression blocker halofuginone [29], as well as with the beta-adrenergic receptor agonist isoproterenol (Figure 2b), known to increase its expression [30]. Notably, this is one of the very few cases of an agonist present in our analysis. The potential involvement of collagen-1 in matrix remodelling, fibrosis and scarring after SCI is a promising area for future investigation.

2.3.2. Upregulated Druggable Proteins without SCI Citations (Figure 2c,g)

In this small network the extensive druggability of PNP (purine nucleoside phosphorylase), an enzyme that converts ribonucleosides into purine bases, is striking. PNP has been implicated as an inflammatory mediator in glia as well as peripheral T and B-cells and is a good target for anti-inflammatory therapies especially with regards to T-cell activity [31–33]. PNP has not been studied in SCI and might represent an interesting drug target given its persistent upregulation, its involvement in inflammatory mechanisms and the sizeable cohort of associated drugs (Figure 2c) that can block its function (i.e. immucillins and forodesine). Interestingly, purine derivatives that associate with PNP (guanosine, inosine, hypoxanthine) are used in experimental SCI as neuroprotective/neurotrophic agents but this is independent to their biological connection to PNP [34].

Unlike cathepsins B and D (CTSB, CTSD) discussed above, the function of upregulated CTSA, CTSH and CTSZ in SCI is unknown (Figure 2c). Similarly, neither specific cathepsin blockers (PPTs: odanacatib, toluenesulfonic acid) nor other protease inhibitors (telaprevir, boceprevir), have been tested in SCI. CTSA, CTSH and CTSZ are all persistently upregulated after SCI and CTSA has high betweenness centrality (Figure 2a). Thus, the availability of cathepsin blockers (Figure 2c) and the lack of knowledge about these cathepsins make them interesting candidates for further investigation. In addition to cathepsins, the role of the proteasome protease PSMB10 (Figure 2c) in the spinal cord is not studied and not much is known about the proteasome-ubiquitin system in SCI [35]. The proteasome inhibitor carfilzomib which interacts with PSMB10 (Figure 2c), was recently shown to exert an acute neuroprotective effect after T10 transection SCI in rats (Figure 2g) but the authors did not implicate PSMB10 to this effect [36].

2.3.3. Downregulated Druggable Proteins with SCI Citations (Figure 2d,h)

This dense network contains few multi-druggable entities (Figure 2d,h). The classic neuronal tubulin beta-3 (TUBB3) is associated with many cytoskeleton-regulating drugs, mainly paclitaxel (taxol) and derivatives (docetaxel, cabazitaxel, epothilone D, patupilone/epothilone B) plus other putative microtubule stabilisers like estramustine, vinblastine and vincristine (Figure 2d). Although mainly used as anti-neoplastic agents, microtubule stabilisers (notably paclitaxel and patupilone/epothilone B) are currently at the forefront of experimental SCI therapies [5,6]. Another microtubule assembly protein, MAP2 (microtubule-associated protein 2) is consistently downregulated after SCI (Figure 1d) and is also predicted to interact with these drugs (Figure 2d). MAP2 is a well-studied neuronal marker. It has been previously shown to be downregulated after SCI and its loss is associated with destabilization and depolymerization of axonal microtubules [37].

The activity of the acidic fibroblast growth factor FGF1 can be blocked by the tyrosine kinase inhibitor pazopanib (FGF1 activates tyrosine kinase signalling) and by the anti-inflammatory amlexanox (Figure 2d) both with no citations in SCI. Nevertheless, the use of drugs that block FGF1 activity is counterintuitive, as it is persistently downregulated in our analysis plus it has been shown to be neurotrophic and neurorestorative after SCI in preclinical studies [38]. Like FGF1, neuron-specific enolase (ENO2/NSE; Figure 2d) has broad neuroprotective function in the central nervous system [39]. ENO2 is a protein with high betweenness centrality (Figure 2a) and potentially high biological importance. The anti-cancer drug fenretinide has been found to interact with enolase (Figure 2d) but the exact pharmacological action is unknown. Interestingly, fenretinide was recently shown to alleviate inflammation in murine contusion SCI but the authors did not connect this effect to ENO2 [40].

Key downregulated sterol synthesis enzymes MVK and HMGCS1 interact with the chemical farnesol (Figure 2d) but potential pharmacological effects are unclear. They also interact with substrates geranyl and farnesyl diphosphate, again with unknown pharmacological benefit. The role of MVK and HMGCS1 is unclear but cholesterol metabolism and the mevalonate cascade are recently gaining attention in the field [41].

2.3.4. Downregulated Druggable Proteins without SCI Citations (Figure 2e,i)

In conjunction with MVK and HMGCS1 from (Figure 2d), farnesyl diphosphate/pyrophosphate synthase (FDPS) is a critical mevalonate synthesis enzyme with multiple established biphosphonates (i.e., alendronate, etidronate, etc.) as well as experimental (NE-10575, NSC724480) inhibitors (Figure 2e) and medium betweenness centrality (Figure 2a). Yet, the enzyme has not been studied in SCI and its function in the brain and spinal cord remains elusive [42]. In contrast, clinical and experimental inhibition of FDPS by biphosphonates is the gold-standard approach to block bone resorption by inhibiting the function of osteoclasts. As a result, biphosphonates are currently used to regulate inactivity-induced bone resorption in SCI patients [43] and this is independent to any potential function of FDPS in the spinal cord. ACSS2 and ACLY are important lipid synthesis mediators with high betweenness centrality but unknown role in SCI (Figure 2a). They are prominent in the drug network (Figure 2e), mainly due to their interaction with adenosine phosphate (and MgATP) and lipid metabolism intermediaries palmitate, succinate and pyruvate. Potential therapeutic effects are unknown. Notably, ACLY is involved in the synthesis of the neurotransmitter acetylcholine in the brain [44]. ACLY is also associated with ME1 (malic enzyme; Figure 2e) which generates NADPH for fatty acid synthesis. The role of ME1 in the spinal cord is also unknown but it was recently shown, together with other lipid synthesis molecules, to have a possible function in white matter development in infants [45].

ATP1A3 (Figure 2e), a sodium/potassium pump ATPase is another enzyme with unknown function in SCI and high betweenness centrality (Figure 2a). The enzyme has a distinct neuronal function as it is involved in the generation of electrical impulses and in the transport of neurotransmitters and calcium ions across the plasma membrane [46,47]. It is associated with the cardiac glycoside digoxin/digitoxin and derivatives, which have not been tested as SCI treatments and are rarely used in modern clinical practice to enhance cardiac function.

Two highly druggable, downregulated proteins with high betweenness centrality are aldehyde dehydrogenase 5A (ALDH5A1) and 4-aminobutyrate aminotransferase (ABAT) (Figure 2a,e) both involved in the catabolism of the inhibitory neurotransmitter GABA [48,49]. Interestingly, although the role of these GABA catabolic enzymes in SCI is unknown, the associated drug valproate (plus associated vigabatrin, chlormerodrin and tiagabine) are used (Figure 2i) to increase GABA and prevent the spasticity and involuntary muscle contractility that affects the majority of SCI patients [50]. Thus, it could be speculated that the persistent downregulation of ALDH5A1 and ABAT described here, might contribute to the molecular mechanisms of post-SCI spasticity which is nevertheless caused by very complex neuronal mechanisms following injury to upper or lower motor neurons.

2.3.5. Transcription Factor Regulation of Persistently Differentially Regulated Proteins

One approach to regulate gene and protein expression in tissues is via interference with relevant transcription factor activity. Given that our combined intersection of transcriptomics and proteomics datasets isolated a filtered list of 40 significantly upregulated and 48 significantly downregulated proteins both at the mRNA and protein level and both at 7 days and 8 weeks post-SCI (Figure 1), we sought to examine likely transcription factor promoter-binding sites for the identified proteins. To do this, we used TRANSFAC-7-based computational prediction for transcription factor promoter binding sites (MSigDB; [51]). This analysis returned 9 transcription factors as potential regulators of the 40 upregulated proteins (Figure 3a) and 5 transcription factors potentially controlling the expression of the 48 downregulated proteins (Figure 3b).

SP1 followed by TCF3 (or TFE2) are predicted to bind to the highest number of upregulated gene promoters (Figure 3a) while MAZ and SP1 are predicted for the highest number of downregulated genes (Figure 3b). These transcription factors are conserved and abundant housekeepers and regulate a plethora of genes, hence their involvement is not surprising. Nevertheless, potential specific role of either MAZ or SP1 in SCI is currently unknown.

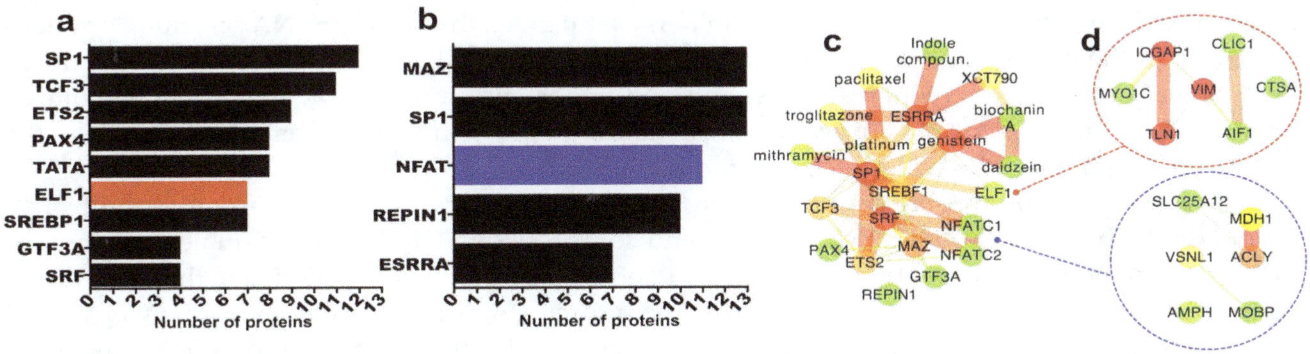

Figure 3. Transcription factor promoter binding site analysis for 40 and 48 persistently differentially regulated proteins: (**a**,**b**) MSigDB was used to identify transcription factors with likely promoter binding sites for the molecules that were consistently upregulated (**a**) or downregulated (**b**) in all 4 transcriptomics and proteomics datasets, at both 7 days and 8 weeks post-SCI. Graphs display the number of proteins (x axis) likely regulated by listed transcription factors. ELF1 is upregulated while NFATC1 is downregulated in both 7 days and 8 weeks transcriptomics datasets. (**c**) Protein-protein-drug interaction network made in StitchDB and Cytoscape depicting interacting transcription factors (from **a**,**b**) and associated drugs. Neither ELF1 nor NFATC1 have predicted drugs with either DGIdb or StitchDB. The upregulated (red) and downregulated proteins with likely promoter binding sites for ELF1 and NFATC1 are highlighted in (**d**).

When we examined the expression profile of these transcription factors in the transcriptomics and proteomics datasets we found that although none were differentially regulated at the protein level (proteomics datasets) ELF1 which was predicted to regulate 7 of the 40 persistently upregulated proteins (Figure 3a), was itself upregulated at the mRNA level both at 7 days and 8 weeks post-SCI (7 days SCI microarray: https://goo.gl/XqbbgN; 8 weeks SCI microarray: https://goo.gl/BXYEeT). On the other hand, NFAT transcription factor complex promoter binding sites were predicted for 11 of the 48 persistently downregulated proteins (Figure 3b) and NFATC1, one of the NFAT components, was downregulated at the mRNA level at both 7 days and 8 weeks post-SCI (7 days SCI microarray: https://goo.gl/XqbbgN; 8 weeks SCI microarray: https://goo.gl/BXYEeT). As for SP1 and MAZ (both upregulated at the mRNA level at 7 days but not 8 weeks), the potential function of either ELF1 or NFATC1 in SCI is unknown. Upregulated proteins with predicted regulation by ELF1 and downregulated proteins with predicted regulation by NFATC1 are depicted in Figure 3d. Predicted transcription factors from Figure 3a,b were also examined using DGIdb and StitchDB for potential association with drugs (Figure 3c). Neither ELF1 nor NFATC1 appear to be druggable. SP1 and ESRRA, are instead associated with anti-cancer compounds (Figure 3c) which have not been tested in SCI thus far. Interestingly, the only transcription factor found in the filtered list of the 40 upregulated molecules at the mRNA and protein level, 7 days and 8 weeks post-SCI, is STAT1 (signal transducer and activator of transcription 1), a key regulator of inflammatory mechanisms and interferon signalling in particular [52,53]. STAT1 is persistently upregulated after SCI and has a high betweenness centrality (Figure 1a–c). Although it has been involved in various inflammatory mechanisms and diseases, its function after SCI is not well-studied, albeit few recent studies have shown that blocking STAT1 activity has a positive effect post-SCI [54,55]. To the best of our knowledge, no approved drugs or inhibitors offer selective inhibition of STAT1.

3. Discussion

In this manuscript combination of transcriptomics, proteomics and bioinformatics provides a comprehensive overview of proteins with persistent differential expression at the mRNA and protein level and from the subacute (7 days) to the chronic (8 weeks) phase of SCI lesion development. To ensure stringent filtering, we accepted only molecules that were significantly differentially regulated in all high-throughput datasets (transcriptomics and proteomics, 7 days and 8 weeks post-SCI). The intersection of transcriptomics and proteomics is useful given that while mRNA screening provides a snapshot of the dynamic gene expression changes following SCI, proteomics confirms functional expression of proteins from regulated transcripts and underscores proteotypic changes in the injured spinal cord. To the best of our knowledge, this is the first attempt to systematically analyse the molecular druggability of SCI in high-throughput.

The intersection of transcriptomics and proteomics at 2 different injury time-points and from 2 independent labs using comparable contusion and compression SCI models in female rats, ensures unbiased validation of the high-throughput data and offers confidence in the filtering of these molecular targets. Nevertheless, it is important to note that the transcriptomics and proteomics data were based on two different SCI models as well as rat strains. More specifically, the transcriptomics analysis by Chamankhah et al. was based on a T7 aneurysm clip (35 g) compression injury (moderate to severe) in female Wistar rats [11], while our proteomics analysis was based on automated 150 kilo-dyne (1.5 Newton) spinal contusion injuries (moderate), performed on female Sprague-Dawley rats (see Section 4 for more details and [7,9,10,56]). It is important to note that different injury models might cause variable tissue pathology and sensorimotor outcomes. Differences and similarities between contusive and compressive injuries have not been studied in detail but both models are considered comparable, as they rely on blunt trauma to the spinal cord and normally involve neither penetration of the meninges, nor sharp severing of axons (as occurs in hemisections and full transections). As a result, they better simulate the biomechanical damage observed in the majority of human injuries (reviewed and summarized in [57–60]). Few studies have directly compared contusions with compressions. Pinzon et al., showed that gross lesion pathological features did not appear to differ greatly between contusion and compression injuries [61]. More recently, Geremia and colleagues concluded that lesion volumes and gross tissue pathology were not significantly different between contusion (severe T12, 200 kilo-dyne) and clip-compression (moderate to severe T12, 35 g aneurysm clip), albeit clearly increased hematoma formation and spreading in the severe contusion group [62]. Differences in contusion/compression forces applied in different studies are clearly important in terms of defining injury severity. Comparison between strains has revealed differences in a number of studies not only between strains but even in same strains obtained from different vendors [63]. 20 years ago Popovich and colleagues focused on differences in inflammation after SCI. They found that while the basic inflammatory reaction after SCI follows similar patterns in Sprague-Dawley and Lewis rats, differences were observed in the magnitude and duration of macrophage activation and T-cell infiltration in lesions. The authors attributed these differences to strain-specific variations in corticosteroid regulation of inflammation [64]. Accordingly, using a neuronal-specific gene array, Schmitt et al., showed that the expression of several genes varies between Sprague-Dawley, Long Evans and Lewis rats after contusive SCI [65] and in a study focusing on post-SCI sensorimotor function, Mills et al., showed that strain selection significantly affects functional recovery in Sprague-Dawley and Wistar rats [57]. Thus, different strains might exhibit pathological or sensorimotor differences. Nevertheless, our focus on proteins that are differentially regulated in both models, both time-points and both at the mRNA and protein level highlights the likely importance of these differentially regulated signatures to SCI.

Our high-throughput intersection returned 40 persistently upregulated and 48 persistently downregulated proteins. To further narrow down the list of target molecules, we applied two-tier computational protein-protein-drug interaction screening combined with literature text-mining. This analysis isolated previously unappreciated druggable proteins and pharmacological substances that could be examined in future experimental and preclinical SCI studies. Notably, excluding a few proteins that have been studied extensively in SCI (i.e., vimentin, IBA1, decorin, ceruloplasmin, CTSB, CTSD, tubulin beta-3, ENO2/NSE, FGF1, MAP2 and others) many proteins and drugs identified in our comparative analysis have received little to no experimental attention and some might be excellent targets for future investigations.

While it would be very difficult within the limits of this manuscript to cover in detail the function of each protein and their potential role in SCI, we have made an effort to describe the bioactivity of multiple druggable proteins and put it in the context of SCI where applicable (see Figure 2 and associated Results). Given that the majority of drugs are antagonists, inhibitors, or function-blockers, upregulated molecules are excellent primary candidates for drug targeting. In contrast, downregulated entities might be modulated with function agonists or over-expression with more complex molecular tools such as viruses or CrispR/CAS9.

Based on biological function, druggability and crucially, lack of knowledge with regards to SCI, we could highlight few interesting proteins that are consistently upregulated or downregulated at the mRNA and protein level, at 7 days and 8 weeks individually depicted in Figure 4. From the upregulated cohort, PNP (purine nucleoside phosphorylase) is a protein with well-documented involvement in T-cell activity and function and PNP inhibitors exert potent immunomodulatory effects against T-cells, especially in diseases with dominant involvement of adaptive immunity [32,66,67]. The role of PNP in B-cell function is also under investigation. Notably, not only the potential function of PNP in SCI is unknown but in addition, the role of T-cells is still unclear, although T-cells infiltrate spinal lesions [64]. Thus, given the importance of inflammation in primary and secondary SCI pathology and the importance of T-cells in immune processes, the highly druggable PNP (Figure 2c) is a very interesting candidate.

Similarly, the role of upregulated lysosomal cathepsin A (CTSA; Figure 4) in SCI is unknown. This serine protease and carboxypeptidase is involved in the activation of sialidase and its deficiency causes the lysosomal storage disease galactosialidosis [68]. It also seems to play an important role in autophagy, which is involved in the regulation of various inflammatory mechanisms including SCI [69]. Recent work in mice showed that CTSA deficiency is associated with a severe neurological phenotype [70]. Similarly, the role of the other consistently upregulated cathepsins CTSH and CTSZ (Figure 4) in SCI is unknown.

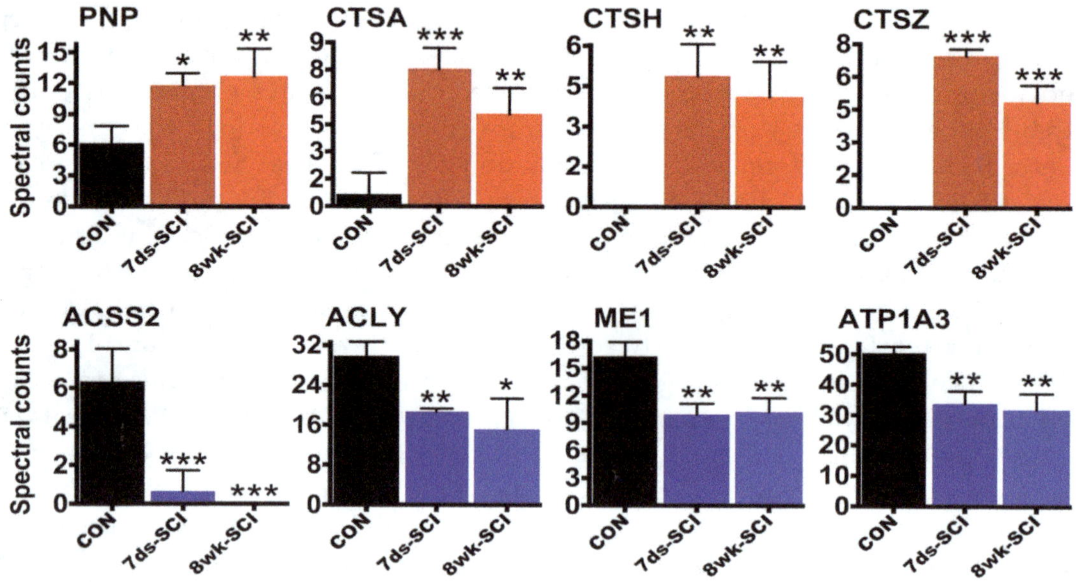

Figure 4. Highlighted differentially regulated proteins after SCI. Graphs depict the differential expression of upregulated purine nucleoside phosphorylase (PNP), cathepsins A, H and Z (CTSA, CTSH, CTSZ) and downregulated ACSS2 (acetyl-CoA synthetase), ATP citrate lyase (ACLY), malic enzyme (ME1) and sodium-potassium ATPase (ATP1A3) proteins using spectral counting values from shotgun liquid chromatography-tandem mass spectrometry (LC-MS/MS). These proteins are amongst the molecules that were consistently upregulated or downregulated at the mRNA and protein level and at 7 days and 8 weeks post-SCI. $n = 3$ per group; mean +SD; ANOVA and Fisher post-hoc test (independent comparison); stars indicate significance versus CON (control intact T10 spinal cord segments); * $p \leq 0.05$, ** $p \leq 0.01$, *** $p \leq 0.001$. CTSA and CTSZ spectral counts are also significantly different from 7 days to 8 weeks.

From the persistently downregulated proteins, lipid and sterol synthesis mediators including ACSS2, ACLY and ME1 (Figure 4) are attractive candidates for further research. They might be involved in lipid and energy homeostasis or in myelin synthesis post-injury. The distinctly neuronal ATP1A3 is another persistently downregulated protein (Figure 4) with very interesting properties given its involvement in neurotransmission [47]. The protein has been studied extensively for its function in the central nervous system but its role in SCI is unknown. Mutations that impair ATP1A3 activity cause rapid-onset dystonia in humans and permanent neurological dysfunction [71]. The enzyme is also downregulated after neonatal cortical injury in rats [46].

In summary, by using a combination of transcriptomics, proteomics and bioinformatics we isolated multiple proteins with drug-targeting potential and unknown function in SCI. While it might be difficult to speculate on the best possible drug target or identify a panacea for SCI, our systematic analysis might stimulate further mechanistic or therapeutic studies in the future.

4. Materials and Methods

4.1. Rat Transcriptomics—Microarray Analysis of Rat SCI

The rat microarray datasets analysed and integrated in this manuscript were recently performed and published by Chamankhah and colleagues. Information about the ethical use of animals in this study and in-depth information about the clinically-relevant compressive SCI model utilised in their study has been published [11]. Briefly, the authors used a clip compression SCI in female Wistar rats using a 35 g aneurysm clip for 60 s producing a moderate to severe T7 SCI. The compression model produces comparable blunt-force gross pathology and lesion characteristics to the contusion model that we used on the thoracic spinal cord (see below). Microarray data is available online via the gene expression omnibus (GEO-NCBI). Microarray data from GEO is qualitatively and statistically curated and MIAME-compliant. Rat T7 spinal clip compression injury microarray $n = 4$ intact versus injured T7 spinal cord samples at 7 days ($n = 4$) and 8 weeks ($n = 4$) post-injury. Microarray experimental information is available here (GEO-NCBI: https://www.ncbi.nlm.nih.gov/geo/query/acc.cgi?acc=GSE45006). Additionally, microarray expression data was downloaded and compiled to excel files (.xlsx) to enable uncomplicated examination of differential mRNA expression between control and injured spinal cord specimens at 7 days and 8 weeks post-SCI and to allow investigation of individual genes. Due to their excessive size, these excel files have been publicly deposited and are free to download from the Mendeley Data public repository. Control versus 7 days post-SCI microarray comparison can be found here: (7 days SCI microarray: https://goo.gl/XqbbgN; 8 weeks SCI microarray: https://goo.gl/BXYEeT). Expression and statistical analysis was performed by GEO-NCBI using standard t-test p-values and multiple p-value error adjustments. We only accepted transcripts that were significant with an adjusted $p \leq 0.05$ and 2-fold change at both 7 days and 8 weeks.

4.2. *Spinal Cord Injury Model in Rats for Proteomics Analysis*

We have previously characterised in detail spinal cord contusion in adult rats [7,9,10,56]. Briefly, adult female Sprague-Dawley rats (~200 g) were anesthetised using breathable isofluorane. 5 mg/kg Baytril (antibiotic) and 5 mg/kg Carprofen (NSAID pain and inflammation control) were given subcutaneously at the time of surgery and the morning after surgery. Spinal laminectomies were performed at vertebral level T10, the vertebral column was stabilised using Adson forceps and the rat-specific impactor probe was positioned 2 mm above the spinal cord. An impact force of 150 kilo-dyne (mean 152.3 kilo-dyne; standard deviation 3.2; $n = 6$ contused animals) was delivered to the exposed spinal cord through the intact dura with an Infinite Horizon impactor (Precision Systems Instrumentation) which generates a moderate severity contusion injury according to our Home Office-approved animal licence. This severity mimics more than 50% of human injuries that are "incomplete" (i.e., where some white matter tissue is spared) containing uninjured axons and the model is generally considered to be relatively clinically-relevant. After injury, all 6 animals used in the study had full bilateral hind limb paralysis and started exhibiting limited spontaneous recovery typically after the first week. After spinal contusion, the overlying muscle and skin were sutured, anaesthesia was reversed using oxygen and animals recovered in cages placed on heated blankets. Saline and Baytril (antibiotic) were given subcutaneously daily for 7 days, after injury. Bladders were manually expressed twice daily until reflexive emptying returned (typically 6–9 days after injury). The study has received approval by the institutional Animal Care and Use Committee (King's College London; PPL 70/8032, 14/11/2016) and all surgical procedures were performed in accordance with the United Kingdom Animals (Surgical Procedures) Act 1996.

4.3. *Shotgun LC-MS/MS Proteomics—Proteomics Analysis of Rat SCI*

We have recently described in detail and published high-resolution shotgun LC-MS/MS proteomics analysis of rat SCI [10]. Prior to proteomics spinal cord tissue from intact ($n = 3$) or injured T10 spinal cord segments 7 days ($n = 3$) and 8 weeks ($n = 3$) post-injury were extracted using a sequential protein extraction protocol previously developed by us [10,12,13]. This approach improves separation of easily soluble cellular proteins (0.08% SDS) followed by isolation of insoluble and cross-linked, extracellular, matrix and matrix-associated extracellular proteins from tissue specimens (4 M guanidine). This method has been published multiple times and is widely used for different tissues including the spinal cord. Following protein extraction shotgun LC-MS/MS was performed as described in depth [10]. Briefly, protein samples were digested by trypsin, tryptic peptides were separated in 2–35%, 120 min acetonitrile gradient and analysed on Q Exactive orbitrap mass spectrometer. Protein identifications were performed using Mascot

Version 2.4.1 (Matrix Science). Scaffold [72] (version 4.2.1) was used to validate MS/MS based peptide and protein identifications. Peptide identifications were accepted only if they could be established at greater than 95.0% probability by the Peptide Prophet algorithm with Scaffold delta-mass correction. Protein identifications were accepted only if they could be established at greater than 95.0% probability and contained at least 2 unique identified peptides. Scaffold was also used to calculate normalised spectral counts for quantitation. All accepted protein spectra (95% probability plus 2 unique peptides minimum) were included in the analysis and no outliers were removed. Although there are multiple different approaches to achieve relative protein quantitation using LC-MS/MS, spectral counting is very simple and less prone to technical errors in comparison to protein-labelling approaches especially when combined with orthogonal validation of findings [10,14]. In this manuscript, extra confidence is obtained from the fact that we focus only on proteins that are common across 2 independent transcriptomics and proteomics datasets and across 2 different time-points. Only proteins with t-test $p \leq 0.05$ at both 7 days and 8 weeks and concomitant significant differential regulation ($p \leq 0.05$) at the transcript level (from microarrays described above) at both 7 days and 8 weeks were accepted. All proteomics identifications and spectral counting quantitation has been deposited online at Mendeley Data: 7 days proteomics: https://goo.gl/k93LwN; 8 weeks proteomics: https://goo.gl/qYoTJz.

4.4. Computational and Bioinformatics Analysis of High-Throughput Data

Hierarchical clustering and heat-maps were created in the MeV TM4 platform [73]. Significantly different ($p \leq 0.05$; t-test) spectral counts were z-normalised (−3; low to +3; high) to obtain a more linear colour representation of the data. Pairwise similarity in spectral counts between different proteins (rows) was computed using Pearson correlation coefficient. Protein-protein interaction networks were created using StringDB v10 (https://string-db.org) [74] of known and predicted protein-protein interactions and inferring protein associations from multiple databases as well as text-mining. For protein-protein interaction networks, a low threshold of association (0.15) was used to capture the largest possible interaction probability. Network parameters were visualised in CytoScape v2.8 [75], which was also used to calculate the betweenness centrality of interacting proteins within networks. Drug candidate analysis was performed using DGIdb (http://www.dgidb.org) [19]. This software is searching multiple different drug databases and uses text-mining to identify drugs matching input proteins. Drug-protein interactions were then validated and filtered using StitchDB v5 (http://stitch.embl.de) [20]. This step resulted in significant filtering of the drug-protein interaction data. StitchDB also creates organic drug-protein and protein-protein interaction networks, the latter using the StringDB platform and generates interaction scores. For protein-drug interactions, a medium threshold of association (0.40) was used to ensure more stringent filtering of drugs and chemicals. As above, network parameters were visualised in CytoScape v2.8, which was also used to calculate the betweenness centrality of interacting proteins and drugs within networks. Transcription factor analysis was performed using MSigDB (http://software.broadinstitute.org/gsea/msigdb) [51], transcription factor targets sub-collection. Mammalian transcriptional regulatory motifs were extracted from v7.4 TRANSFAC database. Each gene set consists of all human genes whose promoters contains at least one conserved instance of the TRANSFAC motif, where a promoter is defined as the non-coding sequence contained within 4-kilobases from the transcription start site.

4.5. Gene and Drug Java Text-Mining Tool

The custom-made text-mining tool was constructed using Java in IntelliJ IDEA community edition. The code used has been publicly deposited in Mendeley Data for Journals and can be found here together with running instructions to operate the tool in IntelliJ for free (https://goo.gl/vRScJ3). Firstly, the nomenclature for the text-mined genes is retrieved using the HGNC REST web-service API (https://www.genenames.org/help/rest-web-service-help). The gene symbol, gene name and synonym identifiers were used in the literature queries. The gene nomenclature is enriched by a set of algorithms that are designed to permute names and omit obsolete name parts. The literature queries are performed using the Europe PubMed Central (EPMC) REST web-service API after nomenclature retrieval. The EPMC database queries are structured into two blocks; the first block contains all gene names, abbreviations, synonyms and accepted protein names from HGNC, whereas the second block contains the keywords of interest including: "spinal cord injury" and "spinal injury" as well as with the words "trauma," "contusion" or "transection" replacing "injury" in the query. The search clause is structured so that at least one search term belonging to each of the search blocks must be present in the abstract or title of the retrieved articles. All search terms were enclosed in quotations to ensure that the terms are searched as is and that individual words within the term are not matched mistakenly. The retrieved articles were manually verified to satisfy search requirements. Drug text-mining was performed similarly. The drugs for the differentially regulated genes were derived manually with the use of DGIdb and StitchDB. Next, EPMC was queried in the same way as for the genes, where the first block of the query contained the primary drug names instead of gene names. This article set contained no false positives. Please note that different text-mining search engines such as Google Scholar might retrieve more or different studies regarding the usage of certain drugs in SCI but in our experience PubMed is more reliable with regards to peer-reviewed research-based studies and in our experience, retrieves fewer false-positives. A deeper text-mining was then performed using all drug synonyms, chemical names and commercial names to ensure a full, in-depth retrieval of literature. Drug synonyms were retrieved using the PubChem REST web-service APIs. The risk for the retrieval of false positive articles was high in this search due to the extensive variety of drug synonyms stored in the PubChem database. To avoid the retrieval of false positives, the results of the deep text mining were overlaid with the "drug name only" results and differences in article numbers between the two datasets were inspected manually and false positives eliminated. URL addresses for all online database queries (PubChem, HGNC, EPMC, UniProt) are output in the console at runtime. The user can verify database query parameters by navigating to these URLs manually. Please not that although every effort was made to minimise retrieval of false-positive associations via text-mining, users must ensure a stringent manual search of target molecules.

Author Contributions: A.D. conceived this work, designed experiments, analysed data, prepared figures and wrote the manuscript; J.T. designed experiments (text-mining), analysed data, prepared figures and wrote the manuscript; E.J.B. supervised part of this work and edited the manuscript.

Acknowledgments: This work was funded by the RoseTrees Trust (M276 and A1384) to Athanasios Didangelos and Elizabeth J. Bradbury; EU 7th framework program (PrimeXS 0220) to Athanasios Didangelos; the Medical Research Council (MRC; SNCF G1002055) to Elizabeth J. Bradbury); MRC and EU funded MR/R005532/1 ERA-NET NEURON to Elizabeth J. Bradbury and Athanasios Didangelos. Athanasios Didangelos was funded by the London Law Trust and King's College London.

Abbreviations

SCI	Spinal cord injury
LC-MS/MS	Liquid-chromatography and tandem mass-spectrometry

References

1. Cregg, J.M.; DePaul, M.A.; Filous, A.R.; Lang, B.T.; Tran, A.; Silver, J. Functional regeneration beyond the glial scar. *Exp. Neurol.* **2014**, *253*, 197–207. [CrossRef] [PubMed]
2. Ramer, L.M.; Ramer, M.S.; Bradbury, E.J. Restoring function after spinal cord injury: Towards clinical translation of experimental strategies. *Lancet Neurol.* **2014**, *13*, 1241–1256. [CrossRef]
3. Fitch, M.T.; Silver, J. CNS injury, glial scars and inflammation: Inhibitory extracellular matrices and regeneration failure. *Exp. Neurol.* **2008**, *209*, 294–301. [CrossRef] [PubMed]
4. Fawcett, J.W.; Schwab, M.E.; Montani, L.; Brazda, N.; Muller, H.W. Defeating inhibition of regeneration by scar and myelin components. *Handb. Clin. Neurol.* **2012**, *109*, 503–522. [PubMed]
5. Hellal, F.; Hurtado, A.; Ruschel, J.; Flynn, K.C.; Laskowski, C.J.; Umlauf, M.; Kapitein, L.C.; Strikis, D.; Lemmon, V.; Bixby, J.; et al. Microtubule stabilization reduces scarring and causes axon regeneration after spinal cord injury. *Science* **2011**, *331*, 928–931. [CrossRef] [PubMed]

6. Ruschel, J.; Hellal, F.; Flynn, K.C.; Dupraz, S.; Elliott, D.A.; Tedeschi, A.; Bates, M.; Sliwinski, C.; Brook, G.; Dobrindt, K.; et al. Axonal regeneration. Systemic administration of epothilone B promotes axon regeneration after spinal cord injury. *Science* **2015**, *348*, 347–352. [CrossRef] [PubMed]
7. Bartus, K.; James, N.D.; Didangelos, A.; Bosch, K.D.; Verhaagen, J.; Yanez-Munoz, R.J.; Rogers, J.H.; Schneider, B.L.; Muir, E.M.; Bradbury, E.J. Large-scale chondroitin sulfate proteoglycan digestion with chondroitinase gene therapy leads to reduced pathology and modulates macrophage phenotype following spinal cord contusion injury. *J. Neurosci.* **2014**, *34*, 4822–4836. [CrossRef] [PubMed]
8. Bradbury, E.J.; Moon, L.D.; Popat, R.J.; King, V.R.; Bennett, G.S.; Patel, P.N.; Fawcett, J.W.; McMahon, S.B. Chondroitinase ABC promotes functional recovery after spinal cord injury. *Nature* **2002**, *416*, 636–640. [CrossRef] [PubMed]
9. Didangelos, A.; Iberl, M.; Vinsland, E.; Bartus, K.; Bradbury, E.J. Regulation of IL-10 by chondroitinase ABC promotes a distinct immune response following spinal cord injury. *J. Neurosci.* **2014**, *34*, 16424–16432. [CrossRef] [PubMed]
10. Didangelos, A.; Puglia, M.; Iberl, M.; Sanchez-Bellot, C.; Roschitzki, B.; Bradbury, E.J. High-throughput proteomics reveal alarmins as amplifiers of tissue pathology and inflammation after spinal cord injury. *Sci. Rep.* **2016**, *6*, 21607. [CrossRef] [PubMed]
11. Chamankhah, M.; Eftekharpour, E.; Karimi-Abdolrezaee, S.; Boutros, P.C.; San-Marina, S.; Fehlings, M.G. Genome-wide gene expression profiling of stress response in a spinal cord clip compression injury model. *BMC Genom.* **2013**, *14*, 583. [CrossRef] [PubMed]
12. Didangelos, A.; Yin, X.; Mandal, K.; Baumert, M.; Jahangiri, M.; Mayr, M. Proteomics characterization of extracellular space components in the human aorta. *Mol. Cell. Proteom.* **2010**, *9*, 2048–2062. [CrossRef] [PubMed]
13. Didangelos, A.; Yin, X.; Mandal, K.; Saje, A.; Smith, A.; Xu, Q.; Jahangiri, M.; Mayr, M. Extracellular matrix composition and remodelling in human abdominal aortic aneurysms: A proteomics approach. *Mol. Cell. Proteom.* **2011**, *10*. [CrossRef] [PubMed]
14. Arike, L.; Peil, L. Spectral counting label-free proteomics. *Methods Mol. Biol.* **2014**, *1156*, 213–222. [PubMed]
15. Koschutzki, D.; Schreiber, F. Centrality analysis methods for biological networks and their application to gene regulatory networks. *Gene Regul. Syst. Biol.* **2008**, *2*, 193–201. [CrossRef]
16. Shree, T.; Olson, O.C.; Elie, B.T.; Kester, J.C.; Garfall, A.L.; Simpson, K.; Bell-McGuinn, K.M.; Zabor, E.C.; Brogi, E.; Joyce, J.A. Macrophages and cathepsin proteases blunt chemotherapeutic response in breast cancer. *Genes Dev.* **2011**, *25*, 2465–2479. [CrossRef] [PubMed]
17. Saher, G.; Brugger, B.; Lappe-Siefke, C.; Mobius, W.; Tozawa, R.; Wehr, M.C.; Wieland, F.; Ishibashi, S.; Nave, K.A. High cholesterol level is essential for myelin membrane growth. *Nat. Neurosci.* **2005**, *8*, 468–475. [CrossRef] [PubMed]
18. Goodrum, J.F. Cholesterol synthesis is down-regulated during regeneration of peripheral nerve. *J. Neurochem.* **1990**, *54*, 1709–1715. [CrossRef] [PubMed]
19. Griffith, M.; Griffith, O.L.; Coffman, A.C.; Weible, J.V.; McMichael, J.F.; Spies, N.C.; Koval, J.; Das, I.; Callaway, M.B.; Eldred, J.M.; et al. DGIdb: Mining the druggable genome. *Nat. Methods* **2013**, *10*, 1209–1210. [CrossRef] [PubMed]
20. Szklarczyk, D.; Santos, A.; von Mering, C.; Jensen, L.J.; Bork, P.; Kuhn, M. STITCH 5: Augmenting protein-chemical interaction networks with tissue and affinity data. *Nucleic Acids Res.* **2016**, *44*, D380–D384. [CrossRef] [PubMed]
21. Perretti, M.; D'Acquisto, F. Annexin A1 and glucocorticoids as effectors of the resolution of inflammation. *Nat. Rev. Immunol.* **2009**, *9*, 62–70. [CrossRef] [PubMed]
22. Nesathurai, S. Steroids and spinal cord injury: Revisiting the NASCIS 2 and NASCIS 3 trials. *J. Trauma* **1998**, *45*, 1088–1093. [CrossRef] [PubMed]
23. Sekhon, L.H.; Fehlings, M.G. Epidemiology, demographics and pathophysiology of acute spinal cord injury. *Spine* **2001**, *26*, S2–S12. [CrossRef] [PubMed]
24. Elkabes, S.; Nicot, A.B. Sex steroids and neuroprotection in spinal cord injury: A review of preclinical investigations. *Exp. Neurol.* **2014**, *259*, 28–37. [CrossRef] [PubMed]
25. Banik, N.L.; Hogan, E.L.; Powers, J.M.; Smith, K.P. Proteolytic enzymes in experimental spinal cord injury. *J. Neurol. Sci.* **1986**, *73*, 245–256. [CrossRef]

26. Guo, Y.; Liu, S.; Wang, P.; Zhang, H.; Wang, F.; Bing, L.; Gao, J.; Yang, J.; Hao, A. Granulocyte colony-stimulating factor improves neuron survival in experimental spinal cord injury by regulating nucleophosmin-1 expression. *J. Neurosci. Res.* **2014**, *92*, 751–760. [CrossRef] [PubMed]
27. Babic, I.; Nurmemmedov, E.; Yenugonda, V.M.; Juarez, T.; Nomura, N.; Pingle, S.C.; Glassy, M.C.; Kesari, S. Pritumumab, the first therapeutic antibody for glioma patients. *Hum. Antib.* **2018**, *26*, 95–101. [CrossRef] [PubMed]
28. Menet, V.; Prieto, M.; Privat, A.; Gimenez y Ribotta, M. Axonal plasticity and functional recovery after spinal cord injury in mice deficient in both glial fibrillary acidic protein and vimentin genes. *Proc. Natl. Acad. Sci. USA* **2003**, *100*, 8999–9004. [CrossRef] [PubMed]
29. Luo, Y.; Xie, X.; Luo, D.; Wang, Y.; Gao, Y. The role of halofuginone in fibrosis: More to be explored? *J. Leukoc. Biol.* **2017**, *102*, 1333–1345. [CrossRef] [PubMed]
30. Jalil, J.E.; Doering, C.W.; Janicki, J.S.; Pick, R.; Shroff, S.G.; Weber, K.T. Fibrillar collagen and myocardial stiffness in the intact hypertrophied rat left ventricle. *Circ. Res.* **1989**, *64*, 1041–1050. [CrossRef] [PubMed]
31. Ciccarelli, R.; Ballerini, P.; Sabatino, G.; Rathbone, M.P.; D'Onofrio, M.; Caciagli, F.; Di Iorio, P. Involvement of astrocytes in purine-mediated reparative processes in the brain. *Int. J. Dev. Neurosci.* **2001**, *19*, 395–414. [CrossRef]
32. Kicska, G.A.; Long, L.; Horig, H.; Fairchild, C.; Tyler, P.C.; Furneaux, R.H.; Schramm, V.L.; Kaufman, H.L. Immucillin H, a powerful transition-state analog inhibitor of purine nucleoside phosphorylase, selectively inhibits human T lymphocytes. *Proc. Natl. Acad. Sci. USA* **2001**, *98*, 4593–4598. [CrossRef] [PubMed]
33. Miles, R.W.; Tyler, P.C.; Furneaux, R.H.; Bagdassarian, C.K.; Schramm, V.L. One-third-the-sites transition-state inhibitors for purine nucleoside phosphorylase. *Biochemistry* **1998**, *37*, 8615–8621. [CrossRef] [PubMed]
34. Rathbone, M.; Pilutti, L.; Caciagli, F.; Jiang, S. Neurotrophic effects of extracellular guanosine. *Nucleosides Nucleotides Nucleic Acids* **2008**, *27*, 666–672. [CrossRef] [PubMed]
35. Gong, B.; Radulovic, M.; Figueiredo-Pereira, M.E.; Cardozo, C. The Ubiquitin-Proteasome System: Potential Therapeutic Targets for Alzheimer's Disease and Spinal Cord Injury. *Front. Mol. Neurosci.* **2016**, *9*, 4. [CrossRef] [PubMed]
36. Sharma, H.S.; Muresanu, D.F.; Lafuente, J.V.; Sjoquist, P.O.; Patnaik, R.; Sharma, A. Nanoparticles Exacerbate Both Ubiquitin and Heat Shock Protein Expressions in Spinal Cord Injury: Neuroprotective Effects of the Proteasome Inhibitor Carfilzomib and the Antioxidant Compound H-290/51. *Mol. Neurobiol.* **2015**, *52*, 882–898. [CrossRef] [PubMed]
37. Wang, X.; Arcuino, G.; Takano, T.; Lin, J.; Peng, W.G.; Wan, P.; Li, P.; Xu, Q.; Liu, Q.S.; Goldman, S.A.; et al. P2X7 receptor inhibition improves recovery after spinal cord injury. *Nat. Med.* **2004**, *10*, 821–827. [CrossRef] [PubMed]
38. Teng, Y.D.; Mocchetti, I.; Wrathall, J.R. Basic and acidic fibroblast growth factors protect spinal motor neurones in vivo after experimental spinal cord injury. *Eur. J. Neurosci.* **1998**, *10*, 798–802. [CrossRef] [PubMed]
39. Haque, A.; Ray, S.K.; Cox, A.; Banik, N.L. Neuron specific enolase: A promising therapeutic target in acute spinal cord injury. *Metab. Brain Dis.* **2015**, *31*, 487–495. [CrossRef] [PubMed]
40. Lopez-Vales, R.; Redensek, A.; Skinner, T.A.; Rathore, K.I.; Ghasemlou, N.; Wojewodka, G.; DeSanctis, J.; Radzioch, D.; David, S. Fenretinide promotes functional recovery and tissue protection after spinal cord contusion injury in mice. *J. Neurosci.* **2010**, *30*, 3220–3226. [CrossRef] [PubMed]
41. Eftekharpour, E.; Nagakannan, P.; Iqbal, M.A.; Chen, Q.M. Mevalonate Cascade and Small Rho GTPase in Spinal Cord Injury. *Curr. Mol. Pharmacol.* **2017**, *10*, 141–151. [PubMed]
42. Abate, M.; Laezza, C.; Pisanti, S.; Torelli, G.; Seneca, V.; Catapano, G.; Montella, F.; Ranieri, R.; Notarnicola, M.; Gazzerro, P.; et al. Deregulated expression and activity of Farnesyl Diphosphate Synthase (FDPS) in Glioblastoma. *Sci. Rep.* **2017**, *7*, 14123. [CrossRef] [PubMed]
43. Nance, P.W.; Schryvers, O.; Leslie, W.; Ludwig, S.; Krahn, J.; Uebelhart, D. Intravenous pamidronate attenuates bone density loss after acute spinal cord injury. *Arch. Phys. Med. Rehabil.* **1999**, *80*, 243–251. [CrossRef]
44. Beigneux, A.P.; Kosinski, C.; Gavino, B.; Horton, J.D.; Skarnes, W.C.; Young, S.G. ATP-citrate lyase deficiency in the mouse. *J. Biol. Chem.* **2004**, *279*, 9557–9564. [CrossRef] [PubMed]

45. Krishnan, M.L.; Wang, Z.; Silver, M.; Boardman, J.P.; Ball, G.; Counsell, S.J.; Walley, A.J.; Montana, G.; Edwards, A.D. Possible relationship between common genetic variation and white matter development in a pilot study of preterm infants. *Brain Behav.* **2016**, *6*, e00434. [CrossRef] [PubMed]
46. Chu, Y.; Parada, I.; Prince, D.A. Temporal and topographic alterations in expression of the alpha3 isoform of Na+, K(+)-ATPase in the rat freeze lesion model of microgyria and epileptogenesis. *Neuroscience* **2009**, *162*, 339–348. [CrossRef] [PubMed]
47. de Carvalho Aguiar, P.; Sweadner, K.J.; Penniston, J.T.; Zaremba, J.; Liu, L.; Caton, M.; Linazasoro, G.; Borg, M.; Tijssen, M.A.; Bressman, S.B.; et al. Mutations in the Na^+/K^+-ATPase alpha3 gene ATP1A3 are associated with rapid-onset dystonia parkinsonism. *Neuron* **2004**, *43*, 169–175. [CrossRef] [PubMed]
48. Besse, A.; Wu, P.; Bruni, F.; Donti, T.; Graham, B.H.; Craigen, W.J.; McFarland, R.; Moretti, P.; Lalani, S.; Scott, K.L.; et al. The GABA transaminase, ABAT, is essential for mitochondrial nucleoside metabolism. *Cell Metab.* **2015**, *21*, 417–427. [CrossRef] [PubMed]
49. Sauer, S.W.; Kolker, S.; Hoffmann, G.F.; Ten Brink, H.J.; Jakobs, C.; Gibson, K.M.; Okun, J.G. Enzymatic and metabolic evidence for a region specific mitochondrial dysfunction in brains of murine succinic semialdehyde dehydrogenase deficiency (Aldh5a1$^{-/-}$ mice). *Neurochem. Int.* **2007**, *50*, 653–659. [CrossRef] [PubMed]
50. Drewes, A.M.; Andreasen, A.; Poulsen, L.H. Valproate for treatment of chronic central pain after spinal cord injury. A double-blind cross-over study. *Paraplegia* **1994**, *32*, 565–569. [CrossRef] [PubMed]
51. Liberzon, A.; Birger, C.; Thorvaldsdottir, H.; Ghandi, M.; Mesirov, J.P.; Tamayo, P. The Molecular Signatures Database (MSigDB) hallmark gene set collection. *Cell Syst.* **2016**, *1*, 417–425. [CrossRef] [PubMed]
52. Durbin, J.E.; Hackenmiller, R.; Simon, M.C.; Levy, D.E. Targeted disruption of the mouse Stat1 gene results in compromised innate immunity to viral disease. *Cell* **1996**, *84*, 443–450. [CrossRef]
53. Meraz, M.A.; White, J.M.; Sheehan, K.C.; Bach, E.A.; Rodig, S.J.; Dighe, A.S.; Kaplan, D.H.; Riley, J.K.; Greenlund, A.C.; Campbell, D.; et al. Targeted disruption of the Stat1 gene in mice reveals unexpected physiologic specificity in the JAK-STAT signaling pathway. *Cell* **1996**, *84*, 431–442. [CrossRef]
54. Profyris, C.; Cheema, S.S.; Zang, D.; Azari, M.F.; Boyle, K.; Petratos, S. Degenerative and regenerative mechanisms governing spinal cord injury. *Neurobiol. Dis.* **2004**, *15*, 415–436. [CrossRef] [PubMed]
55. Wu, Y.; Yang, L.; Mei, X.; Yu, Y. Selective inhibition of STAT1 reduces spinal cord injury in mice. *Neurosci. Lett.* **2014**, *580*, 7–11. [CrossRef] [PubMed]
56. James, N.D.; Bartus, K.; Grist, J.; Bennett, D.L.; McMahon, S.B.; Bradbury, E.J. Conduction failure following spinal cord injury: Functional and anatomical changes from acute to chronic stages. *J. Neurosci.* **2011**, *31*, 18543–18555. [CrossRef] [PubMed]
57. Mills, C.D.; Hains, B.C.; Johnson, K.M.; Hulsebosch, C.E. Strain and model differences in behavioral outcomes after spinal cord injury in rat. *J. Neurotrauma* **2001**, *18*, 743–756. [CrossRef] [PubMed]
58. Kjell, J.; Olson, L. Rat models of spinal cord injury: From pathology to potential therapies. *Dis. Model. Mech.* **2016**, *9*, 1125–1137. [CrossRef] [PubMed]
59. Cheriyan, T.; Ryan, D.J.; Weinreb, J.H.; Cheriyan, J.; Paul, J.C.; Lafage, V.; Kirsch, T.; Errico, T.J. Spinal cord injury models: A review. *Spinal Cord* **2014**, *52*, 588–595. [CrossRef] [PubMed]
60. Sharif-Alhoseini, M.; Khormali, M.; Rezaei, M.; Safdarian, M.; Hajighadery, A.; Khalatbari, M.M.; Meknatkhah, S.; Rezvan, M.; Chalangari, M.; Derakhshan, P.; et al. Animal models of spinal cord injury: A systematic review. *Spinal Cord* **2017**, *55*, 714–721. [CrossRef] [PubMed]
61. Pinzon, A.; Marcillo, A.; Pabon, D.; Bramlett, H.M.; Bunge, M.B.; Dietrich, W.D. A re-assessment of erythropoietin as a neuroprotective agent following rat spinal cord compression or contusion injury. *Exp. Neurol.* **2008**, *213*, 129–136. [CrossRef] [PubMed]
62. Geremia, N.M.; Hryciw, T.; Bao, F.; Streijger, F.; Okon, E.; Lee, J.H.T.; Weaver, L.C.; Dekaban, G.A.; Kwon, B.K.; Brown, A. The effectiveness of the anti-CD11d treatment is reduced in rat models of spinal cord injury that produce significant levels of intraspinal hemorrhage. *Exp. Neurol.* **2017**, *295*, 125–134. [CrossRef] [PubMed]
63. Kjell, J.; Sandor, K.; Josephson, A.; Svensson, C.I.; Abrams, M.B. Rat substrains differ in the magnitude of spontaneous locomotor recovery and in the development of mechanical hypersensitivity after experimental spinal cord injury. *J. Neurotrauma* **2013**, *30*, 1805–1811. [CrossRef] [PubMed]
64. Popovich, P.G.; Wei, P.; Stokes, B.T. Cellular inflammatory response after spinal cord injury in Sprague-Dawley and Lewis rats. *J. Comp. Neurol.* **1997**, *377*, 443–464. [CrossRef]
65. Schmitt, C.; Miranpuri, G.S.; Dhodda, V.K.; Isaacson, J.; Vemuganti, R.; Resnick, D.K. Changes in spinal cord injury-induced gene expression in rat are strain-dependent. *Spine J.* **2006**, *6*, 113–119. [CrossRef] [PubMed]

66. Bantia, S.; Ananth, S.L.; Parker, C.D.; Horn, L.L.; Upshaw, R. Mechanism of inhibition of T-acute lymphoblastic leukemia cells by PNP inhibitor–BCX-1777. *Int. Immunopharmacol.* **2003**, *3*, 879–887. [CrossRef]
67. Somech, R.; Lev, A.; Grisaru-Soen, G.; Shiran, S.I.; Simon, A.J.; Grunebaum, E. Purine nucleoside phosphorylase deficiency presenting as severe combined immune deficiency. *Immunol. Res.* **2013**, *56*, 150–154. [CrossRef] [PubMed]
68. Hiraiwa, M. Cathepsin A/protective protein: An unusual lysosomal multifunctional protein. *Cell. Mol. Life Sci.* **1999**, *56*, 894–907. [CrossRef] [PubMed]
69. Chen, J.; Wang, Z.; Mao, Y.; Zheng, Z.; Chen, Y.; Khor, S.; Shi, K.; He, Z.; Li, J.; Gong, F.; et al. Liraglutide activates autophagy via GLP-1R to improve functional recovery after spinal cord injury. *Oncotarget* **2017**, *8*, 85949–85968. [CrossRef] [PubMed]
70. Calhan, O.Y.; Seyrantepe, V. Mice with Catalytically Inactive Cathepsin A Display Neurobehavioral Alterations. *Behav. Neurol.* **2017**, *2017*, 4261873. [CrossRef] [PubMed]
71. Carecchio, M.; Zorzi, G.; Ragona, F.; Zibordi, F.; Nardocci, N. ATP1A3-related disorders: An update. *Eur. J. Paediatr. Neurol.* **2018**, *22*, 257–263. [CrossRef] [PubMed]
72. Searle, B.C. Scaffold: A bioinformatic tool for validating MS/MS-based proteomic studies. *Proteomics* **2010**, *10*, 1265–1269. [CrossRef] [PubMed]
73. Saeed, A.I.; Bhagabati, N.K.; Braisted, J.C.; Liang, W.; Sharov, V.; Howe, E.A.; Li, J.; Thiagarajan, M.; White, J.A.; Quackenbush, J. TM4 microarray software suite. *Methods Enzymol.* **2006**, *411*, 134–193. [PubMed]
74. Szklarczyk, D.; Franceschini, A.; Wyder, S.; Forslund, K.; Heller, D.; Huerta-Cepas, J.; Simonovic, M.; Roth, A.; Santos, A.; Tsafou, K.P.; et al. STRING v10: Protein-protein interaction networks, integrated over the tree of life. *Nucleic Acids Res.* **2015**, *43*, D447–D452. [CrossRef] [PubMed]
75. Smoot, M.E.; Ono, K.; Ruscheinski, J.; Wang, P.L.; Ideker, T. Cytoscape 2.8: New features for data integration and network visualization. *Bioinformatics* **2010**, *27*, 431–432. [CrossRef] [PubMed]

13

Activity-Based Physical Rehabilitation with Adjuvant Testosterone to Promote Neuromuscular Recovery after Spinal Cord Injury

Dana M. Otzel [1], Jimmy Lee [2], Fan Ye [2], Stephen E. Borst [3] and Joshua F. Yarrow [2,4,*]

1 Brain Rehabilitation Research Center, Malcom Randall Veterans Affairs Medical Center, North Florida/South Georgia Veterans Health System, Gainesville, FL 32608, USA; dana.otzel@va.gov

2 Research Service, Malcom Randall Veterans Affairs Medical Center, North Florida/South Georgia Veterans Health System, Gainesville, FL 32608, USA; jimmylee@ufl.edu (J.L.); 2005evan@gmail.com (F.Y.)

3 Department of Applied Physiology, Kinesiology and University of Florida College of Health and Human Performance, Gainesville, FL 32603, USA; seborst@ufl.edu

4 Division of Endocrinology, Diabetes and Metabolism, University of Florida College of Medicine, Gainesville, FL 32610, USA

* Correspondence: jfyarrow@ufl.edu

Abstract: Neuromuscular impairment and reduced musculoskeletal integrity are hallmarks of spinal cord injury (SCI) that hinder locomotor recovery. These impairments are precipitated by the neurological insult and resulting disuse, which has stimulated interest in activity-based physical rehabilitation therapies (ABTs) that promote neuromuscular plasticity after SCI. However, ABT efficacy declines as SCI severity increases. Additionally, many men with SCI exhibit low testosterone, which may exacerbate neuromusculoskeletal impairment. Incorporating testosterone adjuvant to ABTs may improve musculoskeletal recovery and neuroplasticity because androgens attenuate muscle loss and the slow-to-fast muscle fiber-type transition after SCI, in a manner independent from mechanical strain, and promote motoneuron survival. These neuromusculoskeletal benefits are promising, although testosterone alone produces only limited functional improvement in rodent SCI models. In this review, we discuss the (1) molecular deficits underlying muscle loss after SCI; (2) independent influences of testosterone and locomotor training on neuromuscular function and musculoskeletal integrity post-SCI; (3) hormonal and molecular mechanisms underlying the therapeutic efficacy of these strategies; and (4) evidence supporting a multimodal strategy involving ABT with adjuvant testosterone, as a potential means to promote more comprehensive neuromusculoskeletal recovery than either strategy alone.

Keywords: neuroplasticity; bodyweight-supported treadmill training; estradiol; estrogen; muscle; PI3K; IGF-1; motor neuron; BDNF; FOXO; PGC-1 alpha; PGC-1 beta

---

1. Introduction

Spinal cord injury (SCI) results in profound sensorimotor impairment below the lesion site, which is precipitated by the insult to the spinal cord and exacerbated by a cascade of secondary cellular and molecular processes occurring in the acute and chronic post-injury phases [1–3]. Neuromuscular impairment and muscle loss are hallmarks of the SCI injury cascade that produce substantial impediments to physical therapy regimens intended to restore locomotion [3]. Activity-based physical rehabilitation therapies (ABTs) (e.g., bodyweight-supported treadmill training (BWSTT) or robotic assisted locomotor training with or without electric stimulation) have shown promise in promoting neuromuscular plasticity in humans and rodent models after motor-incomplete SCI [4,5]. However, ABTs are only partially effective in restoring function after SCI and their neuromuscular efficacy declines as injury severity increases [6], indicating the need for adjuvant therapeutic strategies to hasten functional recovery in this population.

Low testosterone (T) is also a secondary consequence of SCI, with hypogonadism being ~ four times more prevalent in men after SCI than in non-injured populations [7]. Non-neurologically impaired men with low T exhibit low muscle mass, impaired muscle function [8], and worsened walking biomechanics [9], while T replacement therapy (TRT) improves muscle mass, neuromuscular function [10], and walking speed in older ambulatory hypogonadal men [11]. To-date, a causal relationship between low T and worsened neuromuscular function after SCI has not been elucidated, although TRT increases sublesional lean mass [12] and muscle cross-sectional area (CSA) in men with motor-complete SCI [13], in a manner completely independent from voluntary muscle contractility. Similarly, in male and female rodent SCI models, androgen treatment attenuates sublesional muscle loss and other phenotypic changes associated with impaired muscle function after SCI [14–20], and may promote slight improvement in locomotor recovery [15]. Herein, we will summarize the (1) molecular deficits underlying muscle loss after SCI; (2) independent influences of T and ABTs on neuromuscular function and musculoskeletal integrity subsequent to SCI; (3) hormonal and molecular mechanisms underlying the therapeutic efficacy of these strategies; and (4) evidence supporting a multimodal strategy involving BWSTT with adjuvant T, as a potential means to promote more comprehensive neuromusculoskeletal recovery after SCI.

2. Neuromuscular Adaptations after SCI

Motoneuron innervation of skeletal muscle fibers influences muscle mass and function, and fiber-type distribution [21]. After SCI, changes to the excitatory and inhibitory inputs to the motor unit (i.e., spinal motoneuron and the innervated fibers) exist [22]. For example, motor units that are dysfunctional after SCI result in a weaker and less fatigue resistant muscle [22,23], with rate of force development and motor axon conduction velocity decreasing [24,25]. These changes may exacerbate functional decline after SCI and can impair locomotor recovery, depending on the injury severity and degree of motor dysfunction [26]. The plethora of anatomical and functional consequences resulting from motor unit impairment after SCI have been detailed elsewhere [22]. Herein, we will focus on somatic motoneuron structural adaptations that influence impaired motor function after SCI [27] and how T administration [17,18] and locomotor training [28,29] may alter these adaptations and ultimately improve muscle function and/or locomotor recovery.

The muscular adaptations to SCI have been detailed previously [30], which we summarize here in brevity. Individuals with SCI exhibit an 18–46% lower sublesional muscle cross-sectional area (CSA) than those without SCI, with the degree of atrophy depending on the injury severity [31] and muscle groups involved [32–34]. Muscle loss is worsened as injury severity progresses [31], a result of more impaired motor function and extended disuse in those with motor-complete SCI. For example, muscle atrophy occurs primarily in the initial six weeks after injury in those with motor-incomplete SCI [32], while whole muscle CSA and muscle fiber (f)CSA continually decline for at least 24 weeks after motor-complete SCI [33,35]. Atrophy of both type I (slow-oxidative) and type II (fast-glycolytic) fibers occurs in humans [35,36] and rodents in response to SCI [37], preceding intramuscular fat accumulation [32] and the well-characterized slow-to-fast fiber transition [38,39]. These structural and physiologic changes impair voluntary force generation and muscle endurance [40,41], factors that are associated with locomotor recovery after SCI [42,43]. However, skeletal muscle retains the ability to reverse the molecular cascade precipitating atrophy [44,45] and to improve contractility after SCI in response to sufficient stimuli [46]. In the sections below, we discuss evidence supporting the involvement of several molecular signaling pathways that likely influence muscle deficits after SCI.

2.1. Ubiquitin-Proteasome Signaling after SCI

Reduced phosphorylation of the forkhead box O (FOXO) proteins FOXO1 and FOXO3a promotes the transcription of muscle atrophy F-box (MAFbx or atrogin-1) and muscle ring finger-1 (MuRF1), muscle-specific E_3 ubiquitin ligases that stimulate atrophy in response to disuse and other catabolic states [47]. The influence of these ubiquitin ligases on skeletal muscle atrophy has been demonstrated by the viral overexpression of MAFbx, which reduced the myotube diameter by ~85% in vitro, and by genetic elimination of MAFbx or MuRF1, which attenuated muscle atrophy in response to sciatic nerve transection [48]. Within several days of SCI, >50 protein ubiquination pathway genes are upregulated in sublesional muscle [49], an effect that likely influences the rapid muscle atrophy in response to injury. In particular, MAFbx and MuRF1 mRNA expressions are increased five- to >40-fold within two to eight days of injury [50–54], with protein expressions elevated >two-fold prior to the initiation of muscle atrophy [55]. Interestingly, the fold inductions of MAFbx and MuRF1 were associated with the rate of skeletal muscle atrophy in response to spinal cord transection [53], suggesting that a higher expression of these genes exacerbates muscle loss after SCI. In this regard, FOXO1 mRNA was 33% higher [54] and MAFbx and MuRF1 mRNA were >two-fold higher in rodents after spinal transection than in animals receiving sciatic nerve transection [53], potentially explaining the more rapid atrophy occurring after SCI than in other disuse conditions [53,56]. However, the increased expressions of these and other ubiquitin proteasome pathway genes do not persist after experimental SCI [49], with FOXO1, MAFbx, and MuRF1 gene expressions and pFOXO1 and pFOXO3 proteins reverting to the level of uninjured controls within two to 10 weeks of spinal cord transection [53,54,57]. Similarly, in humans with motor-complete SCI, MAFbx and MuRF1 expressions are high at one-month post-injury and decline by 50–75% at three- and 12-months, resulting from reductions in pFOXO1 and/or total FOXO3 proteins [58]. Indeed, in cohorts of men with chronic SCI, MAFbx and MuRF1 gene expression appear equal to [59] or less than uninjured controls, with FOXO1, FOXO3a, and MAFbx proteins being >35% lower than controls [60]. While our discussion focused on changes in the ubiquitin-proteasome pathway, it is important to note that other catabolic pathways likely influence muscle atrophy after SCI. For example, calpain 1 mRNA expression is increased as early as day 4 after spinal cord transection, an effect that persists for at least 15 days [50], which is important given the influence of calpain signaling on myofibrillar proteolysis [61].

2.2. *IGF-1 Signaling Pathway after SCI*

IGF-1 mediated activation of the phosphatidylinositol-3 kinase (PI3K)/Akt signaling pathway promotes skeletal muscle anabolism [62]. In the immediate days after SCI, mRNA encoding IGF-1, the IGF-1 receptor (IGF-1R), and several IGF binding proteins (IGFBP) are upregulated in muscle [50,51,63], and muscle IGF-1 protein expression is increased [63]. Despite this, muscle pAkt is reduced within several days of SCI [51,55], while relatively normal total and phosphorylated 4E-BP1 and S6K1 expression persist in the first few weeks after SCI [50,51]. The inability of IGF-1 to increase pAkt and downstream targets acutely after SCI likely occurs because insulin receptor substrate-1 (IRS1) protein expression is rapidly reduced in response to SCI [51]. In this regard, IRS1 expression is required for IGF-1 mediated muscle hypertrophy, evidenced by the inability of genetic IGF-1 overexpression to promote skeletal muscle hypertrophy in IRS1 deficient animals [64]. Subsequently, the downregulation of IGF-1 signaling persists chronically after SCI, evidenced by (1) 25–40% lower circulating IGF-1 [65,66] and 50% lower IGF-1 protein expression in the muscle of individuals with chronic SCI compared with controls [60]; and (2) lower total Akt protein and lower total and phosphorylated mTOR and S6K1 in rodent muscle 10-weeks after spinal cord transection [57,67], accompanying 50% lower immunoprecipitated S6K1 activity [67]. Similarly, in humans with motor-complete SCI, total and phosphorylated mTOR and regulatory-associated protein of mTOR (RPTOR), an mTOR cofactor, were lower at three- and 12-months after injury, when compared with values obtained one-month post-SCI, likely influencing the lower p4E-BP1 and pS6 (subunit of S6K1) protein expression [58] that persists for upwards of 30 years after SCI [60]. In this regard, circulating IGF-1 has been shown to be highly correlated with increased thigh muscle CSA in men with chronic motor-complete SCI [68].

2.3. PGC-1α and PGC-1β Signaling after SCI

In skeletal muscle, peroxisome proliferator-activated receptor gamma co-activator (PGC)-1α regulates type I fiber expression and mitochondrial biogenesis [69], while PGC-1β regulates various aspects of mitochondrial structure and function [70]. As evidence, transgenic PGC-1α expression results in a whole body muscular phenotype that is high in type I oxidative fibers [71] and muscle-specific PGC-1α overexpression increases mitochondrial biogenesis [72]. In comparison, ablation of PGC-1β in skeletal muscle myofibers in adulthood reduced mitochondrial CSA and mitochondrial respiration without altering fiber-type distribution, resulting in increased oxidative stress and impaired exercise performance [70]. Baligand et al. used genome wide analysis and identified that genes associated with mitochondrial dysfunction and impaired oxidative phosphorylation were altered three to 14 days after SCI [49]. In particular, muscle PGC-1α mRNA expression was suppressed to a nearly undetectable level three days after spinal cord transection [54] and within two weeks, muscle PGC-1α protein was dramatically reduced, accompanying reductions in slow myosin heavy chain (MHC) protein expression [73] that is indicative of fewer oxidative fibers. Similarly, at eight-weeks post-transection, muscle PGC-1α gene expression and total and nuclear PGC-1α protein were >50% lower than controls, and slow MHC and slow troponin mRNA and protein were >60% lower [16]. However, at 17-weeks after spinal cord transection, muscle PGC-1α mRNA expression was no longer suppressed in rodents [74]. In this regard, the hallmark slow-to-fast fiber-type shift resulting from spinal cord transection is most pronounced in the first 100 days after injury, with relatively minor changes in type I MHC expression thereafter [38]. Regardless, muscle PGC-1α mRNA was 75% lower in men with chronic motor-complete SCI than in normally active men [75]. In comparison, relatively less is known about the changes in muscle PGC-1β after SCI. Interestingly, PGC-1β mRNA was reduced by 90% within three days of sciatic nerve transection [54], an effect that is mentioned because SCI typically results in relatively larger gene expression changes [76] and more rapid muscle loss than other disuse models [53,56]. Wu et al. also reported that muscle PGC-1β mRNA expression was 50% lower than controls at eight-weeks after spinal transection [74] and Kramer et al. reported 75% lower PGC-1β mRNA in men with chronic motor-complete SCI, when compared with ambulatory controls [75].

3. Androgenic Regulation of Muscle

Maintenance of skeletal muscle mass requires relative balance between muscle protein synthesis (i.e., anabolic processes) and protein degradation (i.e., catabolic processes), with elevated catabolic signaling and/or reduced anabolic signaling influencing muscle loss. Readers are directed to the following in-depth review of the various signaling pathways that influence skeletal muscle anabolism and catabolism in response to disuse [77]. Herein, we will discuss how androgens influence muscle mass via classical AR-mediated signaling and through interactions with other intercellular anabolic and catabolic signaling pathways (Figure 1).

3.1. Testosterone Synthesis and Metabolism

Testosterone is the most abundant bioactive androgen and is primarily synthesized by testicular Leydig cells in males [78] and by the ovaries in females [79], and to a lesser extent in other organs, such as the adrenal cortex [80]. The majority of T circulates are bound to protein transporters (i.e., sex-hormone binding globulin (SHBG) or albumin), with only a small fraction (~1–2%) circulating freely unbound to any protein transporter [81]. The fraction of free (i.e., unbound) T and albumin-bound T is bioavailable [82] because it can bind cell surface or cytosolic androgen receptors (ARs), in the case of free T, or cross the cell membrane and dissociate from its low affinity protein transporter, in the case of albumin, which allows subsequent cytosolic AR binding. In comparison, SHBG-bound T is biologically inactive because it cannot (1) bind cell-surface/plasma-membrane ARs; (2) cross cellular membranes and bind cytosolic ARs [83]; or (3) undergo enzymatic metabolism [84].

As such, elevated SHBG is associated with reduced androgenic action in target tissues expressing ARs, including skeletal muscle [78], bone [84], and spinal motoneurons [85–87], among others.

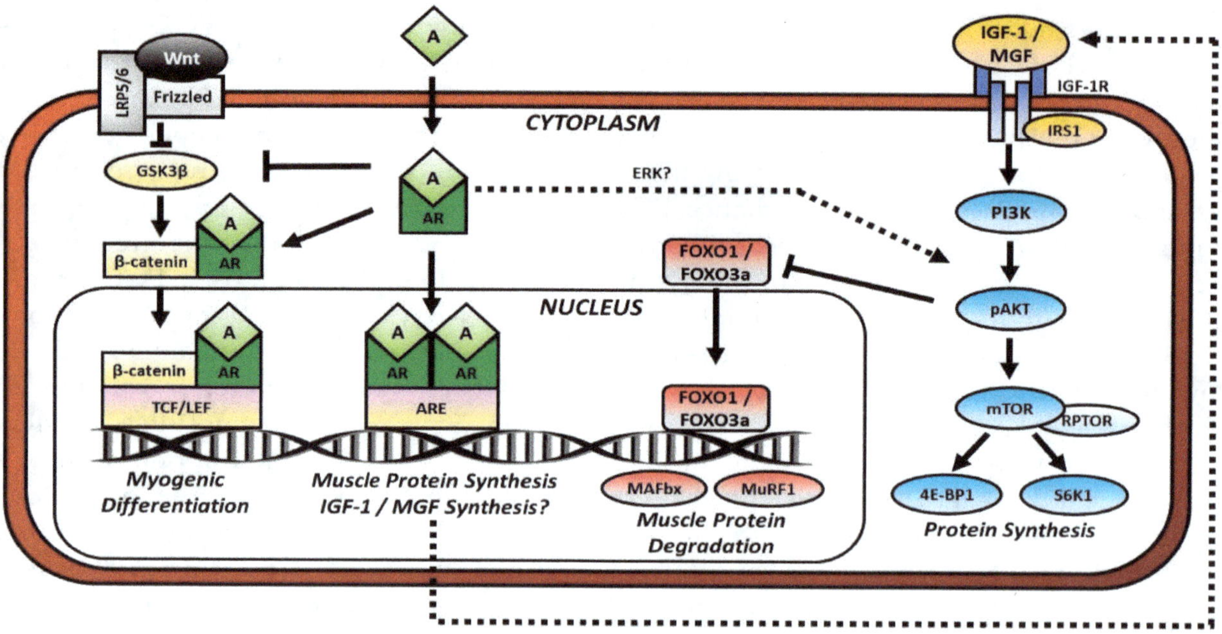

Figure 1. Androgen-mediated Anabolic and Anticatabolic Signaling Pathways in Muscle. Anabolic signaling: Androgens (A) pass through the plasma membrane and bind to cytosolic androgen receptors (AR). Dimerized and phosphorylated ARs pass through the nuclear membrane and bind to a region of the DNA termed the androgen response element (ARE), thereby initiating protein synthesis. Ligand-bound ARs may also enhance Wnt signaling as follows. Wnt binds to Frizzled and in turn disheveled (not shown). Disheveled inhibits the activity of glycogen synthase kinase-3β (GSK3β), which phosphorylates β-catenin and marks it for degradation. When GSK3β is inhibited, β-catenin accumulates and enters the nucleus where it binds to a region of the DNA termed the T-cell factor/lymphoid enhancer factor (TCF/LEF) that regulates genes involved in myogenic differentiation. Ligand-bound ARs enhance Wnt signaling by inhibiting GSK3β and attaching to β-catenin for nuclear shuttling. Androgens may also indirectly stimulate protein synthesis by activating the phosphatidylinositol-3 kinase (PI3K)/Akt signaling through actions of Erk or by promoting synthesis of insulin-like growth factor (IGF)-1 or mechano growth factor (MGF). IGF-1 and MGF bind cell-surface IGF-1 receptors (IGF-1R) and activate PI3K/Akt signaling. Anticatabolic signaling: Activation of PI3K/Akt signaling inhibits the transcription factor forkhead box O (FOXO). FOXO1 and FOXO3a activate muscle atrophy F-box (MAFbx or atrogin-1) and muscle ring finger-1 (MuRF1), and E_3 ubiquitin ligases that prepare proteins for proteasome degradation.

In addition to serving as a hormone, T is a substrate for the tissue-specific synthesis of two bioactive sex-steroid hormones, dihydrotestosterone (DHT) and estradiol (E_2), via actions of the 5α-reductase and aromatase enzymes, respectively [78,84]. The localized conversion of T to DHT, via any of the three 5α-reductase isozymes [78], enhances tissue-specific androgen signaling given that DHT binds to ARs with ~three times the affinity of T [88] and that DHT maintains a longer presence in tissues because it is not aromatized to E_2 nor converted to androstenedione (a weaker androgen), via 17β-hydroxysteroid dehydrogenase (17β-HSD) [78]. Similarly, the aromatization of T to E_2 amplifies estrogen signaling in tissues expressing estrogen receptors (ERs) [89]. In males, this conversion primarily occurs in non-gonadal tissue, with >80% of circulating E_2 derived from localized peripheral metabolism [90]. However, in females, the peripheral aromatization of T to E_2 also amplifies estrogen signaling [79], an effect that is particularly evident after the menopausal transition or in other situations where ovarian estrogen synthesis declines [80].

3.2. Hypogonadism and Testosterone Replacement after SCI

After SCI, 45–60% of men exhibit low T (hypogonadism, T < 300 ng/dL) [91–93] that results, in-part, from secondary testicular dysfunction [94] and impairments in the hypothalamic-pituitary axis [95,96]. Hypogonadism is ~four times more prevalent after SCI than in able-bodied men [7], with T concentrations remaining >25% below that of age-matched healthy men for an extended duration after SCI [91,97]. Additionally, a 50% greater decline in circulating T and >10-fold higher increase in SHBG occurs throughout the age-span in response to SCI [92], indicating that assessment of total T may underestimate hypogonadism incidence after SCI, a concept that we have demonstrated in other populations that exhibit elevated SHBG [81]. A causal relationship between low T and muscle loss after SCI has yet to be identified, although it is interesting to note that Finkelstein et al. reported that healthy men receiving pharmacologic treatment to maintain circulating T in the subphysiologic range (191 $\pm$ 78 ng/dL) exhibited a significant decline in whole body lean mass and thigh muscle area [98]. In this regard, the median T concentrations observed in several SCI cohort studies (i.e., 160–220 ng/dL) [93,99] were similar to that of Finkelstein et al., suggesting that the magnitude of hypogonadism after SCI is sufficient to induce muscle loss.

Our rodent severe contusion SCI model also exhibits 40–55% lower circulating T than controls for at least two months after injury [14,15,37,100] and androgen treatment attenuates muscle loss [14–16] and fCSA atrophy [17–20] in some, but not all, sublesional muscles in rodent SCI models [16,37,101]. In this regard, androgen-induced muscle preservation appears dependent upon muscle-specific AR expression, given that Phillips et al. reported muscle preservation in the sublesional levator ani/bulbocavernosus (LABC) muscle (high AR expression), but not soleus (low AR expression), in response to T treatment after SCI [37]. Importantly, neither E_2 treatment [17] nor the conversion of T to DHT [14] influence muscle preservation in rodent SCI models, suggesting dispensability of aromatase and 5α-reductase activity in muscle. Indeed, Borst et al. [102] demonstrated that co-administration of T with finasteride (type II 5α-reductase inhibitor) to non-neurologically impaired men resulted in dramatically lower DHT, but did not prevent T-induced improvements in lean mass or muscle strength. Several small clinical trials have also assessed TRT in men with motor-complete SCI. For example, Cooper et al. observed ~40% lower urinary protein and creatinine excretion in SCI patients receiving TRT acutely after injury [103,104], indicating reduced whole body and muscle protein catabolism. Additionally, Bauman et al. reported that 12 months of TRT increased upper- and lower-extremity lean mass and resting energy expenditure in hypogonadal men with motor-complete SCI [12], with improvement persisting for at least 12-months after TRT discontinuation [105]. Lastly, a single case-study recently reported that TRT increased thigh muscle CSA in a man with motor-complete SCI [13].

3.3. Classical Androgen Signaling

Classical androgen-mediated genomic signaling is initiated by the binding of T or DHT to cytosolic ARs to form hormone-receptor complexes that translocate to the nucleus and bind androgen response elements (AREs) [106], resulting in the activation or repression of multiple gene pathways that regulate skeletal muscle [107]. Similarly, E_2 stimulates classical estrogen-mediated genomic signaling that is characterized by binding cytoplasmic ERα or ERβ, which stimulates nuclear translocation of the hormone-receptor complex and binding to estrogen response elements (EREs). ER signaling is pronounced in bone [89], although the aromatization of T to E_2 is not obligatory for skeletal muscle maintenance [98].

Androgens also exert actions that are independent of nuclear AREs [78]. For example, androgens [78] and estrogens [108] exert effects by binding non-traditional cell-surface sex-steroid hormone receptors (e.g., G-protein-coupled receptors (GPCR)) that rapidly alter several intracellular signaling pathways [106,109]. In mesenchymal multipotent C3H 10T1/2 cells, ligand-bound ARs also complex with cytosolic β-catenin [110]. This interaction results in the chaperoning and nuclear accumulation of the androgen-AR/β-catenin complex and stimulation of downstream T-cell factor (TCF)-4 genes, an effect that simultaneously promotes myogenic differentiation and suppresses adipogenic differentiation of mesenchymal pluripotent cells [110]. For further discussion on Wnt/β-catenin signaling, readers are directed to the following in-depth review [111]. Similarly, in C2C12 myotubes [112] and rodent skeletal muscle [113], androgens increase the phosphorylation of cytosolic glycogen synthase kinase-3β (GSK3β), which (1) inhibits the phosphorylation, ubiquitination, and degradation of β-catenin; and (2) promotes nuclear β-catenin accumulation and TCF activity. Ligand-bound ARs also interact with cytosolic β-catenin in motoneurons [114] and neuronal gonadotropin-releasing hormone cell lines [115] to promote nuclear shuttling of β-catenin and TCF-4 binding, which influences β-catenin-dependent transcriptional activity. To our knowledge, the functional significance of androgen-AR/β-catenin nuclear shuttling in motoneurons has not been determined. However, the loss of endogenous ARs accelerates motoneuron degeneration [116] and pharmacologically-induced stimulation of β-catenin protein expression in the spinal cord is associated with improved locomotor function after SCI [117–119], suggesting that nuclear β-catenin accumulation may promote motoneuron function.

3.4. Androgenic Crosstalk with IGF-1 and PI3K/Akt Signaling

Ligand-bound ARs activate PI3K/Akt signaling in muscle indirectly by stimulating the expression of (1) IGF-1 [113,120] and/or (2) other intracellular signaling molecules (e.g., Erk) that may activate or suppress components of this pathway independently of IGF-1 [121]. In support of this contention, the upstream promoter of the human *IGF-1* gene exhibits two AREs that activate IGF-1 expression [122]. In rodents, androgen administration increases IGF-1 and mechano growth factor (MGF) mRNA expression by several fold in skeletal muscle within seven days of administration [113], an effect that persists for at least one month [120]. Similarly, within one month of initiating TRT, older men exhibit a >two-fold increase in IGF-1 protein expression in muscle [123]. In cultured rodent myoblasts, T treatment stimulates protein accretion and mammalian target of rapamycin (mTOR) mRNA expression, effects that are abrogated by co-incubation with bicalutamide (competitive AR antagonist), rapamycin (mTOR inhibitor), or LY294002 (PI3K inhibitor) [121,124], indicating that T-induced protein accretion is dependent upon both AR activation and PI3K signaling. Similarly, dose-dependent phosphorylation of Akt, mTOR, S6 (subunit of S6K1), and S6K1 occurs in cultured rodent and C2C12 myotubes in response to increasing concentrations of T [125,126]. Importantly, these effects are also abolished by co-incubation with LY294002, Akt inhibitor VIII, or rapamycin [126], demonstrating dependence upon the PI3K signaling pathway. Further, complete androgen withdrawal was sufficient to reduce muscle IGF-1 mRNA and suppress Akt, mTOR, S6K1, and 4E-BP1 phosphorylation (downstream PI3K targets) by >50% in rodents, with androgen (nandrolone or DHT) treatment increasing these factors two-fold above gonadally-intact animals [125,127]. Interestingly, Serra et al. reported that orchiectomy also increased RPTOR and reduced tuberous sclerosis complex protein 2 (TSC2) phosphorylation by >50%, changes associated with mTOR inhibition, while T treatment reversed these effects [128]. These findings indicate that androgens stimulate various IGF-1/PI3K/Akt signaling components in muscle and suggest that activation PI3K/Akt signaling influences androgen-mediated muscle hypertrophy. This contention is strengthened by the observation that MKR mice, which express a dominant negative IGF-1R in mature muscle fibers, exhibit attenuated hypertrophy of the highly androgen-sensitive LABC muscle in response to T treatment [128]. Regardless, IGF-1 and IGF-1R mRNA expression was not altered in animals receiving nandrolone for eight weeks after spinal cord transection, suggesting that androgens do not chronically stimulate IGF-1 expression in muscle in the absence of descending supraspinal input and/or mechanical strain [16].

3.5. Androgen Crosstalk with the Ubiquitin-Proteasome Pathway

Androgenic influence on FOXO expression and subsequent downstream signaling is evidenced by (1) increased total FOXO1 and FOXO3a protein and lower pFOXO3a in rodent muscle in response to orchiectomy (ORX) [125,128]; (2) 10- to 25-fold higher MAFbx and MuRF-1 mRNA expression in rodent skeletal muscle within seven days of ORX [128,129], an effect that persists for at least one month, albeit to a lesser magnitude over time [120,125]; and (3) the ability of androgen treatment to abolish these changes and prevent ORX-induced muscle atrophy [120,125,128,129]. Similarly, TRT suppresses ubiquitin-proteasome activity in the muscle of older men [130]. In C2C12 myoblasts and myotubes, androgen-induced suppression of MAFbx occurs indirectly via interactions among ligand-bound ARs and octamer binding transcription factor (Oct)-1 or Ankryn repeat domain protein 2 (Ankrd2), co-regulators of sex-steroid hormone induced transcriptional activity in target genes [131,132]. Interestingly, androgen treatment also attenuated muscle atrophy and the increases in FOXO1, MAFbx, and MuRF1 mRNA expression resulting from methylprednisolone administration after SCI [101], an effect that may be mediated by androgenic suppression of glucocorticoid receptor expression [120,133,134]. Alternatively, it is also possible that androgens indirectly influence FOXO signaling by stimulating PI3K/Akt signaling in muscle, given that FOXO1 and FOXO3a are downstream targets of pAkt signaling [62], although we are unaware of any study addressing this interesting possibility.

3.6. Androgenic Influence on PGC-1α and PGC-1β Signaling after SCI

Testosterone stimulates muscle PGC-1α expression via direct AR-mediated and/or ER-mediated pathways following aromatization to E_2. As evidence, (1) castration lowered muscle PGC-1α mRNA by 50% in male rodents and nandrolone treatment increased PGC-1α mRNA >two-fold [125]; (2) ovariectomy lowered muscle PGC-1α >70% in female rodents [135], while one week of E_2 replacement increased PGC-1α mRNA and nuclear protein expression in postmenopausal women [136]; and (3) within eight days of initiating pharmacologic E_2 therapy, muscle PGC-1α mRNA was increased by 30% in men [137]. As discussed above, PGC-1α [16,54] and -1β expressions [74] are suppressed in response to spinal cord transection, an effect that may influence the slow-to-fast fiber transition [30] and/or mitochondrial dysfunction after SCI [138]. In this regard, chronic androgen treatment increased PGC-1α mRNA >three-fold in the muscle of animals receiving spinal cord transection and prevented the SCI-induced reductions in total and nuclear PGC-1α protein, changes that were accompanied by higher slow troponin mRNA and protein expression and lower fast troponin mRNA [16]. Similarly, Gregory et al. reported that androgen treatment attenuated the slow-to-fast fiber transition after spinal cord transection [20]. In addition, Wu et al. observed >two-fold higher PGC-1β mRNA expression in the muscle of spinal cord transected animals receiving nandrolone for eight weeks, although this change did not reach the level of statistical significance [16]. Regardless, the role of aromatase in mediating the influence of androgens on muscle PGC-1α and/or PGC-1β expression remains to be determined after SCI.

4. Androgenic and Estrogenic Regulation of Motoneurons

The influence of SCI on somatic motoneuron structure depends largely upon injury characteristics and the muscle groups innervated (discussed in [27]). For example, Sengelaub et al. [17] and Byers et al. [18] reported no differences in quadriceps motoneuron counts or soma area four-weeks after mid-thoracic contusion SCI, although, dendritic length was decreased 40–50%. Similarly, four-weeks after mid-thoracic spinal transection, fewer dendrites (labeled via sciatic nerve) were present on spinal motoneuron, and dendritic arbor size and dendritic length were reduced in comparison to intact animals [28]. Reduced tibialis anterior and soleus motoneuron dendritic length was also observed four-months after mid-thoracic contusion SCI, with no difference in soma area [29]. Whereas, Bose et al. reported fewer motoneurons innervating the soleus at four-months after mid-thoracic contusion SCI, with residual motoneurons being relatively larger and having fewer total dendrites that exhibited longer dendritic lengths [27]. When taken together, these findings indicate that dendrite length is rapidly reduced after SCI, with the loss of relatively small motoneurons and short dendrites occurring thereafter.

ARs are expressed in the cytoplasm and nuclear regions of spinal motoneurons [86] in a roughly equal distribution among male and female rodents [85]. 5α-reductase type II is highly expressed in several gray- and white-matter areas of the spinal cord [139], including spinal motoneurons [140]. Spinal cord homogenates and cultured NSC34 cells (immortalized motoneurons) actively convert T to DHT [141] in a manner that is ~three-times greater than that occurring in other central nervous system (CNS) regions [142] or the seminal vesicles, an androgen-sensitive tissue that highly expresses 5α-reductase type II [143]. The neuronotrophic effects of androgens are evidenced by the ability of T and DHT to equally preserve motoneuron number and size in cultured rodent lumbosacral spinal cord segments [144]. Indeed, lumbosacral motoneurons innervating the quadriceps and other musculature are androgen responsive [145]. However, the androgen sensitivity of spinal motoneurons appears largely dependent upon the magnitude of AR expression in motoneurons and in the innervated skeletal muscle, given that (1) motoneurons innervating LABC (high AR expression) exhibit robust dendritic atrophy in response to ORX, which is completely prevented by T or DHT administration [146]; (2) motoneurons innervating quadriceps (relatively lower AR expression) do not exhibit dendritic atrophy in response to ORX [147]; and (3) transgenic AR overexpression in skeletal muscle increased somatic motoneuron androgenic responsiveness, evidenced by ORX-induced dendritic atrophy in normally non-androgen responsive motoneurons, which was completely prevented by T administration [147].

ERα and ERβ are also expressed in cytoplasmic and nuclear regions of spinal motoneurons [148,149] and cultured motoneurons actively synthesize E_2 in culture [149], owing to aromatase expression [148,149]. However, cultured rodent embryonic and adult spinal cord homogenates do not appear to synthesize E_2 when incubated with androstenedione [142] or T [141]. Regardless, E_2-mediated preservation of motoneuron dendritic growth [150] is as robust as that resulting from T or DHT treatment [151] and is highly dependent upon motoneuronal ERα expression, at least during development [152]. In culture, E_2 treatment also improves spinal motoneuron cell survival during glutamate-induced toxicity, an effect that was not inhibited by ICI 182,780 (competitive ERα/ERβ agonist) [153], indicating that estrogen-mediated improvement in spinal motoneuron viability occurs independent of nuclear ER-signaling. In this regard, GPCR-30 (or G protein-coupled estrogen receptor-30) has been identified as a cell-surface/transmembrane ER that rapidly stimulates intracellular signaling [108] and E_2 has been shown to improve motoneuron viability during glucose-oxygen deprivation, an effect that was blocked by co-treatment with G15 (GPCR-30 inhibitor) [154].

4.1. *Influence of Androgens and Estrogens on Motoneuron Structure after SCI*

As discussed above, altered dendritic length is a hallmark of SCI that has been observed in motoneurons innervating sublesional vastus lateralis [17,18], tibialis anterior [29], and soleus muscle [27]. In adult female rats, T treatment completely prevented the reduction in dendritic length of quadricep motoneurons resulting from SCI, without altering motoneuron counts, soma volume, or other motoneuron structural variables [18]. Whereas, DHT or E_2 treatment each attenuated the reduction in quadriceps dendritic length by 50–60% [17]. The functional consequences of preserved dendritic length after SCI remains to be determined. However, it is interesting to note that our laboratory has reported that T treatment slightly increased hindlimb locomotor recovery in male rodents subsequent to moderate-severe contusion SCI, with the largest benefit occurring in response to supraphysiologic T [15], while E_2 treatment is known to produce comparatively larger locomotor improvements in both male and female rodents after SCI [155].

4.2. *Molecular Pathways Underlying Androgen-Mediated Motoneuron Protection*

Androgenic regulation of brain-derived neurotrophic factor (BDNF) and tyrosine receptor kinase (Trk)B (BDNF receptor) in spinal motoneurons appears particularly important for motoneuron anatomical preservation [156,157]. As evidence, both somatic motoneurons and the spinal nucleus of the bulbocavernosus (SNB) express BDNF and TrkB mRNA and protein [146,158], with >80% of motoneuron dendrites identified as TrkB-positive [159]. In male rodents, ORX reduced BDNF mRNA and protein expressions in SNB [159] and in motoneurons innervating the quadriceps [158], while T treatment prevented these effects. BDNF regulates soma size independently of T, as evidenced by the ability of exogenous BDNF to maintain SNB motoneuron soma size in ORX male rats after bilateral axotomy [160]. In comparison, both BDNF and T appear necessary for the maintenance of SNB dendritic length, given that neither exogenous BDNF nor T independently prevented the reduction in SNB motoneuron dendritic length resulting from bilateral axotomy in ORX males, while co-treatment with BDNF and T increased dendritic length [161]. In females, T treatment also increased SNB motoneuron count by 50%, an effect that was prevented by the co-administration of TrkB-IgG [162]. These findings are particularly striking and suggest that androgen treatment may represent a means of stimulating BDNF/TrkB signaling, given the prevalence and severity of hypogonadism after SCI [91–93] and that the stimulation of motoneuron BDNF/TrkB signaling enhanced functional recovery in rodent SCI models [163].

In addition, estrogenic activation of GPCR-30 [108] or ERα [164] stimulates intercellular PI3K/Akt signaling, which promotes motoneuron survival [155]. As evidence, treatment of cultured spinal motoneurons with LY294002 (PI3K inhibitor) blocked the anti-apoptotic effects of E_2 treatment during glucose-oxygen deprivation, resulting in a 50% increase in apoptotic motoneurons [154]. Similarly, PC12 cell viability was reduced ~50% upon treatment with rapamycin (mTOR inhibitor), demonstrating the necessity of downstream PI3K/Akt/mTOR signaling for cell survival [165]. Interestingly, LY294002 co-administration suppressed E_2-mediated voluntary locomotor recovery in male rodents after SCI [154], indicating that PI3K/Akt signaling influences locomotor recovery after SCI. Estrogens may also exert neuroprotection via other pathways that have been reviewed by others [155].

5. Activity-Based Physical Rehabilitation after SCI

After SCI, increasing focus has been placed on improving activity-dependent neuromuscular plasticity through the use of BWSTT, a therapy that involves robotic or manual placement of the impaired limbs into normal gait patterns on a slowly moving treadmill, or other ABTs (e.g., passive or functional electric stimulation cycling) [166]. Through intense repetitive practice, it is postulated that ABTs activate sublesional spinal networks that promote beneficial neuromuscular adaptations by retraining the CNS to recover task-specific motor activities, via stimulation of the central pattern generator (CPG) in the lumbosacral region of the spinal cord [166]. Indeed, a number of studies involving persons with motor-incomplete SCI indicate that BWSTT produces several functional benefits, including (1) improved temporal gait parameters associated with walking ability (e.g., increased number of steps, faster cadence, and improved muscle activation patterns) [167–177]; (2) improved muscle strength and rate of torque development in impaired limbs, and reduced detrimental co-activation of antagonist muscle groups [24,169,171,178–180]; and (3) reduced muscle atrophy [24,178,181–184] (Table 1). However, when data from well-controlled randomized clinical trials assessing BWSTT after SCI [179,185–188] are pooled, there appears to be only limited meaningful improvement in overground walking speed or distance [4,189–191], given that the minimal clinically important difference in walking speed is reported as 0.13 m/s in the SCI population [192]. This finding stresses the necessity of testing combinatory therapies that prime the neuromuscular system for better functional recovery when combined with BWSTT.

Preclinical studies also utilize ABTs to evaluate mechanisms underlying activity-dependent neuroplasticity after SCI and have observed locomotor and neuromuscular improvements in response to BWSTT (Table 2) [5]. However, there are considerable differences in the reported effects of BWSTT on locomotor and neuromuscular recovery in SCI rodents, in-part due to the influence of age and gender, the mechanism of producing SCI (i.e., transection, hemisection, or contusion), delay in initiating BWSTT, duration of therapy, and the methods of assessing neuromuscular recovery [5,193]. In general, better outcomes for locomotor recovery are observed in female rats with mild to moderate contusion

SCI, with training that begins seven to 14 days after injury and continues for at least eight weeks [5]. In this regard, female rodents have higher endogenous E_2 than males [194], which is important given that subphysiologic and physiologic E_2 treatment significantly improves open-field locomotor recovery in both male and female rodents after SCI, in-part, by reducing secondary apoptotic and inflammatory damage to the spinal cord [155].

5.1. Effects of ABTs on Muscle

In rodent SCI models, BWSTT produces relatively consistent improvements in muscle integrity, even following complete transection. As evidence, after spinal transection, the incorporation of BWSTT completely preserved the muscle mass:body mass ratio [195,196] and prevented ~55% of soleus fCSA loss [196]. Similarly, in a moderate-contusion SCI model, BWSTT produced 23% higher soleus fCSA and 38% higher soleus peak tetanic force in comparison with untrained SCI animals [197], with analogous effects reported by others [49,197–200]. Similarly, several case-report and cohort-studies have reported muscle responses in individuals with motor-incomplete SCI. For example, in persons with chronic SCI, four to six months of BWSTT increased vastus lateralis muscle fCSA [178,184]. Likewise, Jayaraman et al. reported that nine-weeks of BWSTT enhanced knee extensor and ankle plantar flexion voluntary muscle activation and increased plantar flexion peak torque by 43%, which accompanied a 15% increase in plantar flexor CSA [201], an important finding given that lower extremity strength is positively associated with walking function after SCI [42]. However, others have reported much less robust strength improvements [202,203] or no strength improvement [171] in response to BWSTT.

The structural improvements mentioned above appear to be influenced, in-part, by reduced catabolic signaling resulting from BWSTT. As evidence, in a rodent SCI model, three sessions of BWSTT suppressed >10 protein ubiquitination pathway genes, an effect accompanied by the full preservation of muscle mass [49]. Similarly, after spinal cord transection, five sessions of electrical stimulation of paralyzed muscle suppressed MAFbx and MuRF1 mRNA and myostatin mRNA in muscle [51]. Myostatin is a member of the transforming growth factor (TGF)-β family and a muscle-derived negative regulator of muscle growth, which acts via the activin IIB receptors [204]. Additionally, muscle regeneration occurs in response to BWSTT after SCI, evidenced by the upregulation of myogenic regulatory factors and increased expression of Pax7 positive nuclei (a marker of satellite cell activation) [63,205], suggesting that BWSTT stimulates muscle anabolic signaling pathways. In this regard, IGF-1, MGF, IGF-1R, and several IGFBPs mRNA were increased 1.5 to >10-fold in rodent muscle and IGF-1 protein expression was increased >three-fold within seven days of initiating BWSTT after moderate-contusion SCI [63]. In contrast, other reports indicate that electrical stimulation of paralyzed muscle suppressed IGFBP-4 and -5 mRNA in muscle, without altering IGF-1 or MGF mRNA after spinal transection [51,206]. Similarly, no change in circulating IGF-1 was observed in persons with chronic SCI undergoing a comprehensive physical rehabilitation program involving one to two hours per week of bodyweight-supported locomotor training [207]. As such, the role of IGF-1 signaling in the muscle regenerative response to BWSTT requires further elucidation, especially given that SCI-induced downregulation of IRS1 limits IGF-1 mediated activation of PI3K/Akt signaling in muscle acutely after SCI [51].

In addition to muscle preservation, BWSTT is reported to reduce soleus fatigue and attenuate the slow-to-fast fiber transition occurring in rodent moderate-contusion SCI models [197].

Similarly, in persons with chronic SCI, four to six months of BWSTT partially reversed the slow-to-fast fiber transition, evidenced by increased oxidative fibers and fewer type IIx (glycolytic) fibers compared with the baseline [178,184]. Interestingly, lower *Mhyl*, *Mybph*, and *Myh4* gene expression (fast-twitch fiber markers) was apparent in rodent muscle within five-days of initiating BWSTT [49], indicating that reversal of the slow-to-fast fiber-type switch occurs rapidly with this physical rehabilitation modality. However, to our knowledge, changes in PGC-1α or -1β have not been evaluated in response to BWSTT after SCI. Regardless, a five-fold increase in PGC-1α mRNA in muscle was observed in men with chronic motor-complete SCI within several hours of neuromuscular electrical stimulation of quadriceps [208] and a ~two-fold increase in PGC-1α was present in men with chronic motor-complete SCI undergoing functional electric stimulation for durations of 16-weeks [209] to six-years [210], suggesting that increased PGC-1α expression may underlie the slow-to-fast fiber-type reversal occurring in response to BWSTT.

5.2. *Effects of ABTs on Motoneurons*

In rodent SCI models, ABTs limit injury severity, evidenced by the preservation of myelin, axons, and collagen morphology and decreased lesion volume [198], and produce a host of anatomical and functional improvements to the motor unit [29,198,200,211–213]. For example, after spinal cord transection, BWSTT increases axonal regrowth [212], preserves motoneuron dendritic length, increases neuromuscular junction synaptic density in the lumbar motoneuron pool [29], and produces larger group Ia afferent-evoked monosynaptic excitatory postsynaptic potentials (EPSPs) in the ankle plantar flexors, an effect that is particularly prevalent in rats regaining the greatest stepping ability [213]. Similarly, after moderate-severe contusion SCI, BWSTT produced a beneficial reduction in the sprouting of small caliber afferent fibers and improved stepping patterns while on the treadmill [200], although open-field locomotor activity did not improve in this study, suggesting some limitation to functional recovery in more severe injury scenarios. Interestingly, Singh et al. induced a spinal transection at nine weeks following contusion SCI in a subgroup of rats that previously underwent BWSTT or no training and observed that kinematic improvements were maintained in BWSTT rats and worsened in untrained rats, indicating that functional improvement resulting from BWSTT occurred via neural networks originating below the lesion level [200]. Indeed, Cote el al. reported that after spinal transection, BWSTT facilitated lumbar spine motoneuron pool recruitment via improved reflex pathways resulting from afferent input [211].

In individuals with incomplete SCI, beneficial adaptations to spinal neuronal pathways have been demonstrated in response to BWSTT. For example, the soleus H-reflex phase-dependent modulation during walking normalizes homosynaptic facilitation, reverses homosynaptic depression, and improves the presynaptic inhibition of Ia afferents [214–216]. However, better functional recovery has also been associated with increased ankle dorsiflexor and knee extensor maximal motor-evoked potential, a probe of corticospinal tract excitability, in persons with motor-incomplete SCI undergoing BWSTT [180] and improved ankle dorsiflexor and plantar flexor muscle co-activation patterns accompany improved walking function in response to BWSTT [171], findings that indicate greater descending corticospinal drive. In this regard, improvements in the above-mentioned factors likely stem from the reorganization of both supraspinal and spinal cord neural circuits in response to BWSTT [214,217], with further research needed to resolve whether functional adaptations rely more heavily on improved cortical or spinal circuitry in individuals with SCI.

Table 1. Characteristics of Bodyweight Supported Locomotor Training in Human Spinal Cord Injury Studies.

Study	Intervention	Duration	Population	N	Outcomes
			Studies Assessing Gait		
Dobkin et al., 2007 [185]	Manual-assisted BWSTT vs. OG training	12 wk	38 ASIA B, 107 ASIA C&D	145	BWSTT increased walking speed from ~0.40 m/s at 2 weeks post-entry to 0.85 m/s for ASIA C&D. OG training increased walking speed from ~0.50 at 2 weeks post-entry to 0.84 m/s for ASIA C&D. Poor walking outcomes were observed for ASIA B participants.
Field-Fote et al., 2001 [167]	BWSTT with ES	3 days/wk, 12 wk	ASIA C	19	Walking speed increased from 0.12 to 0.21 m/s. [a]
Alcobendas-Maestro et al., 2012 [218]	Robotic-assisted BWSTT vs. OG training	3–6 mo	ASIA C&D	48 M/32F	Robotic-assisted BWSTT and OG training walking speed remained the same from baseline to post-training. Robotic-assisted BWSTT increased 6 min walk distance from 91 to 169 m. [a]
Alexeeva et al., 2011 [179]	BWS training on a fixed track vs. BWSTT vs. Comprehensive PT	3 days/wk 13 wk	ASIA C&D	30 M/5 F	BWS on a fixed track increased walking speed from 0.33 to 0.44 m/s. [a] BWSTT increased walking speed from 0.30 to 0.46 m/s. [a] PT increased walking speed from 0.41 to 0.51 m/s. [a]
Duffell et al., 2015 [202]	Robotic-assisted BWSTT	3 days/wk, 4 wk	ASIA C&D	19 M/7 F	Walking speed increased from ~0.55 to ~0.58 m/s. [a]
Esclarin-Ruz et al., 2014 [219]	Robotic-assisted BWSTT + OG training (LKOGT) vs. Conventional OG training (OGT)	5 days/wk, 8 wk	ASIA C&D	59 M/24 F	LKOGT increased walking speed from 0.48 to 0.54 m/s and 6 min walk distance from 122 to 187 m [b] in participants with upper motor neuron injury. LKOGT increased walking speed from 0.24 to 0.46 m/s and 6 min walk distance from 82 to 157 m [b] in participants with lower motor neuron injury. OGT increased walking speed from 0.36 to 0.39 m/s and 6 min walk distance from 93 to 119 m in participants with upper motor neuron injury. OGT increased walking speed from 0.28 to 0.45 m/s and 6 min walk distance from 94 to 145 m in participants with lower motor neuron injury.
Field-Fote et al., 2005 [220]	Manual-assisted BWSTT (TM) vs. BWSTT + ES (TS) vs. BWS OG training + ES (OGS) vs. Robotic-assisted BWSTT (LR)	5 days/wk 12 wk	ASIA C&D	22 M/5 F	TM increased walking speed from ~0.07 to ~0.10. TS increased walking speed from ~0.12 to ~0.16 m/s. [a] OG increased walking speed from ~0.14 to ~0.19 m/s. [a] LR increased walking speed from ~0.09 to ~0.11.
Field-Fote & Roach 2011 [186]	Manual-assisted BWSTT (TM) vs. BWSTT + ES (TS) vs. BWS OG training +ES (OGS) vs. Robotic-assisted BWSTT (LR)	5 days/wk, 12 wk	ASIA C&D	52 M/12 F	TM increased walk speed from 0.17 to 0.22 m/s [a] and 2 min distance from 22.1 to 23.0 m. TS increased walk speed from 0.18 to 0.23 m/s [a] and 2 min distance from 20.6 to 24.4 m. [a] OGS increased walk speed from 0.19 to 0.28 m/s [a] and 2 min distance from 24.0 to 38.3 m. [a,b] LR increased walk speed from 0.17 to 0.18 m/s and 2 min distance from 16.8 to 17.9 m.
Gorassini et al., 2009 [169]	Manual-assisted BWSTT	5 days/wk, 14 wk	ASIA C&D	14 M/3 F	In 9 responders, walking speed increased from 0.31 to 0.55 m/s. [a] In 8 non-responders, there was no change in walking speed.
Harkema et al., 2012 [170]	Manual-assisted BWSTT	3 day/wk, 4 to 92 wks	ASIA C&D	148M/48 F	Walking speed increased from 0.31 to 0.51 m/s [a] and 6 min walk distance increased from 91 to 154 m. [a]

Table 1. *Cont.*

Study	Intervention	Duration	Population	N	Outcomes
Kapadia et al., 2014 [221]	Robotic-assisted BWSTT + ES	3 days/wk, 16 wk	ASIA C&D	13 M/3 F	Walking speed increased from 0.23 to 0.28 m/s and 6 min walk distance increased from 187.9 to 217.1 m. [a]
Knikou 2013 [214]	Manual-assisted BWSTT	5 days/wk, 1.5–3.5 mo	ASIA C&D	9 M/3 F	6 min walk distance increased from 36.25 to 39.05 m for ASIA C and from 252 to 279.5 m for ASIA D participants.
Krishnan et al., 2016 [171]	Robotic-assisted BWSTT	3 day/wk, 4 wk	ASIA C&D	8 M/8 F	Median walking speed increased from 0.58 to 0.66 m/s. [a] 6 min walking distance did not change.
Labruyere et al., 2014 [222]	Robotic-assisted BWSTT	4 days/wk, 4 wk	ASIA C&D	5 M/4 F	Walking speed increased from 0.62 to 0.66 m/s.
Lam et al., 2015 [223]	Robotic-assisted BWSTT with resistance (LR) vs. Robotic-assisted BWSTT only (LO)	3 days/wk, 12 wk	ASIA C&D	9 M/6 F	LR increased walking speed from 0.29 to 0.40 m/s. LO increased walking speed from 0.33 to 0.44 m/s.
Lucarelli et al., 2011 [187]	BWSTT vs. Conventional gait training	2 days/wk, 12 wk	ASIA C&D	20 M/10 F	BWSTT increased walking speed from 0.85 to 1.25 m/s [a] as well as increased cadence, distance, step length and swing phase. Conventional training did not improve gait quality or speed.
Morrison et al., 2018 [224]	Manual-assisted BWSTT	120 sessions	ASIA C&D	49 M/20 F	Median walking speed increased by 0.25 m/s. [a] Median 6 min walk distance increased by 66 m. [a]
Niu et al., 2014 [225]	Robotic-assisted BWSTT	3 days/wk, 4 wk	ASIA C&D	27 M/13 F	Walking speed increased in the low-walking capacity group from 0.12 to 0.15 m/s and in the high-walking capacity group from 0.84 to 0.97 m/s. 6 min walk distance did not change.
Nooijen et al., 2009 [172]	Manual-assisted BWSTT vs. Manual-assisted BWSTT with ES vs. OG training with ES vs. Robotic-assisted BWSTT	4 days/wk, 12 wk	ASIA C&D	40 M/11 F	All therapies led to small improvements in gait quality (increased cadence and step length) with no differences among groups.
Potsans et al., 2004 [188]	BWSTT with ES Cross-over design: treatment-control (AB); control-treatment (BA)	5 days/wk, 4 wk	ASIA C&D	12 M/2 F	In AB group, walking speed increased 0.23 m/s and 6 min walk distance increased 72.2 m. In BA group, walking speed increased 0.17 m/s and 6 min walk distance increased 63.8 m.
Thomas et al., 2005 [180]	Manual-assisted BWSTT	4 days/wk, 16 wk	ASIA C&D	8 M/2 F	Walking speed increased from 0.15 to 0.53 m/s [a] and 6 min walk distance increased from 34.2 to 167.6 m.
Varoqui et al., 2014 [203]	Robotic-assisted BWSTT	3 days/wk, 4 wk	ASIA C&D	14 M/ 1 F	Walking speed increased from 0.56 to 0.64 m/s [a] and 6 min walk distance did not change (207 to 209 m).
Winchester et al., 2005 [226]	Robotic-assisted BWSTT	3 days/wk 12 wk	ASIA C&D	4 M	Walking speed increased for 3 participants from 0.0 to 0.11, 0.0 to 0.81, 0.24 to 0.62 m/s and one remained unable to ambulate.
Wirz et al., 2005 [175]	Robotic-assisted BWSTT	4 days/wk, 8 wk	ASIA C&D	18 M/2 F	Walking speed increased from ~0.37 to ~0.48 m/s [a] and 6 min walk distance 120 to 160 m. [a]

Table 1. *Cont.*

Study	Intervention	Duration	Population	N	Outcomes
Wu et al., 2012 [227]	4 wk Robotic-assistance BWSTT + 4 wk Robotic-resistance BWSTT	3 days/wk, 8 wk	ASIA D	8 M/2 F	Walking speed increased from 0.67 to 0.76 m/s [a] and 6 min walk distance increased from 223 to 247 m. Step length and cadence increased. [a]
			Studies Assessing Muscle		
Duffell et al., 2015 [202]	Robotic-assisted BWSTT	3 days/wk, 4 wk	ASIA C&D	19 M/7 F	Maximal isometric ankle dorsiflexion torque increased from 12.3 to 13.2 Nm, [a] but plantar flexion torque did not change (28.1 vs. 28.4 Nm).
Galen et al., 2014 [228]	Robotic-assisted BWSTT	5 days/wk, 6 wk	ASIA C&D	14 M/4 F	Percent peak torque increased 68% for hip flexion, 54% for hip extension, 93% for knee flexion and 71% for knee extension.
Gorassini et al., 2009 [169]	Manual-assisted BWSTT	5 days/wk, 14 wk	ASIA C&D	14 M/3 F	In 9 responders, peak electromyography activity increased from 67 to 135 μV in the tibialis anterior muscle and 36 to 50 μV in the hamstrings. In 8 non-responders, there was no change.
Jayaraman et al., 2008 [201]	Manual-assisted BWSTT	5 days/wk, 9 wk	ASIA C&D	4 M/1 F	Isometric knee extension strength increased 21%. Isometric plantar flexion strength increased 44%. Knee extension and plantar flexion voluntary muscle activation improved. Maximal CSA of the plantar flexors increased and 15%.
Krishnan et al., 2016 [171]	Robotic-assisted BWSTT	3 day/wk, 4 wk	ASIA C&D	8 M/8 F	BWSTT increased isometric ankle dorsiflexion by 20% and ankle plantar flexion by 22%.
Thomas et al., 2005 [180]	Manual-assisted BWSTT	4 days/wk, 16 wk	ASIA C&D	8 M/2 F	Peak electromyography activity averaged from four lower limb muscles increased during treadmill walking from 82.4 to 137.1 μV.
Varoqui et al., 2014 [203]	Robotic-assisted BWSTT	3 days/wk, 4 wk	ASIA C&D	14 M/1 F	Ankle dorsiflexion torque increased from 26.8 to 29.1 Nm[a] and ankle plantar flexion torque increased from 10.9 to 13.5 Nm. [a]

BWSTT = bodyweight supported treadmill training; CSA = cross-sectional area; ES = electrical stimulation; m = meter, min = minute; mo = month; OG = overground; PT = physical therapy; wk = week. Note: [a] indicates statistically different from baseline; [b] indicates statistically different between training groups.

Table 2. Characteristics of Bodyweight Supported Treadmill Training (BWSTT) in Rodent SCI Studies.

Study	Sex/Age	Injury Level	Start of Training	Training Duration	BBB wk 1	BBB End	Gait Outcome	Muscle/Electrophysiology
			Studies Assessing BWSTT after Spinal Hemisection					
Maier et al., 2009 [229]	F/A	T8	1 wk	8 wk	~12	N/R	Stepping ↑	N/R
Battistuzzo et al., 2016 [230]	M/A	T10	1 wk	9 wk	N/R	N/R	Kinematics ↑	N/R
Battistuzzo et al., 2017 [231]	M/A	T10	1 wk	9 wk	N/R	N/R	N/R	G fCSA ↑
Shah et al., 2013 [232]	N/R/N/R	T10	5 days	2.5 wk	N/R	N/R	Stepping ↑	N/R
Goldshmit et al., 2008 [212]	N/R/A	T12	1 wk	4 wk	~3	11T/6C	Kinematics ↑	G-S fCSA ↑
			Studies Assessing BWSTT after Mild Contusion SCI					
Nessler et al., 2006 [233]	F/Y	T9	1 wk	12 wk	13	14T/No C	N/R	N/R
Oh et al., 2009 [234]	M/Y	T9–10	1 wk	4wk	~4	13T/8C	N/R	N/R

Table 2. *Cont.*

Study	Sex/Age	Injury Level	Start of Training	Training Duration	BBB wk 1	BBB End	Gait Outcome	Muscle/Electrophysiology
Studies Assessing BWSTT after Moderate Contusion SCI								
Stevens et al., 2006 [197]	F/Y	T8	1 wk	1 wk	~5	10T/6C	N/R	Sol F ↑/fCSA ↑
Liu et al., 2008 [199]	F/Y	T8	8 days	12 wk	3–7	15T/11C	N/R	G-S CSA ↑
Nessler et al., 2006 [233]	F/Y	T9	1 wk	12 wk	9	11T/No C	N/R	N/R
Shin et al., 2014 [235]	F/Y	T9	1 wk	8 wk	~6	~13T/~10C	N/R	N/R
Wang et al., 2015 [29]	F/Y	T9	1 wk	16 wk	~7	~13T/~11C	N/R	N/R
Singh et al., 2011 [200]	F/Y	T9–10	1 wk	8 wk	~5	~8T/~9C	N/R	mass/bw ↑
Bose et al., 2012 [198]	F/A	T8	1 wk	12 wk	~3	~15T/~11C	Stepping ↑	N/R
Multon et al., 2003 [236]	F/A	T9	2–4 days	12 wk	~2	10T/8C	N/R	N/R
Wu et al., 2016 [237]	F/A	T10	1 wk	4 wk	~5	~13T/~9C	N/R	N/R
Foret et al., 2010 [238]	F/A	T10	1 day	4 wk	~2	~9T/~7C	N/R	N/R
Ward et al., 2014 [239]	M/Y	T8	2 wk	12 wk	~7	~12T/~9C	N/R	Sol EMG ↑
Park et al., 2010 [240]	M/Y	T10	3 days	25 days	~2	11.5	N/R	N/R
Liu et al., 2017 [241]	N/R/N/R	T9	1 wk	2 wk	N/R	N/R	Stepping ↑	N/R
Studies Assessing BWSTT after Severe Contusion SCI								
Hayashibe et al., 2016 [242]	F/Y	T8–9	1 wk	4 wk	<1	16T/10C	N/R	N/R
Heng et al., 2009 [243]	F/Y	T9	42 days	8 wk	N/R	N/R	Stepping ↑	N/R
Nessler et al., 2006 [233]	F/Y	T9	1 wk	12 wk	4.5	~9T/No C	N/R	N/R
Shinozaki et al., 2016 [244]	F/Y	T10	6 wk	8 wk	~1	4T/3C	N/R	N/R
Robert et al., 2010 [245]	F/A	T7–8	2 wk	2 wk	~3	4T/3.5C	N/R	N/R
Ichiyama et al., 2009 [246]	F/A	T10	30 days	8 wk	N/R	N/R	Gait not improved	N/R
Studies Assessing BWSTT after Spinal Transection								
Petruska et al., 2007 [213]	F/N	T6–8	16 days	6 wk	N/R	N/R	Stepping ↑	G EPSP ↑
Tillakaratne et al., 2010 [247]	F/N	T7–8	26 days	8 wk	N/R	N/R	Stepping ↑	N/R
See et al., 2013 [248]	F/N	T8–9	3 wk	4 wk	N/R	N/R	Kinematics ↑	N/R
Timoszyk et al., 2005 [249]	F/N	N/R	64 days	40 days	N/R	N/R	Gait not improved	N/R
Zhang et al., 2007 [250]	F/Y	T8	5 days	40 days	<1	~6.5T/~2C	N/R	N/R
Lee et al., 2010 [251]	F/Y	T8	3 wk	42 wk	N/R	N/R	Gait not improved	N/R
De Leon et al., 2006 [252]	F/Y	T9	3 wk	16 wk	N/R	N/R	Kinematics ↑	N/R
Moshonkina et al., 2004 [253]	F/Y	T9	1 day	9 wk	N/R	N/R	Kinematics ↑	N/R
Kubasak et al., 2008 [254]	F/N/R	T9	4 wk	20 wk	N/R	N/R	Gait not improved	N/R
Fouad et al., 2000 [255]	B/A	T8	3 days	5 wk	~9	14T/14C	Kinematics ↑	N/R
Ihla et al., 2011 [196]	M/A	T8–9	6 days	9 wk	N/R	N/R	N/R	Sol fCSA ↑

Sex: B, both females and males; F, female; M, male; N/R, not reported; Age: A, adult; N, neonate; N/R, not reported; Y, young; Injury Level: T, thoracic; Start of Training: wk, week; BBB end of training: T, trained; C, control SCI untrained; Other gait outcome: ↑ improvement; Muscle/Electrophysiology: bw, bodyweight; EPSP, evoked monosynaptic excitatory postsynaptic potentials F, force; fCSA, fiber cross-sectional area; G, gastrocnemius; G-S, gastrocnemius-soleus; ↑, increased; Sol, soleus, N/R, not reported. Note: The BBB scale ranges from 0–21 and is used to evaluate functional locomotor recovery ranging from no observable movement (0) to consistent weight-supported plantar stepping with coordinated gait (21).

While the molecular signals regulating BWSTT-induced motoneuron recovery after SCI require further elucidation, there is growing evidence that several inducible neurotrophic factors influence neuroplasticity [211]. For example, an upregulation of BDNF and TrkB (BDNF receptor) mRNA and protein has been observed in the skeletal muscle and spinal cord of healthy animals in response to voluntary wheel running or forced treadmill running, with BDNF protein levels increasing to a greater degree in the spinal cord than in the soleus [237,256,257]. In this regard, BDNF and TrkB both undergo retrograde transport from skeletal muscle to the spinal cord [258], an effect that may mediate locomotor recovery after SCI by improving synaptic transmission and plasticity, axon regeneration, and motoneuron survival [259]. Indeed, in rodent SCI models, BWSTT upregulates BDNF mRNA and protein in skeletal muscle and the spinal cord [29,196,198,211,237,260–267] and TrkB protein in the lumbar spinal cord [237,257]. Interestingly, Leech and Hornby also observed increased circulating BDNF in persons with motor-incomplete SCI undergoing treadmill training, with high-intensity treadmill exercise (performed at 100% peak gait speed) resulting in the larger BDNF increases than exercise performed at 33% or 66% peak gait speed [268]. In addition, BSWTT upregulated glial cell derived neurotrophic factor (GDNF) protein in the lumbar spinal cord, which was positively associated with the facilitation of motoneuron excitability [211].

Neurotrophin-3 (NT-3) is another endogenous neurotrophin that regulates synaptic transmission, promotes neuromuscular junction maturation, and improves the survival and function of sensory neurons via the activation of TrkC (receptor), both of which are expressed in the spinal cord [269–273]. Indeed, recent results from Fang et al. indicate that co-treatment with BDNF/TrkB and NT-3/TrkC promoted motor recovery in a rodent SCI model [274]. NT-3 is produced in the spinal cord and NT-3 mRNA and protein levels are upregulated after seven days of voluntary treadmill and wheel running in healthy rodents [256,262,265]. Similarly, following SCI, rodents exhibit increased NT-3 mRNA and protein in the spinal cord within seven days of initiating BWSTT [262,263,265,266]. Interestingly, Ying et al. reported that BWSTT did not increase spinal cord NT-3 protein expression in adult male rats after spinal cord hemisection [266], while Cote et al. observed increased NT-3 protein levels in the lumbar and thoracic spinal cord after four weeks of BWSTT in adult female rats with complete transection [211], suggesting that sex differences may exist in the NT-3 response to BWSTT. In this regard, E_2 treatment increases NT-3 levels in several CNS regions [275], although we are unaware of any study evaluating whether spinal cord NT-3 expression is regulated via E_2-mediated mechanisms. BWSTT is also reported to upregulate genes involved in neuroplasticity (e.g., *Arc* and *Nrcam*) and angiogenesis (e.g., *Adam8* and *Tie1*), which may be important given that improved neurovascular remodeling has the potential to improve locomotor function after SCI [235].

6. Testosterone Adjuvant to BWSTT

We are unaware of published results from any randomized study evaluating T treatment as an adjuvant to BWSTT. However, at least one ongoing study is evaluating TRT as an adjuvant to electric stimulation-based resistance training in men with motor-complete SCI [276]. A single case-report has also indicated that a man with motor-complete SCI exhibited increased thigh muscle CSA in response to twice-weekly neuromuscular electric stimulation-based resistance training, when combined with adjuvant TRT [13]. In addition, our preliminary data indicates that the combination of testosterone-enanthate (TE), a long-acting T ester [277], and quadrupedal BWSTT (consisting of two 20-min bouts performed twice daily, five-days per week for seven-weeks) promoted more complete neuromuscular restoration than TE-alone in our rodent moderate-severe contusion SCI model [278]. Specifically, the incorporation of TE+BWSTT after SCI produced near-complete restoration of the sublesional muscle mass:body mass ratio, completely prevented the slow-to-fast fiber-type transition occurring in the soleus, attenuated the reduction in soleus fCSA by >50%, and maintained isolated soleus muscle force mechanics near the level of intact control animals. Impressively, 100% of SCI animals receiving TE+BWSTT regained the ability to perform occasional voluntary overground weight-supported hindlimb plantar stepping within seven-weeks of initiating therapy, while 0/11 SCI animals and only 2/10 of SCI animals receiving TE-alone regained this ability. As such, our preliminary data appear to support the contention that a combinatory strategy involving BWSTT with adjuvant TE promotes musculoskeletal and neuromuscular improvement in male rodents after moderate-severe contusion SCI.

Potential Side-Effects of TRT

TRT is approved for the treatment of hypogonadism in adult men and has been shown to increase muscle protein synthesis in women [279]. However, given its androgenic potential, chronic TRT remains controversial for women, at least when administered in the doses necessary to produce musculoskeletal benefit in males. This should not detract from TRT research in relation to SCI because men represent ~80% of new SCI cases [280] and many of these men will develop hypogonadism of an indefinite duration [91–93]. Regardless, careful evaluation of TRT safety and efficacy is necessary prior to implementation of this therapy after SCI.

To-date, meta-analyses have confirmed that TRT produces three adverse events (AEs) in non-neurologically impaired adult men: (1) polycythemia, which occurs in ~6% of men treated with TRT; (2) a higher number of cumulative prostate-related events (discussed below); and (3) a slight decrease in HDL cholesterol, which is of unknown clinical significance [281]. The development of polycythemia in men receiving TRT has raised concerns regarding the cardiovascular safety of TRT, especially when taken in context with findings from the Testosterone in Older Men with Mobility Limitations (TOM) trial [282] and from two retrospective studies that indicated increase cardiovascular risk in hypogonadal men receiving TRT [283,284]. In this regard, the TOM trial was discontinued upon recommendation of the Data Safety Monitoring Board due to a higher prevalence of cardiovascular-related AEs in the TRT versus placebo groups [282]. However, this trial received criticism because of the relatively poor classification of cardiovascular AEs [285]. In comparison, the NIH-funded T-trials, which represent the largest randomized clinical trials to-date evaluating the safety and efficacy of TRT, reported no differences in adjudicated cardiovascular AEs in hypogonadal men receiving TRT versus placebo [11]. Similarly, heavy scientific criticism and numerous calls for retraction [286] accompanied the retrospective studies from Vigen et al. [284] and Finkel et al. [283] that reported increased cardiovascular risk in hypogonadal men receiving TRT. Indeed, the aforementioned findings remain in direct conflict with findings from the largest meta-analyses on the topic, which reported that TRT does not increase cardiovascular risk in men enrolled in well-controlled clinical trials [287,288], and with findings from the largest retrospective study (n = 83,010 men with low T) that indicated TRT reduced all-cause mortality by 56% and MI and stroke risk by 24–36% in comparison with untreated hypogonadal men [289]. Of note, the potential cardiovascular responses to TRT have not been extensively evaluated in the SCI population. However, in a small clinical trial, La Fountaine et al. reported that QTa interval variability was higher in hypogonadal men with SCI than in eugonadal men with SCI, and that TRT normalized QTa interval variability, suggestive of reduced arrhythmia risk [290].

The risk for increased cumulative prostate-related events also merits mention because prostate growth and worsened urinary symptoms resulting from TRT have the potential to worsen bladder dysfunction, which is already common in the SCI population [291]. In this regard, the prostate-related AEs associated with TRT appear to be driven primarily by the 5α-reduction of T to DHT [8]. As evidence, we have reported that older hypogonadal men receiving TE-alone exhibited a 43% increase in prostate volume over a period of 12-months, while men receiving TE plus finasteride exhibited no change in prostate volume [102]. In comparison, 5α-reductase inhibition did not prevent the musculoskeletal or lipolytic benefits resulting from TRT in our trial [102] or others [292,293], indicating that finasteride co-treatment improves the prostate-related safety profile of TRT without inhibiting musculoskeletal efficacy in older men. The safety and efficacy of TE plus finasteride treatment in men with SCI currently remains unknown, although an ongoing clinical trial in our laboratory is evaluating this promising combinatory therapy in hypogonadal men with SCI [294].

In addition, it is important to note that a 15-yr retrospective study of 150,000 men reported that TRT was not associated with prostate cancer [295] and that no meta-analysis to-date has reported increased prostate cancer risk resulting from TRT [8].

Several less common risks are also associated with TRT, which we have previously reviewed [296], including: pain or bleeding at injection sites, skin reactions, fluid retention, breast tenderness, gynecomastia, and liver disorders. Importantly, these side-effects remain putative [8] and have not been confirmed by meta-analysis [281]. However, one potential risk that merits mention is the possibility that TRT may cause or worsen obstructive sleep apnea [297], a condition that is relatively common in tetraplegic men with SCI [298]. As such, need exists to determine TRT safety in men with SCI who display obstructive sleep apnea, especially given the higher sleep apnea prevalence in non-neurologically impaired men receiving TRT [297].

7. Conclusions

Upregulation of FOXO signaling occurs in the immediate days to weeks after SCI, an effect that likely influences the rapid muscle loss in this population. Similarly, muscle PGC-1α and -1β are reduced in response to SCI, underlying the slow-to-fast fiber change and impaired mitochondrial function subsequent to SCI. In comparison, downregulation of IGF-1 and PI3K/Akt signaling occurs more chronically after SCI. These molecular changes are precipitated by the spinal injury and subsequent disuse, but may also be exacerbated by low T that occurs in many men with SCI. T promotes muscle anabolism via direct AR-mediated genomic signaling and/or via cross-talk with IGF-1 and the PI3k/Akt signaling pathway. T may also promote anticatabolic effects in muscle by directly or indirectly suppressing FOXO signaling. Further, androgen treatment increases PGC-1α in muscle and attenuates the slow-to-fast muscle fiber-type transition occurring in response to spinal transection. In addition, T improves the preservation of motoneuron dendritic length after SCI directly via AR-mediated mechanisms and/or indirectly, following aromatization to E_2. Regardless, these improvements appear to result in only minor improvement in locomotor recovery in rodents after moderate-severe contusion SCI, likely because only limited descending corticospinal input remains. In comparison, BWSTT improves descending corticospinal drive and/or facilitates reorganization of spinal cord neural circuitry below the lesion, which produces neuromuscular improvement and some restoration of musculoskeletal integrity. However, findings from well-controlled randomized clinical trials indicate that BWSTT only promotes limited clinically meaningful improvement in voluntary locomotor recovery in humans after SCI. Interestingly, activity-mediated neuromuscular plasticity appears to rely, in-part, upon the upregulation of BDNF/TrkB in the spinal cord. Androgen/AR signaling is required for BDNF/TrkB-mediated dendritic restoration in androgen sensitive motoneurons in the lumbosacral spinal cord, suggesting that T treatment may enhance activity-mediated neuromuscular plasticity after SCI. Indeed, our preliminary data supports this contention, given that adult male rodents receiving TE adjuvant to BWSTT exhibited profound musculoskeletal and neuromuscular improvement and recovery of voluntary weight-supported overground plantar stepping after moderate-severe contusion SCI. Elucidation of the molecular mechanisms underlying these neuromusculoskeletal and locomotor improvements will assist in validating our hypothesis and will improve the likelihood for the translation of this promising multimodal therapeutic strategy.

Author Contributions: Conceptualization, D.M.O., J.L., F.Y., S.E.B., and J.F.Y.; Methodology, D.M.O. and J.F.Y.; Formal Analysis, D.M.O. and J.F.Y.; Investigation, D.M.O., J.L., F.Y., S.E.B., and J.F.Y.; Resources, F.Y., S.E.B., and J.F.Y.; Data Curation, D.M.O. and J.F.Y.; Writing—Original Draft Preparation, D.M.O. and J.F.Y.; Writing—Review & Editing, J.L., F.Y., and S.E.B.; Visualization, D.M.O. and J.F.Y.; Supervision, F.Y., S.E.B., and J.F.Y.; Project Administration, D.M.O.; Funding Acquisition, F.Y. and J.F.Y.

Abbreviations

ABT	activity-based therapies
AR	androgen receptor
ARE	androgen response element
BDNF	brain-derived neurotrophic factor
BWSTT	bodyweight-supported treadmill training
CNS	central nervous system
CSA	cross-sectional area
DHT	dihydrotestosterone
E_2	estradiol
EPSP	excitatory postsynaptic potential
ER	estrogen receptor
ERE	estrogen response element
fCSA	fiber cross-sectional area
FOXO	forkhead box O
GPCR	G-protein-coupled receptor
GSK3β	glycogen synthase kinase 3β
IGF-1	insulin-like growth factor
IGF-1R	insulin-like growth factor receptor
IGFBP	insulin-like growth factor binding protein
IRS1	insulin receptor substrate-1
LABC	levator ani/bulbocavernosus
MAFbx	muscle atrophy F-box or atrogin-1
MGF	mechano growth factor
MHC	myosin heavy chain
mTOR	mammalian target of rapamycin
MuRF1	muscle ring finger-1
NT-3	neurotrophin-3
ORX	orchiectomy
PGC-1α	peroxisome proliferator-activated receptor gamma co-activator-1α
PGC-1β	peroxisome proliferator-activated receptor gamma co-activator-1β
PI3K	phosphatidyl inositol-3 kinase
SCI	spinal cord injury
SHBG	sex-hormone binding globulin
SNB	spinal nucleus of the bulbocavernosus
T	testosterone
TCF-4	T-cell factor-4
TE	testosterone enanthate
TrkB	tyrosine receptor kinase B
TrkC	tyrosine receptor kinase C
TRT	testosterone replacement therapy

References

1. Beattie, M.S.; Farooqui, A.A.; Bresnahan, J.C. Review of current evidence for apoptosis after spinal cord injury. *J. Neurotrauma* **2000**, *17*, 915–925. [CrossRef] [PubMed]

2. Hilton, B.J.; Moulson, A.J.; Tetzlaff, W. Neuroprotection and secondary damage following spinal cord injury: Concepts and methods. *Neurosci. Lett.* **2017**, *652*, 3–10. [CrossRef] [PubMed]
3. Kwon, B.K.; Tetzlaff, W.; Grauer, J.N.; Beiner, J.; Vaccaro, A.R. Pathophysiology and pharmacologic treatment of acute spinal cord injury. *Spine J.* **2004**, *4*, 451–464. [CrossRef] [PubMed]
4. Morawietz, C.; Moffat, F. Effects of locomotor training after incomplete spinal cord injury: A systematic review. *Arch. Phys. Med. Rehabil.* **2013**, *94*, 2297–2308. [CrossRef] [PubMed]
5. Battistuzzo, C.R.; Callister, R.J.; Callister, R.; Galea, M.P. A systematic review of exercise training to promote locomotor recovery in animal models of spinal cord injury. *J. Neurotrauma* **2012**, *29*, 1600–1613. [CrossRef] [PubMed]
6. Behrman, A.L.; Ardolino, E.M.; Harkema, S.J. Activity-based therapy: From basic science to clinical application for recovery after spinal cord injury. *J. Neurol. Phys. Ther.* **2017**, *41* (Suppl. S3), S39–S45. [CrossRef] [PubMed]
7. Sullivan, S.D.; Nash, M.S.; Tefera, E.; Tinsley, E.; Blackman, M.R.; Groah, S. Prevalence and etiology of hypogonadism in young men with chronic spinal cord injury: A cross-sectional analysis from two university-based rehabilitation centers. *PM&R* **2017**, *9*, 751–760.
8. Borst, S.E.; Yarrow, J.F. Injection of testosterone may be safer and more effective than transdermal administration for combating loss of muscle and bone in older men. *Am. J. Physiol. Endocrinol. Metab.* **2015**, *308*, E1035–E1042. [CrossRef] [PubMed]
9. Cheung, A.S.; Gray, H.; Schache, A.G.; Hoermann, R.; Lim Joon, D.; Zajac, J.D.; Pandy, M.G.; Grossmann, M. Androgen deprivation causes selective deficits in the biomechanical leg muscle function of men during walking: A prospective case-control study. *J. Cachexia Sarcopenia Muscle* **2017**, *8*, 102–112. [CrossRef] [PubMed]
10. Skinner, J.W.; Otzel, D.M.; Bowser, A.; Nargi, D.; Agarwal, S.; Peterson, M.D.; Zou, B.; Borst, S.E.; Yarrow, J.F. Muscular responses to testosterone replacement vary by administration route: A systematic review and meta-analysis. *J. Cachexia Sarcopenia Muscle* **2018**. [CrossRef] [PubMed]
11. Snyder, P.J.; Bhasin, S.; Cunningham, G.R.; Matsumoto, A.M.; Stephens-Shields, A.J.; Cauley, J.A.; Gill, T.M.; Barrett-Connor, E.; Swerdloff, R.S.; Wang, C.; et al. Effects of testosterone treatment in older men. *N. Engl. J. Med.* **2016**, *374*, 611–624. [CrossRef] [PubMed]
12. Bauman, W.A.; Cirnigliaro, C.M.; La Fountaine, M.F.; Jensen, A.M.; Wecht, J.M.; Kirshblum, S.C.; Spungen, A.M. A small-scale clinical trial to determine the safety and efficacy of testosterone replacement therapy in hypogonadal men with spinal cord injury. *Horm. Metab. Res.* **2011**, *43*, 574–579. [CrossRef] [PubMed]
13. Moore, P.D.; Gorgey, A.S.; Wade, R.C.; Khalil, R.E.; Lavis, T.D.; Khan, R.; Adler, R.A. Neuromuscular electrical stimulation and testosterone did not influence heterotopic ossification size after spinal cord injury: A case series. *World J. Clin. Cases* **2016**, *4*, 172–176. [CrossRef] [PubMed]
14. Yarrow, J.F.; Phillips, E.G.; Conover, C.F.; Bassett, T.E.; Chen, C.; Teurlings, T.; Vasconez, A.; Alerte, J.; Prock, H.; Jiron, J.M.; et al. Testosterone plus finasteride prevents bone loss without prostate growth in a rodent spinal cord injury model. *J. Neurotrauma* **2017**, *34*, 2972–2981. [CrossRef] [PubMed]
15. Yarrow, J.F.; Conover, C.F.; Beggs, L.A.; Beck, D.T.; Otzel, D.M.; Balaez, A.; Combs, S.M.; Miller, J.R.; Ye, F.; Aguirre, J.I.; et al. Testosterone dose dependently prevents bone and muscle loss in rodents after spinal cord injury. *J. Neurotrauma* **2014**, *31*, 834–845. [CrossRef] [PubMed]
16. Wu, Y.; Zhao, J.; Zhao, W.; Pan, J.; Bauman, W.A.; Cardozo, C.P. Nandrolone normalizes determinants of muscle mass and fiber type after spinal cord injury. *J. Neurotrauma* **2012**, *29*, 1663–1675. [CrossRef] [PubMed]
17. Sengelaub, D.R.; Han, Q.; Liu, N.K.; Maczuga, M.A.; Szalavari, V.; Valencia, S.A.; Xu, X.M. Protective effects of estradiol and dihydrotestosterone following spinal cord injury. *J. Neurotrauma* **2018**, *35*, 825–841. [CrossRef] [PubMed]
18. Byers, J.S.; Huguenard, A.L.; Kuruppu, D.; Liu, N.K.; Xu, X.M.; Sengelaub, D.R. Neuroprotective effects of testosterone on motoneuron and muscle morphology following spinal cord injury. *J. Comp. Neurol.* **2012**, *520*, 2683–2696. [CrossRef] [PubMed]
19. Ung, R.V.; Rouleau, P.; Guertin, P.A. Effects of co-administration of clenbuterol and testosterone propionate on skeletal muscle in paraplegic mice. *J. Neurotrauma* **2010**, *27*, 1129–1142. [CrossRef] [PubMed]
20. Gregory, C.M.; Vandenborne, K.; Huang, H.F.; Ottenweller, J.E.; Dudley, G.A. Effects of testosterone replacement therapy on skeletal muscle after spinal cord injury. *Spinal Cord* **2003**, *41*, 23–28. [CrossRef] [PubMed]

21. Schiaffino, S.; Sandri, M.; Murgia, M. Activity-dependent signaling pathways controlling muscle diversity and plasticity. *Physiology* **2007**, *22*, 269–278. [CrossRef] [PubMed]
22. Thomas, C.K.; Bakels, R.; Klein, C.S.; Zijdewind, I. Human spinal cord injury: Motor unit properties and behaviour. *Acta Physiol.* **2014**, *210*, 5–19. [CrossRef] [PubMed]
23. Klein, C.S.; Hager-Ross, C.K.; Thomas, C.K. Fatigue properties of human thenar motor units paralysed by chronic spinal cord injury. *J. Physiol.* **2006**, *573*, 161–171. [CrossRef] [PubMed]
24. Jayaraman, A.; Gregory, C.M.; Bowden, M.; Stevens, J.E.; Shah, P.; Behrman, A.L.; Vandenborne, K. Lower extremity skeletal muscle function in persons with incomplete spinal cord injury. *Spinal Cord* **2006**, *44*, 680–687. [CrossRef] [PubMed]
25. Hager-Ross, C.K.; Klein, C.S.; Thomas, C.K. Twitch and tetanic properties of human thenar motor units paralyzed by chronic spinal cord injury. *J. Neurophysiol.* **2006**, *96*, 165–174. [CrossRef] [PubMed]
26. Barbeau, H.; Nadeau, S.; Garneau, C. Physical determinants, emerging concepts, and training approaches in gait of individuals with spinal cord injury. *J. Neurotrauma* **2006**, *23*, 571–585. [CrossRef] [PubMed]
27. Bose, P.; Parmer, R.; Reier, P.J.; Thompson, F.J. Morphological changes of the soleus motoneuron pool in chronic midthoracic contused rats. *Exp. Neurol.* **2005**, *191*, 13–23. [CrossRef] [PubMed]
28. Gazula, V.R.; Roberts, M.; Luzzio, C.; Jawad, A.F.; Kalb, R.G. Effects of limb exercise after spinal cord injury on motor neuron dendrite structure. *J. Comp. Neurol.* **2004**, *476*, 130–145. [CrossRef] [PubMed]
29. Wang, H.; Liu, N.K.; Zhang, Y.P.; Deng, L.; Lu, Q.B.; Shields, C.B.; Walker, M.J.; Li, J.; Xu, X.M. Treadmill training induced lumbar motoneuron dendritic plasticity and behavior recovery in adult rats after a thoracic contusive spinal cord injury. *Exp. Neurol.* **2015**, *271*, 368–378. [CrossRef] [PubMed]
30. Biering-Sorensen, B.; Kristensen, I.B.; Kjaer, M.; Biering-Sorensen, F. Muscle after spinal cord injury. *Muscle Nerve* **2009**, *40*, 499–519. [CrossRef] [PubMed]
31. Moore, C.D.; Craven, B.C.; Thabane, L.; Laing, A.C.; Frank-Wilson, A.W.; Kontulainen, S.A.; Papaioannou, A.; Adachi, J.D.; Giangregorio, L.M. Lower-extremity muscle atrophy and fat infiltration after chronic spinal cord injury. *J. Musculoskelet. Neuronal Interact.* **2015**, *15*, 32–41. [PubMed]
32. Gorgey, A.S.; Dudley, G.A. Skeletal muscle atrophy and increased intramuscular fat after incomplete spinal cord injury. *Spinal Cord* **2007**, *45*, 304–309. [CrossRef] [PubMed]
33. Castro, M.J.; Apple, D.F., Jr.; Hillegass, E.A.; Dudley, G.A. Influence of complete spinal cord injury on skeletal muscle cross-sectional area within the first 6 months of injury. *Eur. J. Appl. Physiol. Occup. Physiol.* **1999**, *80*, 373–378. [CrossRef] [PubMed]
34. Shah, P.K.; Stevens, J.E.; Gregory, C.M.; Pathare, N.C.; Jayaraman, A.; Bickel, S.C.; Bowden, M.; Behrman, A.L.; Walter, G.A.; Dudley, G.A.; et al. Lower-extremity muscle cross-sectional area after incomplete spinal cord injury. *Arch. Phys. Med. Rehabil.* **2006**, *87*, 772–778. [CrossRef] [PubMed]
35. Castro, M.J.; Apple, D.F., Jr.; Staron, R.S.; Campos, G.E.; Dudley, G.A. Influence of complete spinal cord injury on skeletal muscle within 6 mo of injury. *J. Appl. Physiol.* **1999**, *86*, 350–358. [CrossRef] [PubMed]
36. Gregory, C.M.; Vandenborne, K.; Castro, M.J.; Dudley, G.A. Human and rat skeletal muscle adaptations to spinal cord injury. *Can. J. Appl. Physiol.* **2003**, *28*, 491–500. [CrossRef] [PubMed]
37. Phillips, E.G.; Beggs, L.A.; Ye, F.; Conover, C.F.; Beck, D.T.; Otzel, D.M.; Ghosh, P.; Bassit, A.C.F.; Borst, S.E.; Yarrow, J.F. Effects of pharmacologic sclerostin inhibition or testosterone administration on soleus muscle atrophy in rodents after spinal cord injury. *PLoS ONE* **2018**, *13*, e0194440. [CrossRef] [PubMed]
38. Talmadge, R.J.; Roy, R.R.; Edgerton, V.R. Persistence of hybrid fibers in rat soleus after spinal cord transection. *Anat. Rec.* **1999**, *255*, 188–201. [CrossRef]
39. Talmadge, R.J.; Roy, R.R.; Edgerton, V.R. Prominence of myosin heavy chain hybrid fibers in soleus muscle of spinal cord-transected rats. *J. Appl. Physiol.* **1995**, *78*, 1256–1265. [CrossRef] [PubMed]
40. Thomas, C.K.; Zaidner, E.Y.; Calancie, B.; Broton, J.G.; Bigland-Ritchie, B.R. Muscle weakness, paralysis, and atrophy after human cervical spinal cord injury. *Exp. Neurol.* **1997**, *148*, 414–423. [CrossRef] [PubMed]
41. Gaviria, M.; Ohanna, F. Variability of the fatigue response of paralyzed skeletal muscle in relation to the time after spinal cord injury: Mechanical and electrophysiological characteristics. *Eur. J. Appl. Physiol. Occup. Physiol.* **1999**, *80*, 145–153. [CrossRef] [PubMed]
42. DiPiro, N.D.; Holthaus, K.D.; Morgan, P.J.; Embry, A.E.; Perry, L.A.; Bowden, M.G.; Gregory, C.M. Lower extremity strength is correlated with walking function after incomplete SCI. *Top. Spinal Cord Inj. Rehabil.* **2015**, *21*, 133–139. [CrossRef] [PubMed]

43. Gregory, C.M.; Bowden, M.G.; Jayaraman, A.; Shah, P.; Behrman, A.; Kautz, S.A.; Vandenborne, K. Resistance training and locomotor recovery after incomplete spinal cord injury: A case series. *Spinal Cord* **2007**, *45*, 522–530. [CrossRef] [PubMed]
44. Yarar-Fisher, C.; Bickel, C.S.; Windham, S.T.; McLain, A.B.; Bamman, M.M. Skeletal muscle signaling associated with impaired glucose tolerance in spinal cord-injured men and the effects of contractile activity. *J. Appl. Physiol.* **2013**, *115*, 756–764. [CrossRef] [PubMed]
45. Yarar-Fisher, C.; Bickel, C.S.; Kelly, N.A.; Windham, S.T.; McLain, A.B.; Bamman, M.M. Mechanosensitivity may be enhanced in skeletal muscles of spinal cord-injured versus able-bodied men. *Muscle Nerve* **2014**, *50*, 599–601. [CrossRef] [PubMed]
46. Panisset, M.G.; Galea, M.P.; El-Ansary, D. Does early exercise attenuate muscle atrophy or bone loss after spinal cord injury? *Spinal Cord* **2016**, *54*, 84–92. [CrossRef] [PubMed]
47. Malavaki, C.J.; Sakkas, G.K.; Mitrou, G.I.; Kalyva, A.; Stefanidis, I.; Myburgh, K.H.; Karatzaferi, C. Skeletal muscle atrophy: Disease-induced mechanisms may mask disuse atrophy. *J. Muscle Res. Cell Motil.* **2015**, *36*, 405–421. [CrossRef] [PubMed]
48. Bodine, S.C.; Latres, E.; Baumhueter, S.; Lai, V.K.; Nunez, L.; Clarke, B.A.; Poueymirou, W.T.; Panaro, F.J.; Na, E.; Dharmarajan, K.; et al. Identification of ubiquitin ligases required for skeletal muscle atrophy. *Science* **2001**, *294*, 1704–1708. [CrossRef] [PubMed]
49. Baligand, C.; Chen, Y.W.; Ye, F.; Pandey, S.N.; Lai, S.H.; Liu, M.; Vandenborne, K. Transcriptional pathways associated with skeletal muscle changes after spinal cord injury and treadmill locomotor training. *Biomed. Res. Int.* **2015**, *2015*, 387090. [CrossRef] [PubMed]
50. Haddad, F.; Roy, R.R.; Zhong, H.; Edgerton, V.R.; Baldwin, K.M. Atrophy responses to muscle inactivity. II. Molecular markers of protein deficits. *J. Appl. Physiol.* **2003**, *95*, 791–802. [CrossRef] [PubMed]
51. Kim, S.J.; Roy, R.R.; Kim, J.A.; Zhong, H.; Haddad, F.; Baldwin, K.M.; Edgerton, V.R. Gene expression during inactivity-induced muscle atrophy: Effects of brief bouts of a forceful contraction countermeasure. *J. Appl. Physiol.* **2008**, *105*, 1246–1254. [CrossRef] [PubMed]
52. Urso, M.L.; Chen, Y.W.; Scrimgeour, A.G.; Lee, P.C.; Lee, K.F.; Clarkson, P.M. Alterations in mrna expression and protein products following spinal cord injury in humans. *J. Physiol.* **2007**, *579*, 877–892. [CrossRef] [PubMed]
53. Zeman, R.J.; Zhao, J.; Zhang, Y.; Zhao, W.; Wen, X.; Wu, Y.; Pan, J.; Bauman, W.A.; Cardozo, C. Differential skeletal muscle gene expression after upper or lower motor neuron transection. *Pflugers Arch.* **2009**, *458*, 525–535. [CrossRef] [PubMed]
54. Sacheck, J.M.; Hyatt, J.P.; Raffaello, A.; Jagoe, R.T.; Roy, R.R.; Edgerton, V.R.; Lecker, S.H.; Goldberg, A.L. Rapid disuse and denervation atrophy involve transcriptional changes similar to those of muscle wasting during systemic diseases. *FASEB J.* **2007**, *21*, 140–155. [CrossRef] [PubMed]
55. Thakore, N.P.; Samantaray, S.; Park, S.; Nozaki, K.; Smith, J.A.; Cox, A.; Krause, J.; Banik, N.L. Molecular changes in sub-lesional muscle following acute phase of spinal cord injury. *Neurochem. Res.* **2016**, *41*, 44–52. [CrossRef] [PubMed]
56. Ye, F.; Baligand, C.; Keener, J.E.; Vohra, R.; Lim, W.; Ruhella, A.; Bose, P.; Daniels, M.; Walter, G.A.; Thompson, F.; et al. Hindlimb muscle morphology and function in a new atrophy model combining spinal cord injury and cast immobilization. *J. Neurotrauma* **2013**, *30*, 227–235. [CrossRef] [PubMed]
57. Drummond, M.J.; Glynn, E.L.; Lujan, H.L.; Dicarlo, S.E.; Rasmussen, B.B. Gene and protein expression associated with protein synthesis and breakdown in paraplegic skeletal muscle. *Muscle Nerve* **2008**, *37*, 505–513. [CrossRef] [PubMed]
58. Lundell, L.S.; Savikj, M.; Kostovski, E.; Iversen, P.O.; Zierath, J.R.; Krook, A.; Chibalin, A.V.; Widegren, U. Protein translation, proteolysis and autophagy in human skeletal muscle atrophy after spinal cord injury. *Acta Physiol.* **2018**. [CrossRef] [PubMed]
59. Yarar-Fisher, C.; Bickel, C.S.; Kelly, N.A.; Stec, M.J.; Windham, S.T.; McLain, A.B.; Oster, R.A.; Bamman, M.M. Heightened tweak-nf-kappab signaling and inflammation-associated fibrosis in paralyzed muscles of men with chronic spinal cord injury. *Am. J. Physiol. Endocrinol. Metab.* **2016**, *310*, E754–761. [CrossRef] [PubMed]
60. Leger, B.; Senese, R.; Al-Khodairy, A.W.; Deriaz, O.; Gobelet, C.; Giacobino, J.P.; Russell, A.P. Atrogin-1, murf1, and foxo, as well as phosphorylated gsk-3beta and 4e-bp1 are reduced in skeletal muscle of chronic spinal cord-injured patients. *Muscle Nerve* **2009**, *40*, 69–78. [CrossRef] [PubMed]

61. Huang, J.; Zhu, X. The molecular mechanisms of calpains action on skeletal muscle atrophy. *Physiol. Res.* **2016**, *65*, 547–560. [PubMed]
62. Bikle, D.D.; Tahimic, C.; Chang, W.; Wang, Y.; Philippou, A.; Barton, E.R. Role of IGF-I signaling in muscle bone interactions. *Bone* **2015**, *80*, 79–88. [CrossRef] [PubMed]
63. Liu, M.; Stevens-Lapsley, J.E.; Jayaraman, A.; Ye, F.; Conover, C.; Walter, G.A.; Bose, P.; Thompson, F.J.; Borst, S.E.; Vandenborne, K. Impact of treadmill locomotor training on skeletal muscle IGF1 and myogenic regulatory factors in spinal cord injured rats. *Eur. J. Appl. Physiol.* **2010**, *109*, 709–720. [CrossRef] [PubMed]
64. Pete, G.; Fuller, C.R.; Oldham, J.M.; Smith, D.R.; D'Ercole, A.J.; Kahn, C.R.; Lund, P.K. Postnatal growth responses to insulin-like growth factor i in insulin receptor substrate-1-deficient mice. *Endocrinology* **1999**, *140*, 5478–5487. [CrossRef] [PubMed]
65. Tsitouras, P.D.; Zhong, Y.G.; Spungen, A.M.; Bauman, W.A. Serum testosterone and growth hormone/insulin-like growth factor-i in adults with spinal cord injury. *Horm. Metab. Res.* **1995**, *27*, 287–292. [CrossRef] [PubMed]
66. Bauman, W.A.; Spungen, A.M.; Flanagan, S.; Zhong, Y.G.; Alexander, L.R.; Tsitouras, P.D. Blunted growth hormone response to intravenous arginine in subjects with a spinal cord injury. *Horm. Metab. Res.* **1994**, *26*, 152–156. [CrossRef] [PubMed]
67. Dreyer, H.C.; Glynn, E.L.; Lujan, H.L.; Fry, C.S.; DiCarlo, S.E.; Rasmussen, B.B. Chronic paraplegia-induced muscle atrophy downregulates the mtor/s6k1 signaling pathway. *J. Appl. Physiol.* **2008**, *104*, 27–33. [CrossRef] [PubMed]
68. Gorgey, A.S.; Gater, D.R. Insulin growth factors may explain relationship between spasticity and skeletal muscle size in men with spinal cord injury. *J. Rehabil. Res. Dev.* **2012**, *49*, 373–380. [CrossRef] [PubMed]
69. Kang, C.; Ji, L.L. Role of PGC-1alpha signaling in skeletal muscle health and disease. *Ann. N. Y. Acad. Sci.* **2012**, *1271*, 110–117. [CrossRef] [PubMed]
70. Gali Ramamoorthy, T.; Laverny, G.; Schlagowski, A.I.; Zoll, J.; Messaddeq, N.; Bornert, J.M.; Panza, S.; Ferry, A.; Geny, B.; Metzger, D. The transcriptional coregulator pgc-1beta controls mitochondrial function and anti-oxidant defence in skeletal muscles. *Nat. Commun.* **2015**, *6*, 10210. [CrossRef] [PubMed]
71. Lin, J.; Wu, H.; Tarr, P.T.; Zhang, C.Y.; Wu, Z.; Boss, O.; Michael, L.F.; Puigserver, P.; Isotani, E.; Olson, E.N.; et al. Transcriptional co-activator pgc-1 alpha drives the formation of slow-twitch muscle fibres. *Nature* **2002**, *418*, 797–801. [CrossRef] [PubMed]
72. Kang, C.; Goodman, C.A.; Hornberger, T.A.; Ji, L.L. PGC-1alpha overexpression by in vivo transfection attenuates mitochondrial deterioration of skeletal muscle caused by immobilization. *FASEB J.* **2015**, *29*, 4092–4106. [CrossRef] [PubMed]
73. Higashino, K.; Matsuura, T.; Suganuma, K.; Yukata, K.; Nishisho, T.; Yasui, N. Early changes in muscle atrophy and muscle fiber type conversion after spinal cord transection and peripheral nerve transection in rats. *J. Neuroeng. Rehabil.* **2013**, *10*, 46. [CrossRef] [PubMed]
74. Wu, Y.; Collier, L.; Qin, W.; Creasey, G.; Bauman, W.A.; Jarvis, J.; Cardozo, C. Electrical stimulation modulates wnt signaling and regulates genes for the motor endplate and calcium binding in muscle of rats with spinal cord transection. *BMC Neurosci.* **2013**, *14*, 81. [CrossRef] [PubMed]
75. Kramer, D.K.; Ahlsen, M.; Norrbom, J.; Jansson, E.; Hjeltnes, N.; Gustafsson, T.; Krook, A. Human skeletal muscle fibre type variations correlate with ppar alpha, ppar delta and PGC-1 alpha mrna. *Acta Physiol.* **2006**, *188*, 207–216. [CrossRef] [PubMed]
76. Baldwin, K.M.; Haddad, F.; Pandorf, C.E.; Roy, R.R.; Edgerton, V.R. Alterations in muscle mass and contractile phenotype in response to unloading models: Role of transcriptional/pretranslational mechanisms. *Front. Physiol.* **2013**, *4*, 284. [CrossRef] [PubMed]
77. Atherton, P.J.; Greenhaff, P.L.; Phillips, S.M.; Bodine, S.C.; Adams, C.M.; Lang, C.H. Control of skeletal muscle atrophy in response to disuse: Clinical/preclinical contentions and fallacies of evidence. *Am. J. Physiol. Endocrinol. Metab.* **2016**, *311*, E594–E604. [CrossRef] [PubMed]
78. Yarrow, J.F.; McCoy, S.C.; Borst, S.E. Intracrine and myotrophic roles of 5alpha-reductase and androgens: A review. *Med. Sci. Sports Exerc.* **2012**, *44*, 818–826. [CrossRef] [PubMed]
79. Burger, H.G. Androgen production in women. *Fertil. Steril.* **2002**, *77* (Suppl. S4), S3–S5. [CrossRef]
80. Labrie, F. All sex steroids are made intracellularly in peripheral tissues by the mechanisms of intracrinology after menopause. *J. Steroid Biochem. Mol. Biol.* **2015**, *145*, 133–138. [CrossRef] [PubMed]

81. Conover, C.F.; Yarrow, J.F.; Garrett, T.J.; Ye, F.; Quinlivan, E.P.; Cannady, D.F.; Peterson, M.D.; Borst, S.E. High prevalence of low serum biologically active testosterone in older male veterans. *J. Am. Med. Dir. Assoc.* **2017**, *18*, 366.e17–366.e24. [CrossRef] [PubMed]
82. Laurent, M.R.; Helsen, C.; Antonio, L.; Schollaert, D.; Joniau, S.; Vos, M.J.; Decallonne, B.; Hammond, G.L.; Vanderschueren, D.; Claessens, F. Effects of sex hormone-binding globulin (shbg) on androgen bioactivity in vitro. *Mol. Cell. Endocrinol.* **2016**, *437*, 280–291. [CrossRef] [PubMed]
83. Thaler, M.A.; Seifert-Klauss, V.; Luppa, P.B. The biomarker sex hormone-binding globulin—From established applications to emerging trends in clinical medicine. *Best Pract. Res. Clin. Endocrinol. Metab.* **2015**, *29*, 749–760. [CrossRef] [PubMed]
84. Yarrow, J.F.; Wronski, T.J.; Borst, S.E. Testosterone and adult male bone: Actions independent of 5alpha-reductase and aromatase. *Exerc. Sport Sci. Rev.* **2015**, *43*, 222–230. [CrossRef] [PubMed]
85. Lumbroso, S.; Sandillon, F.; Georget, V.; Lobaccaro, J.M.; Brinkmann, A.O.; Privat, A.; Sultan, C. Immunohistochemical localization and immunoblotting of androgen receptor in spinal neurons of male and female rats. *Eur. J. Endocrinol.* **1996**, *134*, 626–632. [CrossRef] [PubMed]
86. Matsuura, T.; Ogata, A.; Demura, T.; Moriwaka, F.; Tashiro, K.; Koyanagi, T.; Nagashima, K. Identification of androgen receptor in the rat spinal motoneurons. Immunohistochemical and immunoblotting analyses with monoclonal antibody. *Neurosci. Lett.* **1993**, *158*, 5–8. [CrossRef]
87. Cain, M.P.; Kramer, S.A.; Tindall, D.J.; Husmann, D.A. Expression of androgen receptor protein within the lumbar spinal cord during ontologic development and following antiandrogen induced cryptorchidism. *J. Urol.* **1994**, *152*, 766–769. [CrossRef]
88. Bauer, E.R.; Daxenberger, A.; Petri, T.; Sauerwein, H.; Meyer, H.H. Characterisation of the affinity of different anabolics and synthetic hormones to the human androgen receptor, human sex hormone binding globulin and to the bovine progestin receptor. *Acta Pathol. Microbiol. Immunol. Scand.* **2000**, *108*, 838–846. [CrossRef]
89. Almeida, M.; Laurent, M.R.; Dubois, V.; Claessens, F.; O'Brien, C.A.; Bouillon, R.; Vanderschueren, D.; Manolagas, S.C. Estrogens and androgens in skeletal physiology and pathophysiology. *Physiol. Rev.* **2017**, *97*, 135–187. [CrossRef] [PubMed]
90. Gennari, L.; Nuti, R.; Bilezikian, J.P. Aromatase activity and bone homeostasis in men. *J. Clin. Endocrinol. Metab.* **2004**, *89*, 5898–5907. [CrossRef] [PubMed]
91. Durga, A.; Sepahpanah, F.; Regozzi, M.; Hastings, J.; Crane, D.A. Prevalence of testosterone deficiency after spinal cord injury. *PM&R* **2011**, *3*, 929–932.
92. Bauman, W.A.; La Fountaine, M.F.; Spungen, A.M. Age-related prevalence of low testosterone in men with spinal cord injury. *J. Spinal Cord Med.* **2014**, *37*, 32–39. [CrossRef] [PubMed]
93. Clark, M.J.; Schopp, L.H.; Mazurek, M.O.; Zaniletti, I.; Lammy, A.B.; Martin, T.A.; Thomas, F.P.; Acuff, M.E. Testosterone levels among men with spinal cord injury: Relationship between time since injury and laboratory values. *Am. J. Phys. Med. Rehabil.* **2008**, *87*, 758–767. [CrossRef] [PubMed]
94. Bauman, W.A.; La Fountaine, M.F.; Cirnigliaro, C.M.; Kirshblum, S.C.; Spungen, A.M. Testicular responses to hcg stimulation at varying doses in men with spinal cord injury. *Spinal Cord* **2017**, *55*, 659–663. [CrossRef] [PubMed]
95. Bauman, W.A.; La Fountaine, M.F.; Cirnigliaro, C.M.; Kirshblum, S.C.; Spungen, A.M. Provocative stimulation of the hypothalamic-pituitary-testicular axis in men with spinal cord injury. *Spinal Cord* **2016**, *54*, 961–966. [CrossRef] [PubMed]
96. Bauman, W.A.; La Fountaine, M.F.; Cirnigliaro, C.M.; Kirshblum, S.C.; Spungen, A.M. Administration of increasing doses of gonadotropin-releasing hormone in men with spinal cord injury to investigate dysfunction of the hypothalamic-pituitary-gonadal axis. *Spinal Cord* **2018**, *56*, 247–258. [CrossRef] [PubMed]
97. Kostovski, E.; Iversen, P.O.; Birkeland, K.; Torjesen, P.A.; Hjeltnes, N. Decreased levels of testosterone and gonadotrophins in men with long-standing tetraplegia. *Spinal Cord* **2008**, *46*, 559–564. [CrossRef] [PubMed]
98. Finkelstein, J.S.; Lee, H.; Burnett-Bowie, S.A.; Pallais, J.C.; Yu, E.W.; Borges, L.F.; Jones, B.F.; Barry, C.V.; Wulczyn, K.E.; Thomas, B.J.; et al. Gonadal steroids and body composition, strength, and sexual function in men. *N. Engl. J. Med.* **2013**, *369*, 1011–1022. [CrossRef] [PubMed]
99. Schopp, L.H.; Clark, M.; Mazurek, M.O.; Hagglund, K.J.; Acuff, M.E.; Sherman, A.K.; Childers, M.K. Testosterone levels among men with spinal cord injury admitted to inpatient rehabilitation. *Am. J. Phys. Med. Rehabil.* **2006**, *85*, 678–684, quiz 685–677. [CrossRef] [PubMed]

100. Beggs, L.A.; Ye, F.; Ghosh, P.; Beck, D.T.; Conover, C.F.; Balaez, A.; Miller, J.R.; Phillips, E.G.; Zheng, N.; Williams, A.A.; et al. Sclerostin inhibition prevents spinal cord injury-induced cancellous bone loss. *J. Bone Miner. Res.* **2015**, *30*, 681–689. [CrossRef] [PubMed]
101. Wu, Y.; Collier, L.; Pan, J.; Qin, W.; Bauman, W.A.; Cardozo, C.P. Testosterone reduced methylprednisolone-induced muscle atrophy in spinal cord-injured rats. *Spinal Cord* **2012**, *50*, 57–62. [CrossRef] [PubMed]
102. Borst, S.E.; Yarrow, J.F.; Conover, C.F.; Nseyo, U.; Meuleman, J.R.; Lipinska, J.A.; Braith, R.W.; Beck, D.T.; Martin, J.S.; Morrow, M.; et al. Musculoskeletal and prostate effects of combined testosterone and finasteride administration in older hypogonadal men: A randomized, controlled trial. *Am. J. Physiol. Endocrinol. Metab.* **2014**, *306*, E433–E442. [CrossRef] [PubMed]
103. Cooper, I.S.; Rynearson, E.H.; Mac, C.C.; Power, M.H. The catabolic effect of trauma of the spinal cord and its investigative treatment with testosterone propionate; preliminary report. *Proc. Staff Meet. Mayo Clin.* **1950**, *25*, 326–330. [PubMed]
104. Cooper, I.S.; Rynearson, E.H.; Mac, C.C.; Power, M.H. Testosterone propionate as a nitrogen-sparing agent after spinal cord injury. *J. Am. Med. Assoc.* **1951**, *145*, 549–553. [CrossRef] [PubMed]
105. Bauman, W.A.; La Fountaine, M.F.; Cirnigliaro, C.M.; Kirshblum, S.C.; Spungen, A.M. Lean tissue mass and energy expenditure are retained in hypogonadal men with spinal cord injury after discontinuation of testosterone replacement therapy. *J. Spinal Cord Med.* **2015**, *38*, 38–47. [CrossRef] [PubMed]
106. Bennett, N.C.; Gardiner, R.A.; Hooper, J.D.; Johnson, D.W.; Gobe, G.C. Molecular cell biology of androgen receptor signalling. *Int. J. Biochem. Cell Biol.* **2010**, *42*, 813–827. [CrossRef] [PubMed]
107. MacLean, H.E.; Chiu, W.S.; Notini, A.J.; Axell, A.M.; Davey, R.A.; McManus, J.F.; Ma, C.; Plant, D.R.; Lynch, G.S.; Zajac, J.D. Impaired skeletal muscle development and function in male, but not female, genomic androgen receptor knockout mice. *FASEB J.* **2008**, *22*, 2676–2689. [CrossRef] [PubMed]
108. Revankar, C.M.; Cimino, D.F.; Sklar, L.A.; Arterburn, J.B.; Prossnitz, E.R. A transmembrane intracellular estrogen receptor mediates rapid cell signaling. *Science* **2005**, *307*, 1625–1630. [CrossRef] [PubMed]
109. Foradori, C.D.; Weiser, M.J.; Handa, R.J. Non-genomic actions of androgens. *Front. Neuroendocrinol.* **2008**, *29*, 169–181. [CrossRef] [PubMed]
110. Singh, R.; Bhasin, S.; Braga, M.; Artaza, J.N.; Pervin, S.; Taylor, W.E.; Krishnan, V.; Sinha, S.K.; Rajavashisth, T.B.; Jasuja, R. Regulation of myogenic differentiation by androgens: Cross talk between androgen receptor/beta-catenin and follistatin/transforming growth factor-beta signaling pathways. *Endocrinology* **2009**, *150*, 1259–1268. [CrossRef] [PubMed]
111. Rudnicki, M.A.; Williams, B.O. Wnt signaling in bone and muscle. *Bone* **2015**, *80*, 60–66. [CrossRef] [PubMed]
112. Liu, X.H.; Wu, Y.; Yao, S.; Levine, A.C.; Kirschenbaum, A.; Collier, L.; Bauman, W.A.; Cardozo, C.P. Androgens up-regulate transcription of the notch inhibitor numb in c2c12 myoblasts via wnt/beta-catenin signaling to t cell factor elements in the numb promoter. *J. Biol. Chem.* **2013**, *288*, 17990–17998. [CrossRef] [PubMed]
113. Gentile, M.A.; Nantermet, P.V.; Vogel, R.L.; Phillips, R.; Holder, D.; Hodor, P.; Cheng, C.; Dai, H.; Freedman, L.P.; Ray, W.J. Androgen-mediated improvement of body composition and muscle function involves a novel early transcriptional program including igf1, mechano growth factor, and induction of {beta}-catenin. *J. Mol. Endocrinol.* **2010**, *44*, 55–73. [CrossRef] [PubMed]
114. Otto-Duessel, M.; Tew, B.Y.; Vonderfecht, S.; Moore, R.; Jones, J.O. Identification of neuron selective androgen receptor inhibitors. *World J. Biol. Chem.* **2017**, *8*, 138–150. [CrossRef] [PubMed]
115. Pawlowski, J.E.; Ertel, J.R.; Allen, M.P.; Xu, M.; Butler, C.; Wilson, E.M.; Wierman, M.E. Liganded androgen receptor interaction with beta-catenin: Nuclear co-localization and modulation of transcriptional activity in neuronal cells. *J. Biol. Chem.* **2002**, *277*, 20702–20710. [CrossRef] [PubMed]
116. Thomas, P.S., Jr.; Fraley, G.S.; Damian, V.; Woodke, L.B.; Zapata, F.; Sopher, B.L.; Plymate, S.R.; La Spada, A.R. Loss of endogenous androgen receptor protein accelerates motor neuron degeneration and accentuates androgen insensitivity in a mouse model of x-linked spinal and bulbar muscular atrophy. *Hum. Mol. Genet.* **2006**, *15*, 2225–2238. [CrossRef] [PubMed]
117. Gao, K.; Wang, Y.S.; Yuan, Y.J.; Wan, Z.H.; Yao, T.C.; Li, H.H.; Tang, P.F.; Mei, X.F. Neuroprotective effect of rapamycin on spinal cord injury via activation of the wnt/beta-catenin signaling pathway. *Neural Regen. Res.* **2015**, *10*, 951–957. [PubMed]

118. Lu, G.B.; Niu, F.W.; Zhang, Y.C.; Du, L.; Liang, Z.Y.; Gao, Y.; Yan, T.Z.; Nie, Z.K.; Gao, K. Methylprednisolone promotes recovery of neurological function after spinal cord injury: Association with wnt/beta-catenin signaling pathway activation. *Neural Regen. Res.* **2016**, *11*, 1816–1823. [PubMed]
119. Gao, K.; Shen, Z.; Yuan, Y.; Han, D.; Song, C.; Guo, Y.; Mei, X. Simvastatin inhibits neural cell apoptosis and promotes locomotor recovery via activation of wnt/beta-catenin signaling pathway after spinal cord injury. *J. Neurochem* **2016**, *138*, 139–149. [CrossRef] [PubMed]
120. Ye, F.; McCoy, S.C.; Ross, H.H.; Bernardo, J.A.; Beharry, A.W.; Senf, S.M.; Judge, A.R.; Beck, D.T.; Conover, C.F.; Cannady, D.F.; et al. Transcriptional regulation of myotrophic actions by testosterone and trenbolone on androgen-responsive muscle. *Steroids* **2014**, *87*, 59–66. [CrossRef] [PubMed]
121. Wu, Y.; Bauman, W.A.; Blitzer, R.D.; Cardozo, C. Testosterone-induced hypertrophy of l6 myoblasts is dependent upon erk and mtor. *Biochem. Biophys. Res. Commun.* **2010**, *400*, 679–683. [CrossRef] [PubMed]
122. Wu, Y.; Zhao, W.; Zhao, J.; Pan, J.; Wu, Q.; Zhang, Y.; Bauman, W.A.; Cardozo, C.P. Identification of androgen response elements in the insulin-like growth factor i upstream promoter. *Endocrinology* **2007**, *148*, 2984–2993. [CrossRef] [PubMed]
123. Ferrando, A.A.; Sheffield-Moore, M.; Yeckel, C.W.; Gilkison, C.; Jiang, J.; Achacosa, A.; Lieberman, S.A.; Tipton, K.; Wolfe, R.R.; Urban, R.J. Testosterone administration to older men improves muscle function: Molecular and physiological mechanisms. *Am. J. Physiol. Endocrinol. Metab.* **2002**, *282*, E601–E607. [CrossRef] [PubMed]
124. Deane, C.S.; Hughes, D.C.; Sculthorpe, N.; Lewis, M.P.; Stewart, C.E.; Sharples, A.P. Impaired hypertrophy in myoblasts is improved with testosterone administration. *J. Steroid Biochem. Mol. Biol.* **2013**, *138*, 152–161. [CrossRef] [PubMed]
125. White, J.P.; Gao, S.; Puppa, M.J.; Sato, S.; Welle, S.L.; Carson, J.A. Testosterone regulation of akt/mtorc1/foxo3a signaling in skeletal muscle. *Mol. Cell. Endocrinol.* **2013**, *365*, 174–186. [CrossRef] [PubMed]
126. Basualto-Alarcon, C.; Jorquera, G.; Altamirano, F.; Jaimovich, E.; Estrada, M. Testosterone signals through mtor and androgen receptor to induce muscle hypertrophy. *Med. Sci. Sports Exerc.* **2013**, *45*, 1712–1720. [CrossRef] [PubMed]
127. Xu, T.; Shen, Y.; Pink, H.; Triantafillou, J.; Stimpson, S.A.; Turnbull, P.; Han, B. Phosphorylation of p70s6 kinase is implicated in androgen-induced levator ani muscle anabolism in castrated rats. *J. Steroid Biochem. Mol. Biol.* **2004**, *92*, 447–454. [CrossRef] [PubMed]
128. Serra, C.; Sandor, N.L.; Jang, H.; Lee, D.; Toraldo, G.; Guarneri, T.; Wong, S.; Zhang, A.; Guo, W.; Jasuja, R.; et al. The effects of testosterone deprivation and supplementation on proteasomal and autophagy activity in the skeletal muscle of the male mouse: Differential effects on high-androgen responder and low-androgen responder muscle groups. *Endocrinology* **2013**, *154*, 4594–4606. [CrossRef] [PubMed]
129. Pires-Oliveira, M.; Maragno, A.L.; Parreiras-e-Silva, L.T.; Chiavegatti, T.; Gomes, M.D.; Godinho, R.O. Testosterone represses ubiquitin ligases atrogin-1 and murf-1 expression in an androgen-sensitive rat skeletal muscle in vivo. *J. Appl. Physiol.* **2010**, *108*, 266–273. [CrossRef] [PubMed]
130. Ferrando, A.A.; Sheffield-Moore, M.; Paddon-Jones, D.; Wolfe, R.R.; Urban, R.J. Differential anabolic effects of testosterone and amino acid feeding in older men. *J. Clin. Endocrinol. Metab.* **2003**, *88*, 358–362. [CrossRef] [PubMed]
131. Zhao, W.; Pan, J.; Wang, X.; Wu, Y.; Bauman, W.A.; Cardozo, C.P. Expression of the muscle atrophy factor muscle atrophy f-box is suppressed by testosterone. *Endocrinology* **2008**, *149*, 5449–5460. [CrossRef] [PubMed]
132. Wu, Y.; Ruggiero, C.L.; Bauman, W.A.; Cardozo, C. Ankrd1 is a transcriptional repressor for the androgen receptor that is downregulated by testosterone. *Biochem. Biophys. Res. Commun.* **2013**, *437*, 355–360. [CrossRef] [PubMed]
133. MacKrell, J.G.; Yaden, B.C.; Bullock, H.; Chen, K.; Shetler, P.; Bryant, H.U.; Krishnan, V. Molecular targets of androgen signaling that characterize skeletal muscle recovery and regeneration. *Nucl. Recept. Signal.* **2015**, *13*, e005. [PubMed]
134. Zhao, J.; Bauman, W.A.; Huang, R.; Caplan, A.J.; Cardozo, C. Oxandrolone blocks glucocorticoid signaling in an androgen receptor-dependent manner. *Steroids* **2004**, *69*, 357–366. [CrossRef] [PubMed]
135. Barbosa, M.R.; Shiguemoto, G.E.; Tomaz, L.M.; Ferreira, F.C.; Rodrigues, M.F.; Domingues, M.M.; Souza Master, M.V.; Canevazzi, G.H.; Silva-Magosso, N.S.; Selistre-de-Araujo, H.S.; et al. Resistance training and ovariectomy: Antagonic effects in mitochondrial biogenesis markers in rat skeletal muscle. *Int. J. Sports Med.* **2016**, *37*, 841–848. [CrossRef] [PubMed]

136. Park, Y.M.; Pereira, R.I.; Erickson, C.B.; Swibas, T.A.; Kang, C.; Van Pelt, R.E. Time since menopause and skeletal muscle estrogen receptors, PGC-1alpha, and ampk. *Menopause* **2017**, *24*, 815–823. [CrossRef] [PubMed]
137. Maher, A.C.; Akhtar, M.; Tarnopolsky, M.A. Men supplemented with 17beta-estradiol have increased beta-oxidation capacity in skeletal muscle. *Physiol. Genom.* **2010**, *42*, 342–347. [CrossRef] [PubMed]
138. McCully, K.K.; Mulcahy, T.K.; Ryan, T.E.; Zhao, Q. Skeletal muscle metabolism in individuals with spinal cord injury. *J. Appl. Physiol.* **2011**, *111*, 143–148. [CrossRef] [PubMed]
139. Patte-Mensah, C.; Penning, T.M.; Mensah-Nyagan, A.G. Anatomical and cellular localization of neuroactive 5 alpha/3 alpha-reduced steroid-synthesizing enzymes in the spinal cord. *J. Comp. Neurol.* **2004**, *477*, 286–299. [CrossRef] [PubMed]
140. Poletti, A.; Coscarella, A.; Negri-Cesi, P.; Colciago, A.; Celotti, F.; Martini, L. 5 alpha-reductase isozymes in the central nervous system. *Steroids* **1998**, *63*, 246–251. [CrossRef]
141. Hauser, K.F.; MacLusky, N.J.; Toran-Allerand, C.D. Androgen action in fetal mouse spinal cord cultures: Metabolic and morphologic aspects. *Brain Res.* **1987**, *406*, 62–72. [CrossRef]
142. MacLusky, N.J.; Clark, C.R.; Shanabrough, M.; Naftolin, F. Metabolism and binding of androgens in the spinal cord of the rat. *Brain Res.* **1987**, *422*, 83–91. [CrossRef]
143. Pozzi, P.; Bendotti, C.; Simeoni, S.; Piccioni, F.; Guerini, V.; Marron, T.U.; Martini, L.; Poletti, A. Androgen 5-alpha-reductase type 2 is highly expressed and active in rat spinal cord motor neurones. *J. Neuroendocrinol.* **2003**, *15*, 882–887. [CrossRef] [PubMed]
144. Hauser, K.F.; Toran-Allerand, C.D. Androgen increases the number of cells in fetal mouse spinal cord cultures: Implications for motoneuron survival. *Brain Res.* **1989**, *485*, 157–164. [CrossRef]
145. Fargo, K.N.; Foecking, E.M.; Jones, K.J.; Sengelaub, D.R. Neuroprotective actions of androgens on motoneurons. *Front. Neuroendocrinol.* **2009**, *30*, 130–141. [CrossRef] [PubMed]
146. Verhovshek, T.; Buckley, K.E.; Sergent, M.A.; Sengelaub, D.R. Testosterone metabolites differentially maintain adult morphology in a sexually dimorphic neuromuscular system. *Dev. Neurobiol.* **2010**, *70*, 206–221. [CrossRef] [PubMed]
147. Huguenard, A.L.; Fernando, S.M.; Monks, D.A.; Sengelaub, D.R. Overexpression of androgen receptors in target musculature confers androgen sensitivity to motoneuron dendrites. *Endocrinology* **2011**, *152*, 639–650. [CrossRef] [PubMed]
148. Ji, Y.X.; Zhao, M.; Liu, Y.L.; Chen, L.S.; Hao, P.L.; Sun, C. Expression of aromatase and estrogen receptors in lumbar motoneurons of mice. *Neurosci. Lett.* **2017**, *653*, 7–11. [CrossRef] [PubMed]
149. Rakotoarivelo, C.; Petite, D.; Lambard, S.; Fabre, C.; Rouleau, C.; Lumbroso, S.; de Weille, J.; Privat, A.; Carreau, S.; Mersel, M. Receptors to steroid hormones and aromatase are expressed by cultured motoneurons but not by glial cells derived from rat embryo spinal cord. *Neuroendocrinology* **2004**, *80*, 284–297. [CrossRef] [PubMed]
150. Nowacek, A.S.; Sengelaub, D.R. Estrogenic support of motoneuron dendritic growth via the neuromuscular periphery in a sexually dimorphic motor system. *J. Neurobiol.* **2006**, *66*, 962–976. [CrossRef] [PubMed]
151. Cai, Y.; Chew, C.; Munoz, F.; Sengelaub, D.R. Neuroprotective effects of testosterone metabolites and dependency on receptor action on the morphology of somatic motoneurons following the death of neighboring motoneurons. *Dev. Neurobiol.* **2017**, *77*, 691–707. [CrossRef] [PubMed]
152. Rudolph, L.M.; Sengelaub, D.R. Castration-induced upregulation of muscle eralpha supports estrogen sensitivity of motoneuron dendrites in a sexually dimorphic neuromuscular system. *Dev. Neurobiol.* **2013**, *73*, 921–935. [CrossRef] [PubMed]
153. Nakamizo, T.; Urushitani, M.; Inoue, R.; Shinohara, A.; Sawada, H.; Honda, K.; Kihara, T.; Akaike, A.; Shimohama, S. Protection of cultured spinal motor neurons by estradiol. *Neuroreport* **2000**, *11*, 3493–3497. [CrossRef] [PubMed]
154. Chen, J.; Hu, R.; Ge, H.; Duanmu, W.; Li, Y.; Xue, X.; Hu, S.; Feng, H. G-protein-coupled receptor 30-mediated antiapoptotic effect of estrogen on spinal motor neurons following injury and its underlying mechanisms. *Mol. Med. Rep.* **2015**, *12*, 1733–1740. [CrossRef] [PubMed]
155. Elkabes, S.; Nicot, A.B. Sex steroids and neuroprotection in spinal cord injury: A review of preclinical investigations. *Exp. Neurol.* **2014**, *259*, 28–37. [CrossRef] [PubMed]
156. Ottem, E.N.; Bailey, D.J.; Jordan, C.L.; Breedlove, S.M. With a little help from my friends: Androgens tap bdnf signaling pathways to alter neural circuits. *Neuroscience* **2013**, *239*, 124–138. [CrossRef] [PubMed]

157. Verhovshek, T.; Rudolph, L.M.; Sengelaub, D.R. Brain-derived neurotrophic factor and androgen interactions in spinal neuromuscular systems. *Neuroscience* **2013**, *239*, 103–114. [CrossRef] [PubMed]
158. Osborne, M.C.; Verhovshek, T.; Sengelaub, D.R. Androgen regulates trkb immunolabeling in spinal motoneurons. *J. Neurosci. Res.* **2007**, *85*, 303–309. [CrossRef] [PubMed]
159. Ottem, E.N.; Beck, L.A.; Jordan, C.L.; Breedlove, S.M. Androgen-dependent regulation of brain-derived neurotrophic factor and tyrosine kinase b in the sexually dimorphic spinal nucleus of the bulbocavernosus. *Endocrinology* **2007**, *148*, 3655–3665. [CrossRef] [PubMed]
160. Yang, L.Y.; Arnold, A.P. Interaction of bdnf and testosterone in the regulation of adult perineal motoneurons. *J. Neurobiol.* **2000**, *44*, 308–319. [CrossRef]
161. Yang, L.Y.; Verhovshek, T.; Sengelaub, D.R. Brain-derived neurotrophic factor and androgen interact in the maintenance of dendritic morphology in a sexually dimorphic rat spinal nucleus. *Endocrinology* **2004**, *145*, 161–168. [CrossRef] [PubMed]
162. Xu, J.; Gingras, K.M.; Bengston, L.; Di Marco, A.; Forger, N.G. Blockade of endogenous neurotrophic factors prevents the androgenic rescue of rat spinal motoneurons. *J. Neurosci.* **2001**, *21*, 4366–4372. [CrossRef] [PubMed]
163. Gill, L.C.; Gransee, H.M.; Sieck, G.C.; Mantilla, C.B. Functional recovery after cervical spinal cord injury: Role of neurotrophin and glutamatergic signaling in phrenic motoneurons. *Respir. Physiol. Neurobiol.* **2016**, *226*, 128–136. [CrossRef] [PubMed]
164. Cardona-Rossinyol, A.; Mir, M.; Caraballo-Miralles, V.; Llado, J.; Olmos, G. Neuroprotective effects of estradiol on motoneurons in a model of rat spinal cord embryonic explants. *Cell. Mol. Neurobiol.* **2013**, *33*, 421–432. [CrossRef] [PubMed]
165. Lin, C.W.; Chen, B.; Huang, K.L.; Dai, Y.S.; Teng, H.L. Inhibition of autophagy by estradiol promotes locomotor recovery after spinal cord injury in rats. *Neurosci. Bull.* **2016**, *32*, 137–144. [CrossRef] [PubMed]
166. Behrman, A.L.; Harkema, S.J. Physical rehabilitation as an agent for recovery after spinal cord injury. *Phys. Med. Rehabil. Clin.* **2007**, *18*, 183–202. [CrossRef] [PubMed]
167. Field-Fote, E.C. Combined use of body weight support, functional electric stimulation, and treadmill training to improve walking ability in individuals with chronic incomplete spinal cord Injury. *Arch. Phys. Med. Rehabil.* **2001**, *82*, 818–824. [CrossRef] [PubMed]
168. Forrest, G.F.; Sisto, S.A.; Barbeau, H.; Kirshblum, S.C.; Wilen, J.; Bond, Q.; Bentson, S.; Asselin, P.; Cirnigliaro, C.M.; Harkema, S. Neuromotor and musculoskeletal responses to locomotor training for an individual with chronic motor complete ais-b spinal cord injury. *J. Spinal Cord Med.* **2008**, *31*, 509–521. [CrossRef] [PubMed]
169. Gorassini, M.A.; Norton, J.A.; Nevett-Duchcherer, J.; Roy, F.D.; Yang, J.F. Changes in locomotor muscle activity after treadmill training in subjects with incomplete spinal cord injury. *J. Neurophysiol.* **2009**, *101*, 969–979. [CrossRef] [PubMed]
170. Harkema, S.J.; Schmidt-Read, M.; Lorenz, D.J.; Edgerton, V.R.; Behrman, A.L. Balance and ambulation improvements in individuals with chronic incomplete spinal cord injury using locomotor training-based rehabilitation. *Arch. Phys. Med. Rehabil.* **2012**, *93*, 1508–1517. [CrossRef] [PubMed]
171. Krishnan, V.; Kindig, M.; Mirbagheri, M. Robotic-assisted locomotor training enhances ankle performance in adults with incomplete spinal cord injury. *J. Rehabil. Med.* **2016**, *48*, 781–786. [CrossRef] [PubMed]
172. Nooijen, C.F.; Ter Hoeve, N.; Field-Fote, E.C. Gait quality is improved by locomotor training in individuals with sci regardless of training approach. *J. Neuroeng. Rehabil.* **2009**, *6*, 36. [CrossRef] [PubMed]
173. Wernig, A.; Muller, S.; Nanassy, A.; Cagol, E. Laufband therapy based on 'rules of spinal locomotion' is effective in spinal cord injured persons. *Eur. J. Neurosci.* **1995**, *7*, 823–829. [CrossRef] [PubMed]
174. Wirz, M.; Bastiaenen, C.; de Bie, R.; Dietz, V. Effectiveness of automated locomotor training in patients with acute incomplete spinal cord injury: A randomized controlled multicenter trial. *BMC Neurol.* **2011**, *11*, 60. [CrossRef] [PubMed]
175. Wirz, M.; Zemon, D.H.; Rupp, R.; Scheel, A.; Colombo, G.; Dietz, V.; Hornby, T.G. Effectiveness of automated locomotor training in patients with chronic incomplete spinal cord injury: A multicenter trial. *Arch. Phys. Med. Rehabil.* **2005**, *86*, 672–680. [CrossRef] [PubMed]
176. Jones, M.L.; Evans, N.; Tefertiller, C.; Backus, D.; Sweatman, M.; Tansey, K.; Morrison, S. Activity-based therapy for recovery of walking in individuals with chronic spinal cord injury: Results from a randomized clinical trial. *Arch. Phys. Med. Rehabil.* **2014**, *95*, 2239–2246. [CrossRef] [PubMed]

177. Knikou, M. Plasticity of corticospinal neural control after locomotor training in human spinal cord injury. *Neural Plast.* **2012**, *2012*, 254948. [CrossRef] [PubMed]
178. Adams, M.M.; Ditor, D.S.; Tarnopolsky, M.A.; Phillips, S.M.; McCartney, N.; Hicks, A.L. The effect of body weight-supported treadmill training on muscle morphology in an individual with chronic, motor-complete spinal cord injury: A case study. *J. Spinal Cord Med.* **2006**, *29*, 167–171. [CrossRef] [PubMed]
179. Alexeeva, N.; Sames, C.; Jacobs, P.L.; Hobday, L.; Distasio, M.M.; Mitchell, S.A.; Calancie, B. Comparison of training methods to improve walking in persons with chronic spinal cord injury: A randomized clinical trial. *J. Spinal Cord Med.* **2011**, *34*, 362–379. [CrossRef] [PubMed]
180. Thomas, S.L.; Gorassini, M.A. Increases in corticospinal tract function by treadmill training after incomplete spinal cord injury. *J. Neurophysiol.* **2005**, *94*, 2844–2855. [CrossRef] [PubMed]
181. Coupaud, S.; Jack, L.P.; Hunt, K.J.; Allan, D.B. Muscle and bone adaptations after treadmill training in incomplete spinal cord injury: A case study using peripheral quantitative computed tomography. *J. Musculoskelet. Neuronal Interact.* **2009**, *9*, 288–297. [PubMed]
182. Giangregorio, L.; McCartney, N. Bone loss and muscle atrophy in spinal cord injury: Epidemiology, fracture prediction, and rehabilitation strategies. *J. Spinal Cord Med.* **2006**, *29*, 489–500. [CrossRef] [PubMed]
183. Giangregorio, L.M.; Hicks, A.L.; Webber, C.E.; Phillips, S.M.; Craven, B.C.; Bugaresti, J.M.; McCartney, N. Body weight supported treadmill training in acute spinal cord injury: Impact on muscle and bone. *Spinal Cord* **2005**, *43*, 649–657. [CrossRef] [PubMed]
184. Stewart, B.G.; Tarnopolsky, M.A.; Hicks, A.L.; McCartney, N.; Mahoney, D.J.; Staron, R.S.; Phillips, S.M. Treadmill training-induced adaptations in muscle phenotype in persons with incomplete spinal cord injury. *Muscle Nerve* **2004**, *30*, 61–68. [CrossRef] [PubMed]
185. Dobkin, B.; Barbeau, H.; Deforge, D.; Ditunno, J.; Elashoff, R.; Apple, D.; Basso, M.; Behrman, A.; Harkema, S.; Saulino, M.; et al. The evolution of walking-related outcomes over the first 12 weeks of rehabilitation for incomplete traumatic spinal cord injury: The multicenter randomized spinal cord injury locomotor trial. *NeuroRehabil. Neural Repair* **2007**, *21*, 25–35. [CrossRef] [PubMed]
186. Field-Fote, E.C.; Roach, K.E. Influence of a locomotor training approach on walking speed and distance in people with chronic spinal cord injury: A randomized clinical trial. *Phys. Ther.* **2011**, *91*, 48–60. [CrossRef] [PubMed]
187. Lucareli, P.R.; Lima, M.O.; Lima, F.P.; de Almeida, J.G.; Brech, G.C.; D'Andrea Greve, J.M. Gait analysis following treadmill training with body weight support versus conventional physical therapy: A prospective randomized controlled single blind study. *Spinal Cord* **2011**, *49*, 1001–1007. [CrossRef] [PubMed]
188. Postans, N.J.; Hasler, J.P.; Granat, M.H.; Maxwell, D.J. Functional electric stimulation to augment partial weight-bearing supported treadmill training for patients with acute incomplete spinal cord injury: A pilot study. *Arch. Phys. Med. Rehabil.* **2004**, *85*, 604–610. [CrossRef] [PubMed]
189. Mehrholz, J.; Kugler, J.; Pohl, M. Locomotor training for walking after spinal cord injury. *Cochrane Database Syst. Rev.* **2012**, *11*, CD006676. [CrossRef] [PubMed]
190. Nam, K.Y.; Kim, H.J.; Kwon, B.S.; Park, J.W.; Lee, H.J.; Yoo, A. Robot-assisted gait training (lokomat) improves walking function and activity in people with spinal cord injury: A systematic review. *J. Neuroeng. Rehabil.* **2017**, *14*, 24. [CrossRef] [PubMed]
191. Wessels, M.; Lucas, C.; Eriks, I.; de Groot, S. Body weight-supported gait training for restoration of walking in people with an incomplete spinal cord injury: A systematic review. *J. Rehabil. Med.* **2010**, *42*, 513–519. [CrossRef] [PubMed]
192. Lam, T.; Noonan, V.K.; Eng, J.J. A systematic review of functional ambulation outcome measures in spinal cord injury. *Spinal Cord* **2008**, *46*, 246–254. [CrossRef] [PubMed]
193. De Leon, R.D.; Dy, C.J. What did we learn from the animal studies of body weight-supported treadmill training and where do we go from here? *J. Neurotrauma* **2017**, *34*, 1744–1750. [CrossRef] [PubMed]
194. Yarrow, J.F.; Conover, C.F.; Lipinska, J.A.; Santillana, C.A.; Wronski, T.J.; Borst, S.E. Methods to quantify sex steroid hormones in bone: Applications to the study of androgen ablation and administration. *Am. J. Physiol. Endocrinol. Metab.* **2010**, *299*, E841–E847. [CrossRef] [PubMed]
195. Nessler, J.A.; Moustafa-Bayoumi, M.; Soto, D.; Duhon, J.E.; Schmitt, R. Robot applied stance loading increases hindlimb muscle mass and stepping kinetics in a rat model of spinal cord injury. In Proceedings of the 2011 Annual International Conference of the IEEE Engineering in Medicine and Biology Society, Boston, MA, USA, 30 August–3 September 2011; Volume 2011, pp. 4145–4148.

196. Ilha, J.; da Cunha, N.B.; Jaeger, M.; de Souza, D.F.; Nascimento, P.S.; Marcuzzo, S.; Figueiro, M.; Gottfried, C.; Achaval, M. Treadmill step training-induced adaptive muscular plasticity in a chronic paraplegia model. *Neurosci. Lett.* **2011**, *492*, 170–174. [CrossRef] [PubMed]
197. Stevens, J.E.; Liu, M.; Bose, P.; O'Steen, W.A.; Thompson, F.J.; Anderson, D.K.; Vandenborne, K. Changes in soleus muscle function and fiber morphology with one week of locomotor training in spinal cord contusion injured rats. *J. Neurotrauma* **2006**, *23*, 1671–1681. [CrossRef] [PubMed]
198. Bose, P.K.; Hou, J.; Parmer, R.; Reier, P.J.; Thompson, F.J. Altered patterns of reflex excitability, balance, and locomotion following spinal cord injury and locomotor training. *Front. Physiol.* **2012**, *3*, 258. [CrossRef] [PubMed]
199. Liu, M.; Bose, P.; Walter, G.A.; Thompson, F.J.; Vandenborne, K. A longitudinal study of skeletal muscle following spinal cord injury and locomotor training. *Spinal Cord* **2008**, *46*, 488–493. [CrossRef] [PubMed]
200. Singh, A.; Balasubramanian, S.; Murray, M.; Lemay, M.; Houle, J. Role of spared pathways in locomotor recovery after body-weight-supported treadmill training in contused rats. *J. Neurotrauma* **2011**, *28*, 2405–2416. [CrossRef] [PubMed]
201. Jayaraman, A.; Shah, P.; Gregory, C.; Bowden, M.; Stevens, J.; Bishop, M.; Walter, G.; Behrman, A.; Vandenborne, K. Locomotor training and muscle function after incomplete spinal cord injury: Case series. *J. Spinal Cord Med.* **2008**, *31*, 185–193. [CrossRef] [PubMed]
202. Duffell, L.D.; Brown, G.L.; Mirbagheri, M.M. Facilitatory effects of anti-spastic medication on robotic locomotor training in people with chronic incomplete spinal cord injury. *J. Neuroeng. Rehabil.* **2015**, *12*, 29. [CrossRef] [PubMed]
203. Varoqui, D.; Niu, X.; Mirbagheri, M.M. Ankle voluntary movement enhancement following robotic-assisted locomotor training in spinal cord injury. *J. Neuroeng. Rehabil.* **2014**, *11*, 46. [CrossRef] [PubMed]
204. Cardozo, C.P.; Graham, Z.A. Muscle-bone interactions: Movement in the field of mechano-humoral coupling of muscle and bone. *Ann. N. Y. Acad. Sci.* **2017**, *1402*, 10–17. [CrossRef] [PubMed]
205. Jayaraman, A.; Liu, M.; Ye, F.; Walter, G.A.; Vandenborne, K. Regenerative responses in slow- and fast-twitch muscles following moderate contusion spinal cord injury and locomotor training. *Eur. J. Appl. Physiol.* **2013**, *113*, 191–200. [CrossRef] [PubMed]
206. Dupont-Versteegden, E.E.; Murphy, R.J.; Houle, J.D.; Gurley, C.M.; Peterson, C.A. Mechanisms leading to restoration of muscle size with exercise and transplantation after spinal cord injury. *Am. J. Physiol. Cell Physiol.* **2000**, *279*, C1677–C1684. [CrossRef] [PubMed]
207. Astorino, T.A.; Harness, E.T.; Witzke, K.A. Chronic activity-based therapy does not improve body composition, insulin-like growth factor-i, adiponectin, or myostatin in persons with spinal cord injury. *J. Spinal Cord Med.* **2015**, *38*, 615–625. [CrossRef] [PubMed]
208. Petrie, M.; Suneja, M.; Shields, R.K. Low-frequency stimulation regulates metabolic gene expression in paralyzed muscle. *J. Appl. Physiol.* **2015**, *118*, 723–731. [CrossRef] [PubMed]
209. Gorgey, A.S.; Graham, Z.A.; Bauman, W.A.; Cardozo, C.; Gater, D.R. Abundance in proteins expressed after functional electrical stimulation cycling or arm cycling ergometry training in persons with chronic spinal cord injury. *J. Spinal Cord Med.* **2017**, *40*, 439–448. [CrossRef] [PubMed]
210. Adams, C.M.; Suneja, M.; Dudley-Javoroski, S.; Shields, R.K. Altered mrna expression after long-term soleus electrical stimulation training in humans with paralysis. *Muscle Nerve* **2011**, *43*, 65–75. [CrossRef] [PubMed]
211. Cote, M.P.; Azzam, G.A.; Lemay, M.A.; Zhukareva, V.; Houle, J.D. Activity-dependent increase in neurotrophic factors is associated with an enhanced modulation of spinal reflexes after spinal cord injury. *J. Neurotrauma* **2011**, *28*, 299–309. [CrossRef] [PubMed]
212. Goldshmit, Y.; Lythgo, N.; Galea, M.P.; Turnley, A.M. Treadmill training after spinal cord hemisection in mice promotes axonal sprouting and synapse formation and improves motor recovery. *J. Neurotrauma* **2008**, *25*, 449–465. [CrossRef] [PubMed]
213. Petruska, J.C.; Ichiyama, R.M.; Jindrich, D.L.; Crown, E.D.; Tansey, K.E.; Roy, R.R.; Edgerton, V.R.; Mendell, L.M. Changes in motoneuron properties and synaptic inputs related to step training after spinal cord transection in rats. *J. Neurosci.* **2007**, *27*, 4460–4471. [CrossRef] [PubMed]
214. Knikou, M. Neurophysiological characteristics of human leg muscle action potentials evoked by transcutaneous magnetic stimulation of the spine. *Bioelectromagnetics* **2013**, *34*, 200–210. [CrossRef] [PubMed]
215. Knikou, M.; Mummidisetty, C.K. Locomotor training improves premotoneuronal control after chronic spinal cord injury. *J. Neurophysiol.* **2014**, *111*, 2264–2275. [CrossRef] [PubMed]

216. Smith, A.C.; Mummidisetty, C.K.; Rymer, W.Z.; Knikou, M. Locomotor training alters the behavior of flexor reflexes during walking in human spinal cord injury. *J. Neurophysiol.* **2014**, *112*, 2164–2175. [CrossRef] [PubMed]
217. Smith, A.C.; Knikou, M. A review on locomotor training after spinal cord injury: Reorganization of spinal neuronal circuits and recovery of motor function. *Neural Plast.* **2016**, *2016*, 1216258. [CrossRef] [PubMed]
218. Alcobendas-Maestro, M.; Esclarin-Ruz, A.; Casado-Lopez, R.M.; Munoz-Gonzalez, A.; Perez-Mateos, G.; Gonzalez-Valdizan, E.; Martin, J.L. Lokomat robotic-assisted versus overground training within 3 to 6 months of incomplete spinal cord lesion: Randomized controlled trial. *NeuroRehabil. Neural Repair* **2012**, *26*, 1058–1063. [CrossRef] [PubMed]
219. Esclarin-Ruz, A.; Alcobendas-Maestro, M.; Casado-Lopez, R.; Perez-Mateos, G.; Florido-Sanchez, M.A.; Gonzalez-Valdizan, E.; Martin, J.L. A comparison of robotic walking therapy and conventional walking therapy in individuals with upper versus lower motor neuron lesions: A randomized controlled trial. *Arch. Phys. Med. Rehabil.* **2014**, *95*, 1023–1031. [CrossRef] [PubMed]
220. Field-Fote, E.C.; Lindley, S.D.; Sherman, A.L. Locomotor training approaches for individuals with spinal cord injury: A preliminary report of walking-related outcomes. *J. Neurol. Phys. Ther.* **2005**, *29*, 127–137. [CrossRef] [PubMed]
221. Kapadia, N.; Masani, K.; Catharine Craven, B.; Giangregorio, L.M.; Hitzig, S.L.; Richards, K.; Popovic, M.R. A randomized trial of functional electrical stimulation for walking in incomplete spinal cord injury: Effects on walking competency. *J. Spinal Cord Med.* **2014**, *37*, 511–524. [CrossRef] [PubMed]
222. Labruyere, R.; van Hedel, H.J. Strength training versus robot-assisted gait training after incomplete spinal cord injury: A randomized pilot study in patients depending on walking assistance. *J. Neuroeng. Rehabil.* **2014**, *11*, 4. [CrossRef] [PubMed]
223. Lam, T.; Pauhl, K.; Ferguson, A.; Malik, R.N.; Krassioukov, A.; Eng, J.J. Training with robot-applied resistance in people with motor-incomplete spinal cord injury: Pilot study. *J. Rehabil. Res. Dev.* **2015**, *52*, 113–129. [CrossRef] [PubMed]
224. Morrison, S.A.; Lorenz, D.; Eskay, C.P.; Forrest, G.F.; Basso, D.M. Longitudinal recovery and reduced costs after 120 sessions of locomotor training for motor incomplete spinal cord injury. *Arch. Phys. Med. Rehabil.* **2018**, *99*, 555–562. [CrossRef] [PubMed]
225. Niu, X.; Varoqui, D.; Kindig, M.; Mirbagheri, M.M. Prediction of gait recovery in spinal cord injured individuals trained with robotic gait orthosis. *J. Neuroeng. Rehabil.* **2014**, *11*, 42. [CrossRef] [PubMed]
226. Winchester, P.; McColl, R.; Querry, R.; Foreman, N.; Mosby, J.; Tansey, K.; Williamson, J. Changes in supraspinal activation patterns following robotic locomotor therapy in motor-incomplete spinal cord injury. *NeuroRehabil. Neural Repair* **2005**, *19*, 313–324. [CrossRef] [PubMed]
227. Wu, M.; Landry, J.M.; Schmit, B.D.; Hornby, T.G.; Yen, S.C. Robotic resistance treadmill training improves locomotor function in human spinal cord injury: A pilot study. *Arch. Phys. Med. Rehabil.* **2012**, *93*, 782–789. [CrossRef] [PubMed]
228. Galen, S.S.; Clarke, C.J.; McLean, A.N.; Allan, D.B.; Conway, B.A. Isometric hip and knee torque measurements as an outcome measure in robot assisted gait training. *NeuroRehabilitation* **2014**, *34*, 287–295. [PubMed]
229. Maier, I.C.; Ichiyama, R.M.; Courtine, G.; Schnell, L.; Lavrov, I.; Edgerton, V.R.; Schwab, M.E. Differential effects of anti-nogo-a antibody treatment and treadmill training in rats with incomplete spinal cord injury. *Brain* **2009**, *132*, 1426–1440. [CrossRef] [PubMed]
230. Battistuzzo, C.R.; Rank, M.M.; Flynn, J.R.; Morgan, D.L.; Callister, R.; Callister, R.J.; Galea, M.P. Gait recovery following spinal cord injury in mice: Limited effect of treadmill training. *J. Spinal Cord Med.* **2016**, *39*, 335–343. [CrossRef] [PubMed]
231. Battistuzzo, C.R.; Rank, M.M.; Flynn, J.R.; Morgan, D.L.; Callister, R.; Callister, R.J.; Galea, M.P. Effects of treadmill training on hindlimb muscles of spinal cord-injured mice. *Muscle Nerve* **2017**, *55*, 232–242. [CrossRef] [PubMed]
232. Shah, P.K.; Garcia-Alias, G.; Choe, J.; Gad, P.; Gerasimenko, Y.; Tillakaratne, N.; Zhong, H.; Roy, R.R.; Edgerton, V.R. Use of quadrupedal step training to re-engage spinal interneuronal networks and improve locomotor function after spinal cord injury. *Brain* **2013**, *136*, 3362–3377. [CrossRef] [PubMed]

233. Nessler, J.A.; De Leon, R.D.; Sharp, K.; Kwak, E.; Minakata, K.; Reinkensmeyer, D.J. Robotic gait analysis of bipedal treadmill stepping by spinal contused rats: Characterization of intrinsic recovery and comparison with bbb. *J. Neurotrauma* **2006**, *23*, 882–896. [CrossRef] [PubMed]
234. Oh, M.J.; Seo, T.B.; Kwon, K.B.; Yoon, S.J.; Elzi, D.J.; Kim, B.G.; Namgung, U. Axonal outgrowth and erk1/2 activation by training after spinal cord injury in rats. *J. Neurotrauma* **2009**, *26*, 2071–2082. [CrossRef] [PubMed]
235. Shin, H.Y.; Kim, H.; Kwon, M.J.; Hwang, D.H.; Lee, K.; Kim, B.G. Molecular and cellular changes in the lumbar spinal cord following thoracic injury: Regulation by treadmill locomotor training. *PLoS ONE* **2014**, *9*, e88215. [CrossRef] [PubMed]
236. Multon, S.; Franzen, R.; Poirrier, A.L.; Scholtes, F.; Schoenen, J. The effect of treadmill training on motor recovery after a partial spinal cord compression-injury in the adult rat. *J. Neurotrauma* **2003**, *20*, 699–706. [CrossRef] [PubMed]
237. Wu, Q.; Cao, Y.; Dong, C.; Wang, H.; Wang, Q.; Tong, W.; Li, X.; Shan, C.; Wang, T. Neuromuscular interaction is required for neurotrophins-mediated locomotor recovery following treadmill training in rat spinal cord injury. *PeerJ* **2016**, *4*, e2025. [CrossRef] [PubMed]
238. Foret, A.; Quertainmont, R.; Botman, O.; Bouhy, D.; Amabili, P.; Brook, G.; Schoenen, J.; Franzen, R. Stem cells in the adult rat spinal cord: Plasticity after injury and treadmill training exercise. *J. Neurochem.* **2010**, *112*, 762–772. [CrossRef] [PubMed]
239. Ward, P.J.; Herrity, A.N.; Smith, R.R.; Willhite, A.; Harrison, B.J.; Petruska, J.C.; Harkema, S.J.; Hubscher, C.H. Novel multi-system functional gains via task specific training in spinal cord injured male rats. *J. Neurotrauma* **2014**, *31*, 819–833. [CrossRef] [PubMed]
240. Park, K.; Lee, Y.; Park, S.; Lee, S.; Hong, Y.; Kil Lee, S. Synergistic effect of melatonin on exercise-induced neuronal reconstruction and functional recovery in a spinal cord injury animal model. *J. Pineal Res.* **2010**, *48*, 270–281. [CrossRef] [PubMed]
241. Liu, Q.; Zhang, B.; Liu, C.; Zhao, D. Molecular mechanisms underlying the positive role of treadmill training in locomotor recovery after spinal cord injury. *Spinal Cord* **2017**, *55*, 441–446. [CrossRef] [PubMed]
242. Hayashibe, M.; Homma, T.; Fujimoto, K.; Oi, T.; Yagi, N.; Kashihara, M.; Nishikawa, N.; Ishizumi, Y.; Abe, S.; Hashimoto, H.; et al. Locomotor improvement of spinal cord-injured rats through treadmill training by forced plantar placement of hind paws. *Spinal Cord* **2016**, *54*, 521–529. [CrossRef] [PubMed]
243. Heng, C.; de Leon, R.D. Treadmill training enhances the recovery of normal stepping patterns in spinal cord contused rats. *Exp. Neurol.* **2009**, *216*, 139–147. [CrossRef] [PubMed]
244. Shinozaki, M.; Iwanami, A.; Fujiyoshi, K.; Tashiro, S.; Kitamura, K.; Shibata, S.; Fujita, H.; Nakamura, M.; Okano, H. Combined treatment with chondroitinase abc and treadmill rehabilitation for chronic severe spinal cord injury in adult rats. *Neurosci. Res.* **2016**, *113*, 37–47. [CrossRef] [PubMed]
245. Robert, A.A.; Al Jadid, M.S.; Bin Afif, S.; Al Sowyed, A.A.; Al-Mubarak, S. The effects of different rehabilitation strategies on the functional recovery of spinal cord injured rats: An experimental study. *Spine* **2010**, *35*, E1273–E1277. [CrossRef] [PubMed]
246. Ichiyama, R.; Potuzak, M.; Balak, M.; Kalderon, N.; Edgerton, V.R. Enhanced motor function by training in spinal cord contused rats following radiation therapy. *PLoS ONE* **2009**, *4*, e6862. [CrossRef] [PubMed]
247. Tillakaratne, N.J.; Guu, J.J.; de Leon, R.D.; Bigbee, A.J.; London, N.J.; Zhong, H.; Ziegler, M.D.; Joynes, R.L.; Roy, R.R.; Edgerton, V.R. Functional recovery of stepping in rats after a complete neonatal spinal cord transection is not due to regrowth across the lesion site. *Neuroscience* **2010**, *166*, 23–33. [CrossRef] [PubMed]
248. See, P.A.; de Leon, R.D. Robotic loading during treadmill training enhances locomotor recovery in rats spinally transected as neonates. *J. Neurophysiol.* **2013**, *110*, 760–767. [CrossRef] [PubMed]
249. Timoszyk, W.K.; Nessler, J.A.; Acosta, C.; Roy, R.R.; Edgerton, V.R.; Reinkensmeyer, D.J.; de Leon, R. Hindlimb loading determines stepping quantity and quality following spinal cord transection. *Brain Res.* **2005**, *1050*, 180–189. [CrossRef] [PubMed]
250. Zhang, Y.; Ji, S.R.; Wu, C.Y.; Fan, X.H.; Zhou, H.J.; Liu, G.L. Observation of locomotor functional recovery in adult complete spinal rats with bwstt using semiquantitative and qualitative methods. *Spinal Cord* **2007**, *45*, 496–501. [CrossRef] [PubMed]
251. Lee, Y.S.; Zdunowski, S.; Edgerton, V.R.; Roy, R.R.; Zhong, H.; Hsiao, I.; Lin, V.W. Improvement of gait patterns in step-trained, complete spinal cord-transected rats treated with a peripheral nerve graft and acidic fibroblast growth factor. *Exp. Neurol.* **2010**, *224*, 429–437. [CrossRef] [PubMed]

252. De Leon, R.D.; Acosta, C.N. Effect of robotic-assisted treadmill training and chronic quipazine treatment on hindlimb stepping in spinally transected rats. *J. Neurotrauma* **2006**, *23*, 1147–1163. [CrossRef] [PubMed]
253. Moshonkina, T.R.; Gilerovich, E.G.; Fedorova, E.A.; Avelev, V.D.; Gerasimenko, Y.P.; Otellin, V.A. Morphofunctional basis for recovery of locomotor movements in rats with completely crossed spinal cord. *Bull. Exp. Biol. Med.* **2004**, *138*, 198–201. [CrossRef] [PubMed]
254. Kubasak, M.D.; Jindrich, D.L.; Zhong, H.; Takeoka, A.; McFarland, K.C.; Munoz-Quiles, C.; Roy, R.R.; Edgerton, V.R.; Ramon-Cueto, A.; Phelps, P.E. Oeg implantation and step training enhance hindlimb-stepping ability in adult spinal transected rats. *Brain* **2008**, *131*, 264–276. [CrossRef] [PubMed]
255. Fouad, K.; Metz, G.A.; Merkler, D.; Dietz, V.; Schwab, M.E. Treadmill training in incomplete spinal cord injured rats. *Behav. Brain Res.* **2000**, *115*, 107–113. [CrossRef]
256. Gomez-Pinilla, F.; Ying, Z.; Roy, R.R.; Molteni, R.; Edgerton, V.R. Voluntary exercise induces a bdnf-mediated mechanism that promotes neuroplasticity. *J. Neurophysiol.* **2002**, *88*, 2187–2195. [CrossRef] [PubMed]
257. Skup, M.; Dwornik, A.; Macias, M.; Sulejczak, D.; Wiater, M.; Czarkowska-Bauch, J. Long-term locomotor training up-regulates trkb(fl) receptor-like proteins, brain-derived neurotrophic factor, and neurotrophin 4 with different topographies of expression in oligodendroglia and neurons in the spinal cord. *Exp. Neurol.* **2002**, *176*, 289–307. [CrossRef] [PubMed]
258. Koliatsos, V.E.; Clatterbuck, R.E.; Winslow, J.W.; Cayouette, M.H.; Price, D.L. Evidence that brain-derived neurotrophic factor is a trophic factor for motor neurons in vivo. *Neuron* **1993**, *10*, 359–367. [CrossRef]
259. Blum, R.; Konnerth, A. Neurotrophin-mediated rapid signaling in the central nervous system: Mechanisms and functions. *Physiology* **2005**, *20*, 70–78. [CrossRef] [PubMed]
260. De Leon, R.D.; See, P.A.; Chow, C.H. Differential effects of low versus high amounts of weight supported treadmill training in spinally transected rats. *J. Neurotrauma* **2011**, *28*, 1021–1033. [CrossRef] [PubMed]
261. Dupont-Versteegden, E.E.; Houle, J.D.; Dennis, R.A.; Zhang, J.; Knox, M.; Wagoner, G.; Peterson, C.A. Exercise-induced gene expression in soleus muscle is dependent on time after spinal cord injury in rats. *Muscle Nerve* **2004**, *29*, 73–81. [CrossRef] [PubMed]
262. Gomez-Pinilla, F.; Ying, Z.; Opazo, P.; Roy, R.R.; Edgerton, V.R. Differential regulation by exercise of bdnf and nt-3 in rat spinal cord and skeletal muscle. *Eur. J. Neurosci.* **2001**, *13*, 1078–1084. [CrossRef] [PubMed]
263. Hutchinson, K.J.; Gomez-Pinilla, F.; Crowe, M.J.; Ying, Z.; Basso, D.M. Three exercise paradigms differentially improve sensory recovery after spinal cord contusion in rats. *Brain* **2004**, *127*, 1403–1414. [CrossRef] [PubMed]
264. Macias, M.; Nowicka, D.; Czupryn, A.; Sulejczak, D.; Skup, M.; Skangiel-Kramska, J.; Czarkowska-Bauch, J. Exercise-induced motor improvement after complete spinal cord transection and its relation to expression of brain-derived neurotrophic factor and presynaptic markers. *BMC Neurosci.* **2009**, *10*, 144. [CrossRef] [PubMed]
265. Ying, Z.; Roy, R.R.; Edgerton, V.R.; Gomez-Pinilla, F. Voluntary exercise increases neurotrophin-3 and its receptor trkc in the spinal cord. *Brain Res.* **2003**, *987*, 93–99. [CrossRef]
266. Ying, Z.; Roy, R.R.; Edgerton, V.R.; Gomez-Pinilla, F. Exercise restores levels of neurotrophins and synaptic plasticity following spinal cord injury. *Exp. Neurol.* **2005**, *193*, 411–419. [CrossRef] [PubMed]
267. Ying, Z.; Roy, R.R.; Zhong, H.; Zdunowski, S.; Edgerton, V.R.; Gomez-Pinilla, F. Bdnf-exercise interactions in the recovery of symmetrical stepping after a cervical hemisection in rats. *Neuroscience* **2008**, *155*, 1070–1078. [CrossRef] [PubMed]
268. Leech, K.A.; Hornby, T.G. High-intensity locomotor exercise increases brain-derived neurotrophic factor in individuals with incomplete spinal cord injury. *J. Neurotrauma* **2017**, *34*, 1240–1248. [CrossRef] [PubMed]
269. Farinas, I.; Jones, K.R.; Backus, C.; Wang, X.Y.; Reichardt, L.F. Severe sensory and sympathetic deficits in mice lacking neurotrophin-3. *Nature* **1994**, *369*, 658–661. [CrossRef] [PubMed]
270. Frisen, J.; Arvidsson, U.; Lindholm, T.; Fried, K.; Verge, V.M.; Cullheim, S.; Hokfelt, T.; Risling, M. Trkc expression in the injured rat spinal cord. *Neuroreport* **1993**, *5*, 349–352. [CrossRef] [PubMed]
271. Lohof, A.M.; Ip, N.Y.; Poo, M.M. Potentiation of developing neuromuscular synapses by the neurotrophins nt-3 and bdnf. *Nature* **1993**, *363*, 350–353. [CrossRef] [PubMed]
272. Scarisbrick, I.A.; Isackson, P.J.; Windebank, A.J. Differential expression of brain-derived neurotrophic factor, neurotrophin-3, and neurotrophin-4/5 in the adult rat spinal cord: Regulation by the glutamate receptor agonist kainic acid. *J. Neurosci.* **1999**, *19*, 7757–7769. [CrossRef] [PubMed]

273. Wang, T.; Xie, K.; Lu, B. Neurotrophins promote maturation of developing neuromuscular synapses. *J. Neurosci.* **1995**, *15*, 4796–4805. [CrossRef] [PubMed]
274. Fang, H.; Liu, C.; Yang, M.; Li, H.; Zhang, F.; Zhang, W.; Zhang, J. Neurotrophic factor and trk signaling mechanisms underlying the promotion of motor recovery after acute spinal cord injury in rats. *Exp. Ther. Med.* **2017**, *14*, 652–656. [CrossRef] [PubMed]
275. Bimonte-Nelson, H.A.; Nelson, M.E.; Granholm, A.C. Progesterone counteracts estrogen-induced increases in neurotrophins in the aged female rat brain. *Neuroreport* **2004**, *15*, 2659–2663. [CrossRef] [PubMed]
276. Gorgey, A.S.; Khalil, R.E.; Gill, R.; O'Brien, L.C.; Lavis, T.; Castillo, T.; Cifu, D.X.; Savas, J.; Khan, R.; Cardozo, C.; et al. Effects of testosterone and evoked resistance exercise after spinal cord injury (terex-sci): Study protocol for a randomised controlled trial. *BMJ Open* **2017**, *7*, e014125. [CrossRef] [PubMed]
277. Yarrow, J.F.; Conover, C.F.; Purandare, A.V.; Bhakta, A.M.; Zheng, N.; Conrad, B.; Altman, M.K.; Franz, S.E.; Wronski, T.J.; Borst, S.E. Supraphysiological testosterone enanthate administration prevents bone loss and augments bone strength in gonadectomized male and female rats. *Am. J. Physiol. Endocrinol. Metab.* **2008**, *295*, E1213–E1222. [CrossRef] [PubMed]
278. Yarrow, J.F.; Phillips, E.G.; Kok, H.J.; Conover, C.F.; Basset, T.E.; Vasconez, A.; Alerte, J.; Prock, H.; Flores, M.; Borst, S.E.; et al. Locomotor training with adjuvant testosterone promotes activity-mediated neuromuscular plasticity in spinal cord injured rats. *Med. Sci. Sports Exerc.* **2017**, *49*, 1038. [CrossRef]
279. Wang, X.; Smith, G.I.; Patterson, B.W.; Reeds, D.N.; Kampelman, J.; Magkos, F.; Mittendorfer, B. Testosterone increases the muscle protein synthesis rate but does not affect very-low-density lipoprotein metabolism in obese premenopausal women. *Am. J. Physiol. Endocrinol. Metab.* **2012**, *302*, E740–746. [CrossRef] [PubMed]
280. Spinal Cord Injury (SCI) Facts and Figures at a Glance. Available online: https://www.nscisc.uab.edu/Public/Facts%202016.pdf (accessed on 25 May 2018).
281. Calof, O.M.; Singh, A.B.; Lee, M.L.; Kenny, A.M.; Urban, R.J.; Tenover, J.L.; Bhasin, S. Adverse events associated with testosterone replacement in middle-aged and older men: A meta-analysis of randomized, placebo-controlled trials. *J. Gerontol. A Biol. Sci. Med. Sci.* **2005**, *60*, 1451–1457. [CrossRef] [PubMed]
282. Basaria, S.; Coviello, A.D.; Travison, T.G.; Storer, T.W.; Farwell, W.R.; Jette, A.M.; Eder, R.; Tennstedt, S.; Ulloor, J.; Zhang, A.; et al. Adverse events associated with testosterone administration. *N. Engl. J. Med.* **2010**, *363*, 109–122. [CrossRef] [PubMed]
283. Finkle, W.D.; Greenland, S.; Ridgeway, G.K.; Adams, J.L.; Frasco, M.A.; Cook, M.B.; Fraumeni, J.F., Jr.; Hoover, R.N. Increased risk of non-fatal myocardial infarction following testosterone therapy prescription in men. *PLoS ONE* **2014**, *9*, e85805. [CrossRef] [PubMed]
284. Vigen, R.; O'Donnell, C.I.; Baron, A.E.; Grunwald, G.K.; Maddox, T.M.; Bradley, S.M.; Barqawi, A.; Woning, G.; Wierman, M.E.; Plomondon, M.E.; et al. Association of testosterone therapy with mortality, myocardial infarction, and stroke in men with low testosterone levels. *JAMA* **2013**, *310*, 1829–1836. [CrossRef] [PubMed]
285. Morgentaler, A.; Lunenfeld, B. Testosterone and cardiovascular risk: World's experts take unprecedented action to correct misinformation. *Aging Male* **2014**, *17*, 63–65. [CrossRef] [PubMed]
286. Traish, A.M.; Guay, A.T.; Morgentaler, A. Death by testosterone? We think not! *J. Sex. Med.* **2014**, *11*, 624–629. [CrossRef] [PubMed]
287. Borst, S.E.; Shuster, J.J.; Zou, B.; Ye, F.; Jia, H.; Wokhlu, A.; Yarrow, J.F. Cardiovascular risks and elevation of serum dht vary by route of testosterone administration: A systematic review and meta-analysis. *BMC Med.* **2014**, *12*, 211. [CrossRef] [PubMed]
288. Onasanya, O.; Iyer, G.; Lucas, E.; Lin, D.; Singh, S.; Alexander, G.C. Association between exogenous testosterone and cardiovascular events: An overview of systematic reviews. *Lancet Diabetes Endocrinol.* **2016**, *4*, 943–956. [CrossRef]
289. Sharma, R.; Oni, O.A.; Gupta, K.; Chen, G.; Sharma, M.; Dawn, B.; Parashara, D.; Savin, V.J.; Ambrose, J.A.; Barua, R.S. Normalization of testosterone level is associated with reduced incidence of myocardial infarction and mortality in men. *Eur. Heart J.* **2015**, *36*, 2706–2715. [CrossRef] [PubMed]
290. La Fountaine, M.F.; Wecht, J.M.; Cirnigliaro, C.M.; Kirshblum, S.C.; Spungen, A.M.; Bauman, W.A. Testosterone replacement therapy improves qtavi in hypogonadal men with spinal cord injury. *Neuroendocrinology* **2013**, *97*, 341–346. [CrossRef] [PubMed]
291. Hamid, R.; Averbeck, M.A.; Chiang, H.; Garcia, A.; Al Mousa, R.T.; Oh, S.J.; Patel, A.; Plata, M.; Del Popolo, G. Epidemiology and pathophysiology of neurogenic bladder after spinal cord injury. *World J. Urol.* **2018**. [CrossRef] [PubMed]

292. Page, S.T.; Amory, J.K.; Bowman, F.D.; Anawalt, B.D.; Matsumoto, A.M.; Bremner, W.J.; Tenover, J.L. Exogenous testosterone (T) alone or with finasteride increases physical performance, grip strength, and lean body mass in older men with low serum T. *J. Clin. Endocrinol. Metab.* **2005**, *90*, 1502–1510. [CrossRef] [PubMed]
293. Amory, J.K.; Watts, N.B.; Easley, K.A.; Sutton, P.R.; Anawalt, B.D.; Matsumoto, A.M.; Bremner, W.J.; Tenover, J.L. Exogenous testosterone or testosterone with finasteride increases bone mineral density in older men with low serum testosterone. *J. Clin. Endocrinol. Metab.* **2004**, *89*, 503–510. [CrossRef] [PubMed]
294. Clinicaltrials.Gov. Available online: https://clinicaltrials.gov/ct2/show/NCT02248701 (accessed on 25 May 2018).
295. Kaplan, A.L.; Hu, J.C. Use of testosterone replacement therapy in the united states and its effect on subsequent prostate cancer outcomes. *Urology* **2013**, *82*, 321–326. [CrossRef] [PubMed]
296. Jia, H.; Sullivan, C.T.; McCoy, S.C.; Yarrow, J.F.; Morrow, M.; Borst, S.E. Review of health risks of low testosterone and testosterone administration. *World J. Clin. Cases* **2015**, *3*, 338–344. [CrossRef] [PubMed]
297. Cole, A.P.; Hanske, J.; Jiang, W.; Kwon, N.K.; Lipsitz, S.R.; Kathrins, M.; Learn, P.A.; Sun, M.; Haider, A.H.; Basaria, S.; et al. Impact of testosterone replacement therapy on thromboembolism, heart disease and obstructive sleep apnoea in men. *BJU Int.* **2018**, *121*, 811–818. [CrossRef] [PubMed]
298. Chiodo, A.E.; Sitrin, R.G.; Bauman, K.A. Sleep disordered breathing in spinal cord injury: A systematic review. *J. Spinal Cord Med.* **2016**, *39*, 374–382. [CrossRef] [PubMed]

Permissions

All chapters in this book were first published by MDPI; hereby published with permission under the Creative Commons Attribution License or equivalent. Every chapter published in this book has been scrutinized by our experts. Their significance has been extensively debated. The topics covered herein carry significant findings which will fuel the growth of the discipline. They may even be implemented as practical applications or may be referred to as a beginning point for another development.

The contributors of this book come from diverse backgrounds, making this book a truly international effort. This book will bring forth new frontiers with its revolutionizing research information and detailed analysis of the nascent developments around the world.

We would like to thank all the contributing authors for lending their expertise to make the book truly unique. They have played a crucial role in the development of this book. Without their invaluable contributions this book wouldn't have been possible. They have made vital efforts to compile up to date information on the varied aspects of this subject to make this book a valuable addition to the collection of many professionals and students.

This book was conceptualized with the vision of imparting up-to-date information and advanced data in this field. To ensure the same, a matchless editorial board was set up. Every individual on the board went through rigorous rounds of assessment to prove their worth. After which they invested a large part of their time researching and compiling the most relevant data for our readers.

The editorial board has been involved in producing this book since its inception. They have spent rigorous hours researching and exploring the diverse topics which have resulted in the successful publishing of this book. They have passed on their knowledge of decades through this book. To expedite this challenging task, the publisher supported the team at every step. A small team of assistant editors was also appointed to further simplify the editing procedure and attain best results for the readers.

Apart from the editorial board, the designing team has also invested a significant amount of their time in understanding the subject and creating the most relevant covers. They scrutinized every image to scout for the most suitable representation of the subject and create an appropriate cover for the book.

The publishing team has been an ardent support to the editorial, designing and production team. Their endless efforts to recruit the best for this project, has resulted in the accomplishment of this book. They are a veteran in the field of academics and their pool of knowledge is as vast as their experience in printing. Their expertise and guidance has proved useful at every step. Their uncompromising quality standards have made this book an exceptional effort. Their encouragement from time to time has been an inspiration for everyone.

The publisher and the editorial board hope that this book will prove to be a valuable piece of knowledge for researchers, students, practitioners and scholars across the globe.

List of Contributors

Margot Bergmann, Anna Zahharova, Helena Gapeyeva and Doris Vahtrik
Institute of Sport Sciences and Physiotherapy, University of Tartu, 51008 Tartu, Estonia

Märt Reinvee
Institute of Technology, Estonian University of Life Sciences, 51006 Tartu, Estonia

Toomas Asser
Institute of Clinical Medicine, University of Tartu, 50406 Tartu, Estonia

Inês M. Pereira, Ana Marote, António J. Salgado and Nuno A. Silva
Life and Health Sciences Research Institute (ICVS), School of Medicine, University of Minho, Campus de Gualtar, 4710-057 Braga, Portugal
ICVS/3B's—PT Government Associate Laboratory, Braga/Guimarães, Portugal

Kyriakos Dalamagkas
The Institute for Rehabilitation and Research, Memorial Hermann Texas Medical Centre, Houston, TX 77030, USA
Centre for Nanotechnology & Regenerative Medicine, Division of Surgery and Interventional Science, University College of London (UCL), London NW3 2QG, UK

Magdalini Tsintou
Centre for Nanotechnology & Regenerative Medicine, Division of Surgery and Interventional Science, University College of London (UCL), London NW3 2QG, UK
Center for Neural Systems Investigations, Massachusetts General Hospital/HST Athinoula A., Martinos Centre for Biomedical Imaging, Harvard Medical School, Boston, MA 02129, USA

Amelia Seifalian
Faculty of Medical Sciences, UCL Medical School, London WC1E 6BT, UK

Alexander M. Seifalian
NanoRegMed Ltd. (Nanotechnology & Regenerative Medicine Commercialization Centre), The London BioScience Innovation Centre, London NW1 0NH, UK

Aleš Hejčl
Institute of Experimental Medicine, Academy of Sciences of the Czech Republic, Vídeňská 1083, 142 20 Prague, Czech Republic
Department of Neurosurgery, J. E. Purkinje University, Masaryk Hospital, Sociální Péče 12A, 401 13 Ústí nad Labem, Czech Republic

Jiří Růžička, Kristýna Kekulová, Barbora Svobodová, Lucia Machová Urdziková and Šárka Kubinová
Institute of Experimental Medicine, Academy of Sciences of the Czech Republic, Vídeňská 1083, 142 20 Prague, Czech Republic

Vladimír Proks, Hana Macková and Daniel Horák
Institute of Macromolecular Chemistry, Academy of Sciences of the Czech Republic, Heyrovského nám.2, 162 06 Praha, Czech Republic

Kateřina Jiránková
Second Faculty of Medicine, Charles University, V Úvalu 84, 150 06 Prague, Czech Republic

Kristýna Kárová and Pavla Jendelová
Institute of Experimental Medicine, Academy of Sciences of the Czech Republic, Vídeňská 1083, 142 20 Prague, Czech Republic
Department of Neuroscience, 2nd Faculty of Medicine, Charles University, V Úvalu 84, 150 06 Prague, Czech Republic

Jiří Cihlář
Department of Mathematics, Faculty of Science, J. E. Purkyně University, České Mládeže 8, 400 96 Ústí nad Labem, Czech Republic

Marina Gazdic
Faculty of Medical Sciences, Department of Genetics, University of Kragujevac, 34000 Kragujevac, Serbia

Vladislav Volarevic and Nebojsa Arsenijevic
Faculty of Medical Sciences, Department of Microbiology and immunology, Center for Molecular Medicine and Stem Cell Research, University of Kragujevac, 34000 Kragujevac, Serbia

C. Randall Harrell and Crissy Fellabaum
Regenerative Processing Plant, LLC, 34176 US Highway 19 N Palm Harbor, Palm Harbor, FL 34684, USA

Nemanja Jovicic
Faculty of Medical Sciences, Department of Histology and embryology, University of Kragujevac, 34000 Kragujevac, Serbia

Miodrag Stojkovic
Faculty of Medical Sciences, Department of Genetics, University of Kragujevac, 34000 Kragujevac, Serbia
Spebo Medical, 16 Norvezanska, 16000 Leskovac, Serbia

Jian Wang and Yang Liu
Division of Genetics and Development, Toronto Western Research Institute, University Health Network, Toronto, ON M5T 2S8, Canada

James Hong, Alex Chang and Mohammad-Masoud Zavvarian
Division of Genetics and Development, Toronto Western Research Institute, University Health Network, Toronto, ON M5T 2S8, Canada
Institute of Medical Science, University of Toronto, Toronto, ON M5S 1A8, Canada

Michael G. Fehlings
Division of Genetics and Development, Toronto Western Research Institute, University Health Network, Toronto, ON M5T 2S8, Canada
Spinal Program, University Health Network, Toronto Western Hospital, Toronto, ON M5T 2S8, Canada

Ana Alastrue-Agudo, Francisco Javier Rodriguez-Jimenez, Eric López Mocholi, Francesca De Giorgio, and Victoria Moreno-Manzano
Neuronal and Tissue Regeneration Laboratory, Príncipe Felipe Research Center, 46012 Valencia, Spain

Slaven Erceg
Stem Cell Therapies in Neurodegenerative Diseases Laboratory, Centro de Investigación Príncipe Felipe, 46012 Valencia, Spain

Masahiko Hatano
Department of Biomedical Science, Graduate School of Medicine, Chiba University, Chiba City, Chiba 260-8670, Japan

Yoshitoshi Kasuya
Department of Biomedical Science, Graduate School of Medicine, Chiba University, Chiba City, Chiba 260-8670, Japan
Department of Biochemistry and Molecular Pharmacology, Graduate School of Medicine, Chiba University, Chiba City, Chiba 260-8670, Japan

Hiroki Umezawa
Department of Biomedical Science, Graduate School of Medicine, Chiba University, Chiba City, Chiba 260-8670, Japan
Department of Biochemistry and Molecular Pharmacology, Graduate School of Medicine, Chiba University, Chiba City, Chiba 260-8670, Japan
Department of Respirology, Graduate School of Medicine, Chiba University, Chiba City, Chiba 260-8670, Japan

Sian F. Irvine
School of Biomedical Sciences, University of Leeds, Leeds LS2 9JT, UK

Jessica C. F. Kwok
School of Biomedical Sciences, University of Leeds, Leeds LS2 9JT, UK
Centre of Reconstructive Neurosciences, Institute of Experimental Medicine, The Czech Academy of Sciences, Prague 4, Czech Republic

Katarina Bimbova, Maria Bacova, Alexandra Kisucka, Jaroslav Pavel, Jan Galik, Andrea Stropkovska, Jana Fedorova, Stefania Papcunova, Jana Jachova and Nadezda Lukacova
Institute of Neurobiology of Biomedical Research Centre of Slovak Academy of Sciences, Soltesovej 4,6, 040 01 Kosice, Slovakia

Peter Zavacky
1st Department of Surgery, Louis Pasteur University Hospital, Faculty of Medicine University of Pavol Jozef Safarik, Trieda SNP 1, 041 66 Kosice, Slovakia

Martin Marsala
Institute of Neurobiology of Biomedical Research Centre of Slovak Academy of Sciences, Soltesovej 4,6, 040 01 Kosice, Slovakia
Neuroregeneration Laboratory, Department of Anesthesiology, University of California, 9500 Gilman Drive, San Diego, CA 92092-0100, USA

Svatopluk Rehak
Department of Neurosurgery, Charles University, Medical Faculty and University Hospital Hradec Králové, Sokolska 581, 50005 Hradec Kralove, Czech Republic

Petr Krupa
Department of Neurosurgery, Charles University, Medical Faculty and University Hospital Hradec Králové, Sokolska 581, 50005 Hradec Kralove, Czech Republic
Institute of Experimental Medicine, Czech Academy of Sciences, Vídeňská 1083, 14220 Prague 4, Czech Republic

Irena Vackova, Jiri Ruzicka, Karolina Turnovcova, Lucia Machova Urdzikova and Sarka Kubinova
Institute of Experimental Medicine, Czech Academy of Sciences, Vídeňská 1083, 14220 Prague 4, Czech Republic

Kristyna Zaviskova, Jana Dubisova, Zuzana Koci and Pavla Jendelova
Institute of Experimental Medicine, Czech Academy of Sciences, Vídeňská 1083, 14220 Prague 4, Czech Republic
Department of Neuroscience, Charles University, Second Faculty of Medicine, 15006 Prague 5, Czech Republic

Jure Tica
Imperial College London, Alexander Fleming Building, London SW7 2AZ, UK

Elizabeth J. Bradbury
King's College London, Wolfson CARD, Institute of Psychiatry, Psychology & Neuroscience, London SE1 1UL, UK

Athanasios Didangelos
Department of Infection, Immunity and Inflammation, University of Leicester, Leicester LE1 7RH, UK

Dana M. Otzel
Brain Rehabilitation Research Center, Malcom Randall Veterans Affairs Medical Center, North Florida/South Georgia Veterans Health System, Gainesville, FL 32608, USA

Jimmy Lee and Fan Ye
Research Service, Malcom Randall Veterans Affairs Medical Center, North Florida/South Georgia Veterans Health System, Gainesville, FL 32608, USA

Stephen E. Borst
Department of Applied Physiology, Kinesiology and University of Florida College of Health and Human Performance, Gainesville, FL 32603, USA

Joshua F. Yarrow
Research Service, Malcom Randall Veterans Affairs Medical Center, North Florida/South Georgia Veterans Health System, Gainesville, FL 32608, USA
Division of Endocrinology, Diabetes and Metabolism, University of Florida College of Medicine, Gainesville, FL 32610, USA

Index

www.ingramcontent.com/pod-product-compliance
Lightning Source LLC
LaVergne TN
LVHW080947210926
848485LV00004B/796